Biomechanics in Ergonomics

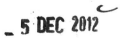

DEDICATION

To my parents – Tribeni and Dhairyavati Shankar – with profound love, respect and gratitude and to my wife, son and daughter – Rita, Rajesh and Sheela – with fond love and appreciation.

Biomechanics in Ergonomics

EDITED BY

SHRAWAN KUMAR, PhD, DSc, FErgS
Department of Physical Therapy,
University of Alberta,
Edmonton, Alberta,
Canada

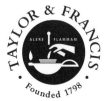

TAYLOR & FRANCIS
ALERE FLAMMAM
Founded 1798

UK   Taylor & Francis Ltd, 11 New Fetter Lane, London EC4P 4EE
USA   Taylor & Francis Inc., 325 Chestnut Street, Philadelphia, PA 19106

Copyright © Taylor & Francis 1999

British Library Cataloguing in Publication Data

A catalogue record for this book is available from the British Library.
ISBN 0–7484–0704–9

Library of Congress Cataloguing in Publication Data are available

Cover design by Jim Wilkie
Typeset in 10/12pt Times by Graphicraft Limited, Hong Kong
Printed and bound by T.J. International Ltd, Padstow, UK
Cover printed by Flexiprint, Lancing, West Sussex

Contents

Biographical sketch

SHRAWAN KUMAR

Shrawan Kumar is currently a Professor in Physical Therapy in the Faculty of Rehabilitation Medicine and in the Division of Neuroscience, Faculty of Medicine at the University of Alberta. He joined the Faculty of Rehabilitation Medicine in 1977 and rose to the ranks of Associate and Full Professor in 1979 and 1982 respectively. Dr Kumar holds BSc (Biology and Chemistry) and MSc (Zoology) degrees from the University of Allahabad, India, and a PhD (Human Biology) degree from the University of Surrey, UK. Following his PhD, he did his post-doctoral work at Trinity College, Dublin, in Engineering, and worked as a Research Associate at the University of Toronto in the Department of Physical Medicine and Rehabilitation. For his life-time work, Dr Kumar was recognised by the University of Surrey, UK, with the award of a peer reviewed DSc Degree in 1994. Dr Kumar was invited to be a Visiting Professor for the year 1983–84 at the University of Michigan, Department of Industrial Engineering. He was a McCalla Professor 1984–85. He is a Fellow of the Human Factors Association of Canada, the Human Factors and Engineering Society of the USA, and the Ergonomics Society of the UK. Dr Kumar was awarded the Sir Fredéric Bartlett Medal for excellence in ergonomics research by the Ergonomics Society of the UK in 1997. During the 48 years of existence of the Society, Dr Kumar is the 17th recipient of this highest honour of the society. For his distinguished research the University of Alberta awarded Dr Kumar one of the seven Killam Annual Professorships for the year 1997–98. The Human Factors and Ergonomics Society of the USA also bestowed its top honour on Dr Kumar by awarding him the most prestigious award for 1997 entitled 'Distinguished International Colleague'. Dr Kumar has been an invited keynote/plenary speaker at several international scientific meetings held in Canada, Brazil, Taiwan, India, Malaysia, New Zealand and South Africa.

Dr Kumar has authored over 250 scientific peer-reviewed publications and works in the area of musculoskeletal injury causation/prevention with special emphasis on low-back pain. He has edited/authored seven books/monographs. He currently holds a grant from NSERC. In addition to the above, his work has been supported by MRC, WCB and NRC. He has supervised or is supervising ten MSc students, three PhD students and three post-doctoral students. He is Editor of the *International Journal of Industrial Ergonomics*, Consulting Editor of *Ergonomics*, Advisory Editor of *Spine*, and Assistant Editor of the *Transactions of Rehabilitation Engineering*. He serves as a reviewer for several other international peer-reviewed journals. He also acts as a grant reviewer for NSERC, MRC, Alberta Occupational Health and Safety, and BC Research.

Shrawan Kumar has organised and chaired regional, national and international conferences. He has served as the Chair of the Graduate Program in Physical Therapy from 1979–87, Director of Research, 1985–90, Chair of the Doctoral Program Development Committee – Faculty of Rehabilitation Medicine, and on several other committees. He has served on Chairs and Deans selection committees. Dr Kumar has served as a member of the University of Alberta Planning and Priority Committee and the Academic Development Committee. As Chair of the 'Code of Ethics' committee of the International Ergonomics Association, he has had additional valuable experience in larger and global issues. He therefore has had experience in local, university-wide, and global (international) issues in professional and managerial arenas.

Preface

Two of the three main goals of ergonomics are 'comfort' and 'health and safety' of workers. These two goals are mutually complimentary and represent a progression of potential undesirable consequences of hazards. If health and safety are in jeopardy the feeling, in most cases, will pass through a zone of discomfort. In a large number of occupational settings such progression is commonplace. Work is unavoidable as it is essential to maintain the socioeconomic fabric. With the advent, permeation, and proliferation of technology in ever increasing complexity of sociological structures the magnitude and duration of work related activities and hence stresses have progressively increased. In order to meet the increasing needs and demands of people the work activities need to be increasingly repeated for enhanced productivity. This hybrid evolutionary context (biological and socioeconomic) poses hazards of overexertion and injury by stressing the same structures repeatedly. The precipitation of all injuries, in final analysis, is a biomechanical perturbation of the tissue or the organ involved. Therefore for physical ergonomics, biomechanics is an essential and integral part of the discipline. Application of biomechanics in ergonomics has been commonly at the entire organ or whole body level. Less commonly it has been applied at the tissue level. Therefore, this book has taken the approach of progressing from tissue to organ/structure, and finally to the whole body aspects.

In the introductory chapter, Kumar presents some of his thinking with respect to theories of injury causation. It is hoped that Chapter 1 will put the forthcoming material in perspective by discussing various variables which may have a role to play in injury causation. He distinguishes between 'injuries' and 'disorders', indicating how genetic predisposition, morphological vulnerability and psychosocial susceptibility may facilitate the causation of injury but only the biomechanical hazards help precipitate it. Following on from this theme, he proposes a methodology to assess quantitatively the biomechanical factors and their impact on risk of injury. The same methodology can be used as a tool for control of these occupational injuries. Such an initial conceptual perspective will help the reader to piece together information in subsequent chapters for an integrated understanding.

Part I deals with tissue biomechanics. Woo *et al.*, in their chapter on tissue mechanics of ligaments and tendons, describe their structure and mechanics. These are the most commonly injured connective tissues. While they mostly deal with complete injuries to these tissues they also mention the significance of partial injuries. Timmermann *et al.*, on the other hand, in describing and discussing ligament sprains, deal with partial injuries in greater detail along with the mechanical behaviour of partially injured tissues. A valuable component of this chapter is clinical management options. The next chapter by Judex *et al.* describes the structure and mechanical properties of bones and reviews biomechanical concepts and testing procedures. Finally, in this section, Bobet discusses muscle mechanics in the ergonomic context. He reviews and explains the properties of muscles and their implications in solving workplace problems.

Part II is dedicated to the upper extremity. In the first chapter Feldman describes the functional anatomy of the upper extremity, starting with the hand and progressing proximally to the elbow. Imrhan provides a more detailed function of the hand and focuses on grasping, pinching and squeezing. Mital and Pennathur further extend the discussion of the use of hands with hand tools in industrial applications. They describe their association with the musculoskeletal injuries of upper extremities. More importantly they provide guidelines and recommendations for design, selection and use of hand tools based on ergonomic considerations. Wells and Keir discuss work and activity-related musculoskeletal disorders of the upper extremity. In the last chapter, Hughes and An describe biomechanical models of the hand, wrist and elbow. They include optimisation, electromyography and belt-pulley models as well as strength prediction models. They also deal with multiple segment arm models and hand-arm vibration models. Clearly models do have a special use in ergonomic application.

Part III deals with the shoulder and neck complex. Jensen *et al.* present the anatomy and mechanics of the shoulder and neck from a physiological and ergonomic perspective. In their chapter they also deal with muscle activity, posture, biomechanical modelling and motor control. The next chapter, by Panjabi *et al.*, deals with whiplash injuries to the neck. They describe the biomechanical background, current perspective and understanding of whiplash and its ergonomic significance. It is fair to say that understanding of whiplash is still relatively incomplete and several efforts to understand it are underway.

Part IV is concerned with problems of the low back. Pope *et al.* consider the impact of whole body vibration on low back pain. They describe physiological measures, electromyographic measures, creep and unexpected loads. Goel *et al.* consider in detail the impact of workplace factors on disc degeneration, which has been linked to many low-back problems. Most of the jobs requiring strength and use of the human trunk, such as manual materials handling, have been thought to be the biggest contributing factor in low-back pain problems. Ayoub and Woldstad describe several models which have been developed to understand and control low-back pain problems due to manual materials handling including biomechanical, physiological and psychophysical models.

In Part V the whole body biomechanics are discussed in some of the most common activities involved in occupational settings. Konz considers the pervasive role of posture and its impact on the health and safety of workers. He describes static and dynamic postures of the human body, measuring of posture, and the external factors affecting it. Sitting is the most common posture employed at work. Eklund presents a biomechanical perspective of sitting postures and their analysis. Based on the literature he proposes a generic seat design. Bloswick discusses climbing, which is a common activity requiring the whole body. He describes the epidemiology, biomechanics and ergonomic significance of climbing activities. In the last chapter, Grönqvist deals with a common hazardous event in many workplaces – slip and fall. He focuses on the biomechanics and prevention of falls initiated by foot slip-ups. He also discusses the criteria for safe friction, and assessment of slip resistance of shoes and floors.

SHRAWAN KUMAR

List of contributors

Kai-Nan An
Professor and Associate Chair
Department of Orthopaedic Surgery
Orthopaedic Biomechanics Lab
Rochester, MN 55905
USA

Maria Apreleva
University of Pittsburgh
Department of Orthopaedic Surgery
Liliane Kaufmann Building, Suite 1011
3471 Fifth Avenue
Pittsburgh, PA 15213
USA

M.M. Ayoub
Horn Professor
Texas Tech. University
Department of Industrial Engineering
Lubbock, TX 79409–3061
USA

Donald S. Bloswick
Associate Professor
University of Utah
Department of Mechanical Engineering
50 S Central Campus Dr.
Rm 2202
Salt Lake City, UT 84112
USA

Jacques Bobet
Associate Professor
Department of Physical Therapy
Rm 2–50 Corbett Hall
University of Alberta
Edmonton, Alberta
T6G 2E1
Canada

R. Boorman
Division of Orthopaedic Surgery
Department of Surgery
Faculty of Medicine
University of Calgary
3330 Hospital Drive NW
Calgary, Alberta
T2N 4N1
Canada

Jacek Cholewicki
Biomechanics Laboratory
Department of Orthopaedics and
Rehabilitation
Yale University School of Medicine
PO Box 208071
New Haven, CT 06520–8071
USA

Jörgen Eklund
Division of Industrial Ergonomics
Department of Mechanical Engineering
Linköping University of Technology
S-581 83 Linköping
Sweden

Reuben Feldman
604 College Plaza
8215–112 Street
Edmonton, Alberta
T6G 2C8
Canada

C.B. Frank
Professor
Division of Orthopaedic Surgery
Department of Surgery
Faculty of Medicine
University of Calgary
3330 Hospital Drive NW
Calgary, Alberta
T2N 4N1
Canada

Vijay K. Goel
Iowa Spine Research Center
Departments of Biomedical Engineering
and Orthopaedics
University of Iowa
Iowa City, Iowa 52242
USA

Jonathan N. Grauer
Biomechanics Laboratory
Department of Orthopaedics and
Rehabilitation
Yale University School of Medicine
PO Box 208071
New Haven, CT 06520–8071
USA

Raoul Grönqvist
Finnish Institute of Occupational Health
Department of Physics
Laajaniitytie 1
SS-1520 Vantaa
Finland

Nicole M. Grosland
Iowa Spine Research Center
Departments of Biomedical Engineering
and Orthopaedics
University of Iowa
Iowa City, Iowa 52242
USA

Jürgen Höher
University of Pittsburgh
Department of Orthopaedic Surgery
Liliane Kaufmann Building, Suite 1011
3471 Fifth Avenue
Pittsburgh, PA 15213
USA

Richard E. Hughes
Orthopaedic Biomechanics Lab
Mayo Clinic/Mayo Foundation
Rochester, MN 55905
USA

Sheik N. Imrhan
Associate Professor
Department of Industrial and
Manufacturing Systems Engineering
The University of Texas at Arlington
Box 19017
Arlington, TX 76013
USA

Chris Jensen
Department of Physiology
National Institute of Occupational
Health
Lersø Parkallé 105
DK-2100 Copenhagen Ø
Denmark

Stefan Judex
McCaig Centre for Joint Injury and
Arthritis Research
Department of Mechanical Engineering
University of Calgary
3330 Hospital Drive NW
Calgary, Alberta
T2N 4N1
Canada

Peter Keir
Occupational Biomechanics Laboratory
Department of Kinesiology
University of Waterloo
Waterloo, Ontario
N2L 3G1
Canada

Stephan Konz
Professor
Department of Industrial and
Manufacturing Systems Engineering
Kansas State University
Manhattan, KS 66506
USA

Shrawan Kumar
Department of Physical Therapy
Rm 3–75 Corbett Hall
University of Alberta
Edmonton, Alberta
T6G 2G4
Canada

Bjarne Laursen
Department of Physiology
National Institute of Occupational
Health
Lersø Parkallé 105
DK-2100 Copenhagen Ø
Denmark

Marianne Magnusson
Iowa Spine Research Center
01090 JPP
University of Iowa Hospitals and Clinics
200 Hawkins Drive
Iowa City, IA 52242–1088
USA

Anil Mital
Professor of Industrial Engineering
Ergonomics and Engineering Controls
Research Laboratory
Industrial Engineering
University of Cincinnati
Cincinnati, OH 45221–0116
USA

Robert E. Montgomery
Iowa Spine Research Center
Departments of Biomedical Engineering
and Orthopaedics
University of Iowa
Iowa City, Iowa 52242
USA

Kimio Nibu
Department of Orthopaedics
Yamaguchi University School of
Medicine
Yamaguchi
Japan

Manohar M. Panjabi
Biomechanics Laboratory
Department of Orthopaedics and
Rehabilitation
Yale University School of Medicine
PO Box 208071
New Haven, CT 06520–8071
USA

Arunkumar Pennathur
Doctoral Student in Industrial
Engineering
Ergonomics and Engineering Controls
Research Laboratory
Industrial Engineering
University of Cincinnati
Cincinnati, OH 45221–0116
USA

Malcolm H. Pope
Professor and Chairman
Iowa Spine Research Center
01090 JPP
University of Iowa Hospitals and Clinics
200 Hawkins Drive
Iowa City, IA 52242–1088
USA

Gisela Sjøgaard
Department of Physiology
National Institute of Occupational
Health
Lersø Parkallé 105
DK-2100 Copenhagen Ø
Denmark

S.A. Timmermann
Division of Orthopaedic Surgery
Department of Surgery
Faculty of Medicine
University of Calgary
3330 Hospital Drive NW
Calgary, Alberta
T2N 4N1
Canada

S.P. Timmermann
Division of Orthopaedic Surgery
Department of Surgery
Faculty of Medicine
University of Calgary
3330 Hospital Drive NW
Calgary, Alberta
T2N 4N1
Canada

Richard Wells
Occupational Biomechanics Laboratory
Department of Kinesiology
University of Waterloo
Waterloo, Ontario
N2L 3G1
Canada

William Whiting
Department of Kinesiology
California State University, Northridge
18111 Nordhoff Street
Northridge, CA 91330–8287
USA

David G. Wilder
Iowa Spine Research Center
01090 JPP
University of Iowa Hospitals and Clinics
200 Hawkins Drive
Iowa City, IA 52242–1088
USA

Jeffrey C. Woldstad
Texas Tech. University
Department of Industrial Engineering
Lubbock, TX 79409–3061
USA

Savio L.-Y. Woo
University of Pittsburgh
Department of Orthopaedic Surgery
Liliane Kaufmann Building, Suite 1011
3471 Fifth Avenue
Pittsburgh, PA 15213
USA

Ronald Zernicke
McCaig Centre for Joint Injury and
Arthritis Research
Departments of Surgery, Mechanical
Engineering and Kinesiology
University of Calgary
3330 Hospital Drive NW
Calgary, Alberta
T2N 4N1
Canada

General

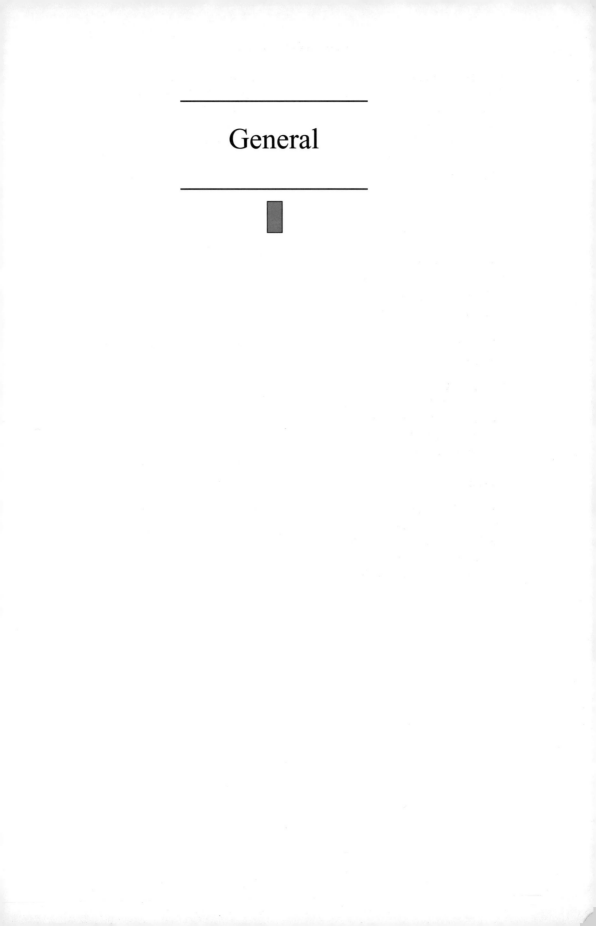

CHAPTER ONE

Selected theories of musculoskeletal injury causation

SHRAWAN KUMAR

INTRODUCTION

According to the World Health Organisation (WHO) (1995) about 58 per cent of the world's population over the age of 10 years spend one-third of their time at work. This collective work generates US $21.6 trillion as gross domestic product which sustains the socioeconomic fabric worldwide. While there are many beneficial aspects of work approximately 30–50 per cent of workers are exposed to significant physical occupational hazards, and an equal number of working people report psychological overload resulting in stress symptoms (WHO, 1995). Globally about 120 million occupational accidents and 200 000 fatalities were estimated to occur annually in addition to 68–157 million new cases of occupational diseases due to various exposures (WHO, 1995). Only 5–10 per cent of workers in developing countries and 20–50 per cent of workers in industrialised countries (with very few exceptions) have access to occupational health services. Where present, they may assist workers and organisations in remediation and management of manifested problems. An approach of primary prevention will be more appropriate to attack the root of the problem. Given that work is essential to our society and the nature of work is largely predetermined, it may appear that little can be done to change the situation. However, an understanding of the mechanism of causation of occupational injuries and accidents will put us in a better position to design effective strategies of control and prevention. All work is designed for productivity with efficiency; accidents and injuries are unplanned events, and are hence avoidable in some measure with appropriate planning and design of the work.

A large majority of the Workers' Compensation Board (WCB) compensated cases are regional musculoskeletal problems. Workers in different economic sectors generally have injuries which are characteristic of those sectors. People in forestry, construction, and manufacturing have a higher proportion of back injuries. Those working in office type jobs involving keyboarding have cumulative trauma disorders (also called repetitive strain injuries). Since it does not happen the other way round, i.e. the heavy physical workers developing cumulative trauma disorder and the office workers injuring their backs, this offers credence to the argument that the nature of the physical stress and the region enduring the load largely determine the affected area and probably the nature of injury. If, therefore, one is able to delineate the mechanism of injuries and the quantitative details of the relevant variables one may be able to develop a more effective intervention. An effective intervention will result in a better control of injuries which clearly has a signific-ant pay-off. Thus, the long term success in controlling these injuries depends on under-standing their causation. A clear understanding and establishment of the mechanism of injury causation has been somewhat elusive. Therefore, an appropriate starting point is to examine and construct theories of musculoskeletal injury causation.

INJURY: NATURE, BASIS AND RISK FACTORS

Nature of injury

An injury, by definition, means mechanical disruption of tissues. Thus, it is a traumatic event in which the integrity of the tissue in question is violated and its mechanical order has been perturbed. The latter leads to pain in addition to inflammation and other bio-chemical responses, hence the difficulty in deploying these structures in any activity including occupational. The term 'injury' is distinguished from that of 'disorder' which is frequently used in any malfunctioning of an organ or an organism. Contrary to injury, a disorder can result without a mechanical perturbation of the tissues involved. Examples of disorders can be myopathies, neuropathies or several central nervous system problems resulting in improper functioning of the musculoskeletal system. Whereas an injury may result in a functional disorder which can be remedied by healing the injury, the injury in itself is not a disorder.

Another difference between injury and disorder is that while the onset of a disorder may be gradual and mediated by a pathogen or prepathological progression, the onset of an injury is sudden and does not involve prepathogenesis. It may, however, involve mechanical degradation of the tissue due to overuse. Subsequent to injury inflammation and pathology of healing sets in. In the case of occupational musculoskeletal injuries the organs or tissues are invariably exposed to factors which place mechanical stresses on the tissues. Most frequently such exposure is repetitive and prolonged and hence is con-sidered a hazard or risk factor. The exposure to risk factors and subsequent injury pre-cipitation does not follow a known dose response relationship, at least in the short term. In the long term, however, numerous studies have reported a strong association between exposure to risk factors and precipitation of injury (for neck and shoulder region – Fine et al., 1986; Hagberg, 1984; Herberts et al., 1984; Silverstein et al., 1986; Westgaard et al., 1986; for low back region – Anderssen, 1981; Chaffin, 1974; Heliovaara, 1987; Hult, 1954; Kumar, 1990a; Magora, 1970, 1972, 1973; and others).

A clear and undisputable causal relationship between any of the risk factors and precipitation of injuries has not been demonstrated for any risk factor. Factors which are likely to confound this situation are the tissue's ability to undergo adaptation to stress and recover from the stress exposure. Repeated exposure over a prolonged period may impede complete recovery, causing residual strain. This is most likely to occur when the balance between adaptive changes is insufficient to offset the adverse biomechanical effects of stress exposure. An accumulation of residual strain over years may set the stage for injury even if the stress does not rise extraordinarily. The latter is due to progressive reduction

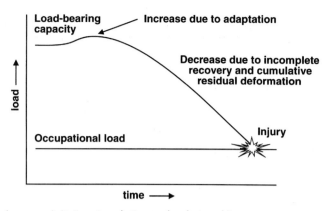

Figure 1.1 Injury precipitation in relation to load–time history.

in stress tolerance capacity due to steadily increasing residual strain (Figure 1.1). Kumar (1990a) reported this concept of threshold level of cumulative exposure prior to injury precipitation. He demonstrated in an age, height, weight, recreation and occupational activity matched sample that the workers with injury and pain had to reach a threshold range of cumulative load exposure not reached by the sample without injury and pain.

The tissues which frequently get injured as a result of exposure to occupational bio-mechanical hazards are ligaments, tendons, muscles, and nerves. Other structures which are affected less frequently are cartilage and bones. All biological tissues are viscoelastic in nature, hence their mechanical properties are time and strain rate dependent. The tissue viscoelastic property determines the duration required for complete mechanical recovery. Any deformation or residual deformation alters the mechanical response characteristics of the tissue in question, most frequently lowering its stress bearing capacity and raising the injury potential. On the contrary muscles are active organs and undergo voluntary con-traction and relaxation rapidly to generate force. Therefore, muscles are rarely affected by unrecovered deformation. It is the passive structures of muscles, e.g. the sarcolemma, which can tear due to very rapid contraction or excessive force generation.

Biomechanical basis of injury

The most frequently injured connective tissues are ligaments and tendons. Both these tissues are made of the same protein – collagen. The difference between them lies largely in the arrangement of the collagen fibres. In ligaments the arrangement of collagen fibres is largely in the form of a flat sheet, generally well supplied with blood vessels and nerve fibres. The tendons on the other hand are densely packed collagen fibres in the form of a rope. Tendons are proportionately less vascular. Due to the common building block they have similar mechanical properties with a difference in magnitude. A brief description of their mechanical properties is given here to emphasise the aspects needed for integrating the hypotheses of injury.

Collagenous tissues are viscoelastic in nature and they transmit and endure forces in tensile mode. Tendons provide rigid attachment of muscles to bones. Therefore, they must transmit the muscle force with a minimum loss. For this reason they have a high modulus of elasticity and high tensile strength. Ligaments on the other hand provide joint support and stability, and hence have a sheet like arrangement of fibres. They are designed to accommodate the normal range of joint motion and bear considerable load. High density collagen tissues such as tendons and many ligaments have a physiological and reversible range of deformation up to 4 per cent. Deformations beyond this value, even upon full recovery, show residual deformation. Rupture of these tissues occurs at around 8 per cent to 10 per cent of deformation. These collagenous tissues also have an ultimate tensile strength at which the tissues fail. Being viscoelastic, their mechanical properties are strain rate dependent. Thus for the same load if applied slowly one obtains significantly greater deformation. Conversely if the load is applied rapidly the tissue behaves as a much stiffer structure allowing significantly smaller deformation. Finally, another immediately relevant property of collagen is that under prolonged loading it continues to deform allowing creep to set in. Combination of the foregoing basic properties of collagen serves to explain most of the common occupational injuries to the musculoskeletal system. Uncommonly, the magnitude of one time load is so high that it exceeds the ultimate tensile strength of collagenous structure and causes failure of the rested tissue. More commonly repetitive exertions set the scene for occupational injuries. With repeated exertions and inadequate time for recovery of the deformation there will be reduction in the cross sectional area of the connective tissue stressed, thereby increasing the stress concentration. The latter will lower the stress tolerance of the tissue and heighten the chances of injury. Prolonged static loading resulting in creep will also render these tissues vulnerable in a similar way.

Occupational activities are generally kinesiologically complex and involve a large number of muscles. Not all muscles may share load proportional to their capacity by the nature of activity and the job demand. Such situations will require differential loading. This frequently occurs in asymmetric activities (Kumar and Narayan, 1998). With repeated or prolonged activity there will be differential fatigue of the muscles involved (Kumar and Narayan, 1998; Kumar et al., 1998) and differential straining of the connective tissue. More fatigued muscle may become incoordinated before less fatigued ones, causing variable and jerky forces to be generated. The connective tissue of these muscles, due to prior strain and reduced cross sectional area, is therefore likely to suffer variable and jerky stress concentration. Such a situation would clearly set the stage for injury precipitation. It is probably for these reasons that over 60 per cent of all injuries to the back involve rotation of the trunk (Manning et al., 1984). Other authors have also reported trunk rotation to be the predominant mechanical factor in low-back pain (Duncan and Ahmed, 1991; Frymoyer et al., 1980, 1983; Ralston et al., 1974; Schaffer, 1982; Snook et al., 1978, 1980; and others).

Evidence for the foregoing theory can be seen from a couple of studies conducted by the author. Kumar and Narayan (1998) studied upright axial rotation of the human trunk in young and healthy subjects in fatiguing contraction. These subjects were seated in an axial rotation tester (Kumar, 1996) in an upright posture, stabilising their lower body hip down. Their shoulders were coupled with the shoulder harness of the device which allowed only axial rotation and coupled lateral flexion, preventing any motion in the sagittal plane. These subjects were required to attempt axial rotation at the 60 per cent level of their maximal voluntary contraction (MVC) for a period of two minutes. The electromyogram (EMG) was recorded from their erector spinae at the tenth thoracic and third lumbar vertebral levels, latissimus dorsi, external and internal obliques, rectus abdominis, and pectoralis major muscles bilaterally. Spectral analysis of EMG signals was carried out at every ten percentile points of the task cycle. The median frequency

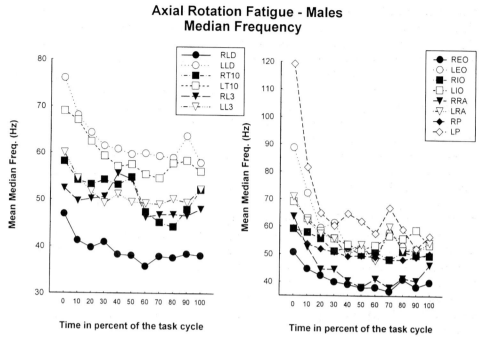

Figure 1.2 Median frequencies of trunk muscles during a fatiguing axial rotation contraction. RLD, right latissimus dorsi; LLD, left latissimus dorsi; RT10, right erector spinae at 10th thoracic vertebra; LT10, left erector spinae at 10th thoracic vertebra; RL3, right erector spinae at 3rd lumber vertebra; LL3, left erector spinae at 3rd lumbar vertebra; REO, right external oblique; LEO, left external oblique; RIO, right internal oblique; LIO, left internal oblique; RRA, right rectus abdominis; LRA, left rectus abdominis; RP, right pectoralis major; LP, left pectoralis major.

plots through the task cycle revealed that the overall slopes of decline of the median frequency (an index of physiological fatigue) of different muscles were significantly different (p < 0.01) (Figure 1.2). The latter clearly indicates a differential fatiguing rate. The decline in median frequency however cannot be quantitatively equated to force fatigue but a qualitative implication is obvious. In another experiment Kumar *et al.* (1998) studied the complex motion of simultaneous flexion and rotation among 18 young and normal subjects. The subjects were required to perform an isometric flexion–rotation or extension–rotation from 40° flexed and 40° right rotated postures. The subjects maintained 80 per cent of their MVC. EMGs from the same muscles were similarly processed. A differential decline in median frequencies of these muscles was also obvious (Figure 1.3).

Risk factors and back injuries

Hildebrandt (1987) identified from published literature 73 individual factors and 25 work-related factors which were considered as risk or potential risk factors for low-back pain (LBP). Taking the degree of agreement between sources as a measure of significance of the cited factors only 11 per cent of the individual factors (six) and 25 per cent of the

Female: Flexion - Rotation

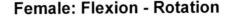

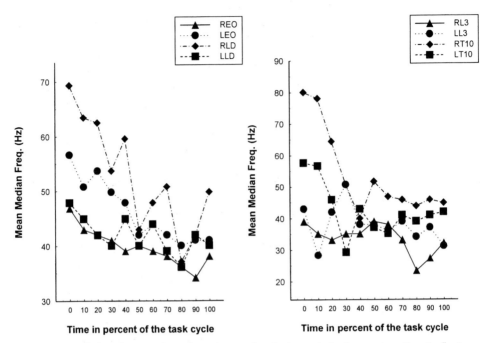

Figure 1.3   Median frequencies of trunk muscles during a fatiguing contraction in flexion–rotation. REO, right external oblique; LEO, left external oblique; RLD, right latissimus dorsi; LLD, left latissimus dorsi; RL3, right erector spinae at 3rd lumbar vertebra; LL3, left erector spinae at 3rd lumbar vertebra; RT10, right erector spinae at 10th thoracic vertebra; LT10, left erector spinae at 10th thoracic vertebra.

work related factors (six) emerged as important factors. Therefore, it appears that the epidemiological literature can be quite diverse in its factor selection and conclusions drawn therefrom. Millard (1988) reported fall as a cause of back injury. Kumar (1990a) reported cumulative load or life-time exposure to biomechanical loads as an important risk factor for low back pain. Most epidemiological studies are cross-sectional and do not allow a conclusive assessment of cause and effect; hence they do not have predictive value. Low-back pain is under multifactorial control. Whereas most risk factors identified may influence its causation (some directly and others indirectly), the one which precipitates the problem must reach its threshold level for the given individual. Since the life style occupation, leisure activity, nutrition, and anthropometry all vary for different people an array of results have been reported with a variety of conclusions.

All risk factors can be placed in one of four categories: genetic; morphological; psychosocial; and biomechanical. While not much can be done about genetic and morphological factors, knowledge of their role in causation or association with LBP, combined with the management strategies of biomechanical and psychosocial factors, could allow a significant and effective control strategy. Unfortunately, however, a comprehensive study of these factors with a view to controlling the LBP problem has not been undertaken. The genetic and morphological factors (as non-manipulatable factors) and psychosocial and biomechanical factors (as manipulatable factors) can be used for prediction. Such a combined approach is necessary, especially when no single test or a small battery of tests can be used to identify the potential LBP patient.

Disc herniation has been shown to have a genetic association (Lawrence, 1977; Varlotta and Brown, 1988). Varlotta and Brown found evidence to support the Mendelian pattern of inheritance in disc herniation cases. Annular fissure and disc protrusion was also reported to have a genetic association (Porter, 1987). Some of the many common morphological factors are age, body size and spinal canal size. An increasing risk of low-back pain with age has been reported in numerous epidemiological studies (Biering-Sorenson, 1982; Burton et al., 1989; Frymoyer et al., 1980). Similarly several workers have reported a disproportionate amount of back pain among taller men (Gyntelberg, 1974; Hrubec and Nashbold, 1975; Tauber, 1970; Weir, 1979; and others). However, it has been refuted by Pope et al. (1985) and Heliovaara (1988). A reduced vertebral canal size has been attributed as an important predictor of low back pain (Ehni, 1969; Heliovaara et al., 1988; Porter et al., 1980; Rothman and Simone, 1982; Verbiest, 1954; and others).

Job dissatisfaction has been reported as an important psychosocial factor which has a strong association with low-back pain (Andersson et al., 1983; Vallfors, 1985). Lloyd et al. (1979) and Frymoyer et al. (1985) have reported increased anxiety, neurosis, depression and heightened somatic awareness among low-back pain patients. Biering-Sorenson (1984) found previous hospitalisation, surgery, restlessness, frequent headaches, living alone, stomach ache, and fatigue were among the factors of psychosocial stress found among low-back pain patients. Whether these multiple psychosocial factors are causes or symptoms of low-back pain remains largely speculative. However, Bigos et al. (1988) indicate that a significant portion of the problem antedates the actual disability.

A large array of variables constitute biomechanical factors. Strength relative to job demand has been reported to be a risk factor for low back pain (Chaffin and Park, 1973; Keyserling et al., 1980). Biering-Sorenson (1984) reported the protective effect of good isometric endurance for back problems. Porter (1987) stated that strength protects an individual from disc protrusion. However, heavy manual work has been widely reported to be associated with low-back pain (Ayoub and Mital, 1989; Frymoyer et al., 1983; Gyntelberg, 1974; Heliovaara, 1987; Kumar, 1990a; Snook, 1978; and others). Bending and twisting have also been linked to low back pain (Frymoyer et al., 1980, 1983; Manning et al., 1984; Schaffer, 1982; Snook et al., 1978; and others). Exposure to vibration is reported to be contributory to low back pain problems (Frymoyer et al., 1983, Svensson and Andersson, 1983.)

THEORY OF INJURY PRECIPITATION

From the foregoing consideration of the nature of injury, the biomechanical basis of injury, and the risk factors one may state that a precipitation of low-back injury is an interactive process between genetic, morphological, psychosocial and biomechanical factors (Figure 1.4). Within each of these categories are numerous variables which potentiate and may effect precipitation of the low-back pain. Since the permutation and combination of so many variables is extensive there are numerous ways in which such an undesirable event may happen. However, it is speculated that an interaction between the relative weighting of the variables and the extent to which they have been stressed in any given individual determines the final outcome as depicted in Figure 1.4.

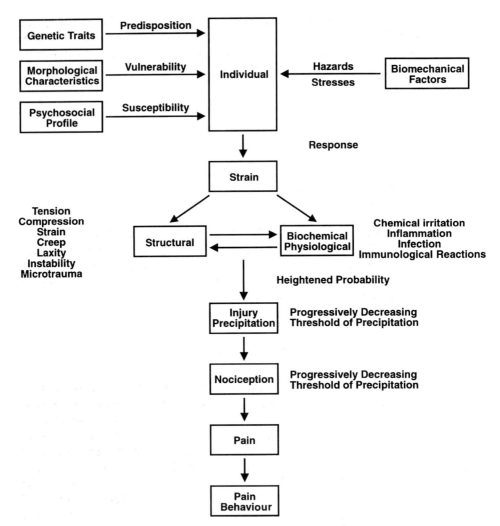

Figure 1.4 A global theory of musculoskeletal injury precipitation (modified from Kumar, 1991).

OVEREXERTION THEORY OF INJURY

A generic concept of overexertion

By definition exertion is an activity in which physical efforts are made. Therefore, overexertion will be a physical activity in which the level of effort would exceed the normal physiological and physical tolerance limits. It is however, unclear as to what may be considered normal physical and physiological standards. Should it be peak maximal voluntary contraction (MVC) or average strength over a five-second period, or 40 per cent of MVC, or 15 per cent of MVC? The answer to this question is further complicated when the activity concerned is either performed over some time or repeated periodically/ frequently. Such a scenario adds another dimension of frequency and duration in addition to the magnitude. Lastly, the range of the available inventory of motion in which the activity takes place is an important variable. Thus, overexertion can be created by exceeding the normal physical and physiological limits in any one of the foregoing criteria. Furthermore, a weighting of their function also remains obscure. Conceptually, however, overexertion can be symbolically represented as follows:

$$OE = \int (F_x, D_y, M_z) \tag{1.1}$$

where,

OE = overexertion
F_x = weight adjusted force magnitude
D_y = weight adjusted effective exposure
M_z = weight adjusted motion for the job.

All of these variables entered in determination of overexertion are complex in themselves and deserve further discussion in order to understand their impact and obtain a meaningful grasp of overexertion. This in turn may enable the development of a valid and manageable preventative strategy. However, prior to dealing with these variables an account of the association between exertion and injuries will be presented.

Overexertion injuries

A plethora of epidemiological studies reported in the literature reveal beyond doubt a strong association between exertion and injuries to the various regions of the human body. Statistics Canada (1991) reported that the largest portion of all occupational injuries (48 per cent) were overexertion injuries. A number of cross-sectional and case studies have shown that various disorders were caused in the neck and shoulder regions by increased muscle contraction. Onishi et al. (1976) reported shoulder muscle tenderness, and Bjelle et al. (1979, 1981) and Hagberg (1984) showed degenerative tendinitis of the rotator cuff tendons and chronic myalgia due to such exertions. Similarly, neck and shoulder pain and tense necks were reported due to exertion (Herberts and Kadefors, 1976; Hunting et al., 1981; Kukkonen et al., 1983; Kumar and Scaife, 1979). Other conditions have also been reported associated with exertion, such as supraspinatus tendinitis, myofascial syndrome and cervicobrachial disorders (Hagberg and Kvarnström, 1984; Herberts et al., 1984; Sällström and Schmidt, 1984), and neck and shoulder regional muscle disorders (Blader et al., 1987; Fine et al., 1986; Westgaard et al., 1986). The argument of association is supported by the observation that when muscle and joint loads were reduced or eliminated the incidence and severity of neck and shoulder disorders also decreased (Hagberg, 1984; Westgaard and Aaras, 1984; Westgaard et al., 1986).

The rapid increase of upper limb repetitive strain injury (RSI) or cumulative trauma disorders (CTD) has been largely attributed to the loads of posture (Armstrong, 1986), force levels (Armstrong et al., 1982; Silverstein et al., 1986), and repetition of posture and/or force application (Hymovich and Lyndholm, 1966; Kaplan, 1983; Silverstein et al., 1986). All three factors which have been reported to be causally associated, cause exertion of the structures. Awkward, fixed, constrained or deviated postures can overload the muscles, ligaments, and tendons and also load the joints in an asymmetrical manner. Smith et al. (1977) and Armstrong et al. (1982) have reported extreme flexion or extension associated with CTD of the wrist. In a cross-sectional study, Silverstein et al. (1986)

reported that industrial jobs involving low force and little repetition had the fewest CTD cases and that those involving high force and frequent repetition had approximately 30 times greater morbidity, indicating an interactive behaviour of the risk factors. Jobs requiring high force and little repetition or low force and frequent repetition had morbidity rates in between the extremes.

The magnitude of the mechanical load has been associated with low-back pain incidence by numerous authors (Andersson, 1981; Chaffin, 1974; Chaffin and Park, 1973; Heliovaara et al., 1987; Hult, 1954; Kumar, 1990a; Magora, 1970, 1972, 1973; NIOSH, 1981; Statistics Canada, 1991; and others). In the United States overexertion was claimed to have caused low-back pain in more than 60 per cent of low-back pain patients (Jensen, 1988). Forty-five per cent of all heavy load handlers were reported to have sought medical help for low-back pain in a ten year study by Rowe (1969).

Forceful static or repetitive contraction of muscles causes their corresponding tendons to stretch, thereby compressing their vascular epitenon, peritenon and endotenon microstructures. This in turn causes ischaemia, fibrillar tearing, and inflammation (Rathburn and MacNab, 1970). Frictional damage to the sheaths can occur with repetitive motion (Lamphier et al., 1965). Awkward postures contribute to muscle tendon inflammation by compression of the microstructure and by increasing the force requirements of the tasks (Tichauer, 1973). Tissue injuries are known to occur in maximal exertions; tissue tolerance characteristics are therefore considered to be factors of paramount importance. Evans and Lissner (1959) and Sonoda (1962) reported that mean ultimate compressive strengths of human spinal units are age dependent (3400 N for those 60 years and older, and 6700 N for those 40 years or younger). On this basis the National Institute for Occupational Safety and Health developed its *Work Practices Guide for Manual Lifting* (1981) which was updated by Waters et al. (1993). Brinckmann et al. (1988) demonstrated an interaction between the magnitude and repetition of loading on tissue failure of spinal structures. They also reported mechanical fatigue fractures of spinal units due to repetitive loading. Thus, an association of injuries with exertion is supported by many reports in the literature.

Components of the overexertion theory

Force of exertion

A reliable measure of strength is a single maximal voluntary contraction exerted over a period of up to five seconds (Chaffin, 1975). The value of strength varies in different activities (Ayoub et al., 1978; Chaffin et al., 1978; Kumar, 1990b, 1991; Kumar and Garand, 1992; Kumar et al., 1988, 1991; Snook, 1978; and others). Different levels of strength exertion have different levels of physiological demand. Rohmert, as early as 1973, demonstrated that the duration for which a muscular contraction can be sustained depends on the level of contraction. Contractions of the levels of 15 to 20 per cent only can be held indefinitely as a continuous hold. Higher levels of contraction impede the blood supply and thereby availability of nutrients and oxygen to the muscles doing the work. Furthermore, such an occlusion of the blood supply also interferes with the removal of metabolites, which results in a sensation of pain. Industrial jobs are not prolonged static holds; rather they generally require short time repetitive exertions. These exertions remain constant for the task in hand (constant work level, CWL) though they may represent a different proportion of the MVC for different workers. Ayoub et al. (1978) and Chaffin

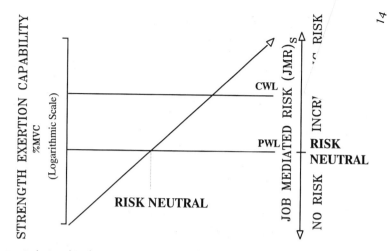

Figure 1.5 Relationship between exertion and risk of overexertion injuries.

et al. (1978) have reported that as the strength required on the job increases the injury incidence also increases. It is, however, unclear as to what level of strength requirement may be considered risk neutral. It has been suggested that due to an integrative capacity, the human perception of a preferred level of work may optimise the balance of physical and physiological factors in favour of system safety (Kumar and Mital, 1992). Kumar and Simmonds (1992) have also reported that people underestimate precision and power as well as gross motor efforts under 40 per cent of MVC and overestimate efforts greater than that value. The pattern of perception was repeatable and reliable. It may, therefore, follow that an assessment of a preferred work level (PWL) based on the perceptual sense may provide a level of exertion which may be risk neutral. An exertion above PWL will increase and below PWL will maintain the job mediated risk (JMR) for overexertion injuries at risk neutral level (Figure 1.5). Though the quantitative nature of this relationship is unclear a logarithmic association is assumed. Thus according to this conceptual model any exertion above the PWL would be considered overexertion. Taking MVC as maximal capability and PWL as risk neutral, the range can be considered to represent 100 to 0 per cent of the strength component of the JMR. For scoring the margin of safety (MOS), a scale from 0 (to represent maximum risk) to 1 (to represent no risk) can be used. Thus, the risk neutral level of exertion will have an MOS of 1 and an exertion at the level of MVC will have an MOS of 0. The range will be proportionally divided between 0 and 1.

Duration of exertion

The significance of the time variable of exertion is dependent upon the type of contraction, the magnitude of contraction, the recovery period and the repetition of the activity in question. With any activity there will be phosphagen and glycogen depletion from the intrinsic muscular sources before the aerobic glycolysis ensues, depending on the circumstances. Such metabolic response will also result in accumulation of lactate. Following high intensity activity, although up to 70 per cent replenishment of phosphagen on the one hand and removal of lactate on the other may take place in 30 seconds (Hultman *et al.*, 1967) near complete replenishing may take up to five minutes (Astrand and Rodahl, 1977). Though the endurance times of submaximal contractions as a percentage of MVC

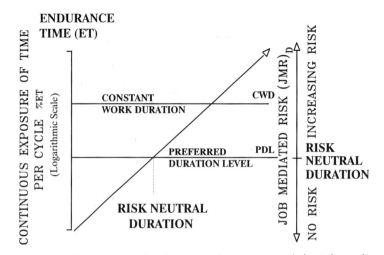

Figure 1.6 Relationship between the duration of exposure and the job mediated risk of overexertion injuries.

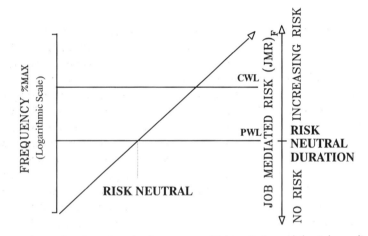

Figure 1.7 Relationship between the frequency of job activity and the job mediated risk of overexertion injuries.

are widely reported (Rohmert, 1973) the exact time required for near full recovery is unclear. What is also unclear is the duration of submaximal contractions at different levels of MVC and the corresponding time durations by which time no significant adverse physiological and metabolic change has taken place. However, in an occupationally less relevant study Molbech (1963) reported that the strength of isometric exertions (MVC) declined from 85 to 60 per cent of MVC as the frequency of exertion was increased from five to 30 per minute.

In the absence of clear quantitative data, a subjective estimation of the preferred duration and frequency of the activity at the level of contraction required by the job may be the most appropriate design variable to consider. Thus, the duration and frequency risk of activity can be represented as in Figures 1.6 and 1.7.

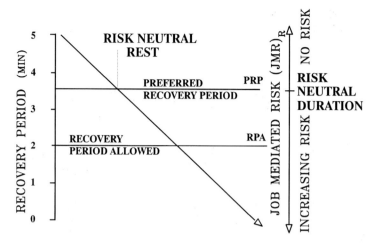

Figure 1.8 Empirical relationship between the inter-cycle rest and the job mediated risk of overexertion injuries.

Taking the endurance time and maximum possible frequency for the level of contraction as maximal duration and frequency achievable with maximal risk and 0 MOS and preferred duration and frequency levels of the activity as the risk neutral duration with an MOS of 1, various levels of safety and risk can be calculated on a logarithmic scale. However, the exact quantitative relationship may be different and is currently unknown.

The period of recovery following an activity is an important variable which may determine the pacing of the task without accumulation of stress which eventually leads to overexertion injuries. Though there are data available regarding recovery of the central system following maximal exercise (at VO_2 max), similar information is unavailable for submaximal activity and for local factors. Due to the paucity of such information a subjective assessment of an optimum rest period for the combination of the individual and the task may be an appropriate methodology to adopt. Therefore, the preferred rest period may be assumed to be the same as the required rest period. Based on these presuppositions and the rationale used for other variables the recovery from stress (RS) may be depicted as in Figure 1.8.

Even though the magnitude and duration of contractions are at or below the preferred level, if sufficient recovery time is unavailable there will be a residual effect from each contraction. These may then accumulate over the work period and predispose the worker to an occupational overexertion injury. The risk of injury will tend to grow with the residual stress. Thus, the MOS at risk neutral rest duration and above will be 1, and below this value continue to decrease. With continuous activity, i.e. no rest, it will be zero. Due to a lack of quantitative information the relationship between lack of rest and job mediated risk is presumed logarithmic.

In cases where rest and recovery is not a factor, either due to a very short duration and/ or low grade contraction the frequency of operation may be an important variable to constitute a risk factor of the job. For this variable as well, a preferred frequency of the job or job simulated activity and the frequencies below may be considered as the risk neutral frequency with an MOS of 1. The frequencies above this level will increase the JMR. With activities being performed at a continuous pace the MOS will be zero.

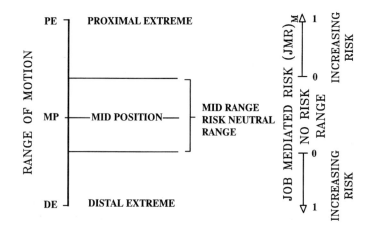

Figure 1.9 Empirical relationship between the job range of motion and the job mediated risk of overexertion injuries.

Job range of motion

The geometric relationships of the muscle, tendon, and bones with respect to the joint vary with the degree of motion at the joint. At the extremes of their ranges the joints are at the greatest mechanical and physiological disadvantage. Though the exact angle at which the best mechanical and physiological advantage is available may vary somewhat from joint to joint, generally the mid position of the range is perceived to require low effort for performance. This will be designated the risk neutral position. Deviations from the mid range position to either side will represent increasing hazard. The range around the mid position which may either be subjectively considered as the comfortable zone or which increases the effort required (by virtue of the position) by 20 per cent may be designated the risk neutral zone. Deviations from this or motion in excess of the mid range may constitute a job mediated motion risk, rising from 0 to 1 on either side of the range as shown in Figure 1.9. Deviation to either side of the mid range beyond the risk neutral zone will be considered hazardous independently on a 0 to 1 scale. Deviations on both sides in a given job are expected to have a multiplicative effect, but are finally represented by one value on a 0 to 1 scale as the product of the proximal and distal scores.

A global model of safety and hazard

All musculoskeletal injuries have a biomechanical basis, which is affected by three variables: force application; effective exposure to the force exertion; and the extent and range of motion in these activities. It is, therefore, important to integrate these three ingredients of injury causation in order to arrive at a meaningful composite index. It is also proposed here that the sum of the MOS and the JMR will always be unity. Such a relationship is based on the logic that if the MOS is 100 per cent, there is no risk of injury. Conversely, if the risk is 100 per cent, there can be no safety. If, however, the MOS is 40 per cent then the risk will be 60 per cent. Therefore,

$$MOS + JMR = 1 \tag{1.2}$$

Thus, it follows that,

$$MOS = 1 - JMR. \tag{1.3}$$

The composite index (CI) of JMR can be obtained by subtracting the total safety from 1. Thus, if there are three risk factors, R_1, R_2, and R_3, their corresponding safety, S_1, S_2, and S_3 can be expressed as follows:

$$S_1 = (1 - R_1)$$
$$S_2 = (1 - R_2)$$
$$S_3 = (1 - R_3)$$

The MOS of the system will be proportional to the product of the individual safety components. Such a multiplicative model accounts for interaction among the variables in question, which is the case in life. When force is applied, it is done so for varying periods. Furthermore, it could be applied through a varying range of motion. Also, the multiplicative model will ensure that as the number of risk factors increases, even with smaller risks, the safety margin will decline. Such is the case in any phenomenon affected by many variables, as reported by Kumar (1990a) for low back pain. Therefore,

$$MOS \propto S1 \cdot S2 \cdot S3.$$

However, different safety factors may have different weight because of the structure, geometry, size, strength, material property, strength, or any other relevant factor. There-fore, a more reliable relationship can be obtained by multiplying the individual safety components by their respective weighting factors as shown below:

$$MOS \propto S1_a \cdot S2_b \cdot S3_c,$$

where,

a = weighting factor for S1
b = weighting factor for S2, and
c = weighting factor for S3.

Inserting the proportionality constant, the exact quantitative relationship can be expressed as:

$$MOS = K \cdot S1_a \cdot S2_b \cdot S3_c, \tag{1.4}$$

where,

K = proportionality constant for safety factors.

These weighting factors and proportionality constants are unknown and will have to be obtained through various *in vivo* and *in vitro* experimentations and epidemiological stud-ies carried out to specifically deduce these values. Furthermore, because each of these individual variables of stress, duration and motion is a complex entity, they may poten-tially be affected by more than one variable. Therefore, they will need a specific internal proportionality constant. Rewriting the above equation in terms of risk factors and in its expanded form we get:

$$MOS = K \, (1 - \alpha_1 R1_x)(1 - \alpha_2 R2_y)(1 - \alpha_3 R3_z) \tag{1.5}$$

where,

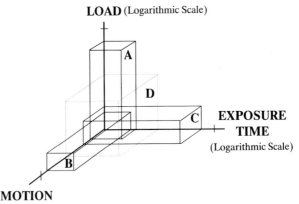

Figure 1.10   Depiction of job mediated risk indices of four different jobs – A, B, C, and D. Jobs A, B, and C have predominantly load, motion and duration risks. Job D has a similar magnitude of risk all around.

K = proportionality constant for MOS
α_1 = proportionality constant for R1
x = weighting factor for R1
α_2 = proportionality constant for R2
y = weighting factor for R2
α_3 = proportionality constant for R3
z = weighting factor for R3

Therefore, the CI of JMR can be expressed as follows:

$$CI = [1 - K\,(1 - \alpha_1 R1_x)(1 - \alpha_2 R2_y)(1 - \alpha_3 R3_y)] \tag{1.6}$$

Bringing the foregoing concept into the context of overexertion injuries, the overall job-mediated risk can be obtained through the risks posed by the indices for stress, effective exposure, and motion. The higher the composite index score, the greater the risk. Although a composite index of the JMR may not provide an indication of the variable most at risk, it does indicate the extent of the potential problem. In order to quantify the risk, one should list the stress, effective exposure, and motion indices separately as shown below and in Figure 1.10 for a hypothetical example:

$$CI \text{ of } JMR = 0.957 \;(SI - 0.87, \; EI - 0.2, \; MI - 0.25) \tag{1.7}$$

where,

SI is stress index
EI is exposure index, and
MI is motion index.

Using the relationship depicted in Equation 1.1 and integrating the job mediated risks, one can express the margin of safety as follows:

$$MOS = K\,(1 - \alpha_1 SI_x)(1 - \alpha_2\,EI_y)(1 - \alpha_3 MI_z) \tag{1.8}$$

where x, y, and z are weighting factors for SI, EI and MI respectively.

Expanding Equation 1.2 by substituting for SI, EI and MI, one will get the following:

$$\text{MOS} = K \left[1 - \alpha_1 \left(\frac{\text{CWL} - \text{PWL}}{\text{MVC} - \text{PWL}} \right)_X \right]_X$$

$$\left[1 - \alpha_2 \left\{ \left(1 - \frac{\text{CWD} - \text{PDL}}{\text{ET} - \text{PDL}} \right) \left(1 - \frac{\text{CF} - \text{PF}}{\text{MF} - \text{PF}} \right) \left(1 - \frac{\text{RR} - \text{AR}}{\text{RR}} \right) \right\}_Y \right]_X$$

$$\left[1 - \alpha_3 \left\{ \left(1 - \frac{\text{MRQ}_p - \text{MDR}_p}{\text{PE} - \text{MDR}_p} \right) \left(1 - \frac{\text{MRQ}_d - \text{MDR}_d}{\text{DE} - \text{MDR}_d} \right) \right\}_Z \right]_X \qquad (1.9)$$

where,

K = proportionality constant for margin of safety
α_1 = a constant for stress index
MOS = margin of safety
CWL = constant work level
PWL = preferred work level
MVC = maximum voluntary contraction
x = weighting factor of the stress index
α_2 = constant for the duration index
CWD = constant work duration
PDL = preferred duration level
ET = endurance time
CF = constant job frequency
PF = preferred job frequency
MF = maximum frequency possible for the job activity
AR = allowed recovery period
RR = required recovery period
y = weighting factor of the duration index
α_3 = constant for the motion index
MRQ_p = motion required in proximal direction
MDR_p = mid range in proximal direction
PE = proximal extreme motion
MRQ_d = motion required in distal direction
MDR_d = mid range in distal motion
DE = distal extreme motion
z = weighting factor of the motion index (Kumar, 1994; quoted with permission).

Thus the overexertion theory of musculoskeletal injury causation incorporates different variables which affect the load on the system by means of force, duration or posture. All three factors may be operative at the same time in varying degrees. Any of these variables or their combination, when they exceed the natural margin of safety will potentiate injury. Musculoskeletal injuries are multivariate phenomena and they can be explained and thus controlled only through multivariate approaches. The overexertion theory addresses only the internal physical factors and their role in injury causation. Direct trauma to the tissues through external agents and devices is excluded from this approach. Furthermore, the role of psychosocial factors, if any, has not been explored and explained in this theory. Are psychosocial factors causal in musculoskeletal injury precipitation? Although

many opinions are floating in scientific circles, the literature has only reported an association. Questions have been asked as to whether the psychosocial traits are the result
of musculoskeletal injuries or whether they have been instrumental in their causation.
It would appear that certain psychosocial traits may facilitate physical overexertion,
causing injury. In this sense their role may be an important one. Nonetheless, injuries
have biomechanical bases and their occurrence under most circumstances, if not all, will
require overexertion.

SUMMARY

Occupational activities result in occupational musculoskeletal injuries. Injuries have a
biomechanical basis and occur as a result of mechanical disruption of tissues. Tissues
have material properties and exceeding their limits results in tissue failure. Tissue load
bearing capacity changes in time or due to its loading history as all biological materials
are viscoelastic. Almost all identified risk factors affect the material properties of the
tissues determining their vulnerability. Genetic predisposition and psychosocial susceptibility contribute to the innate characteristics, physical preparedness and mental alertness
to negotiate biomechanical hazards. An interaction of these factors may determine safety
or injury precipitation. The biomechanical hazards comprising force, effective exposure
and postural load interact to create a composite job mediated risk of injury. When the
magnitude of this risk exceeds the tissue tolerance capacity, an injury is precipitated.

References

ANDERSSON, G.B.J., 1981, Epidemiologic aspects on low-back pain in industry, *Spine*, **6**, 53–60.
ANDERSSON, G.B.J., SVENSSON, H.O. and ODEN, A., 1983, The intensity of work recovery in
    low back pain, *Spine*, **8**, 880–884.
ARMSTRONG, T.J., 1986, Ergonomics and cumulative trauma disorders, *Hand Clinics*, **2**, 533–565.
ARMSTRONG, T.J., FOULKE, J.A., JOSEPH, B.S. and GOLDSTEIN, S.A., 1982, Investigation of
    cumulative trauma disorders in a poultry processing plant. *American Industrial Hygiene Asso-
    ciation Journal*, **43**, 103–116.
ASTRAND, P.O. and RODAHL, K., 1977, *Textbook of Work Physiology*, New York: McGraw-Hill
    Book Co.
AYOUB, M.M. and MITAL, A., 1989, *Manual Materials Handling*, London: Taylor & Francis.
AYOUB, M.M., BETHEA, N.J., DEIVANYAGAM, S., *et al.*, 1978, Determination and modeling of
    lifting capacity, Final Report, DHEW/NIOSH Grant No. 5 R01 OH DO545-02.
BIERING-SORENSON, F., 1982, Low back trouble in a general population of 30-, 40-, 50-, and 60-
    year old men and women: study design, representativeness and basic results, *Danish Medical
    Bulletin*, **29**, 289–299.
BIERING-SORENSON, F., 1984, Physical measurements as risk indicators for low-back trouble
    over a one-year period, *Spine*, **9**, 106–119.
BIGOS, S.J., BATTIÉ, M.C., FISHER, L.D., *et al.*, 1988, The prospective study of risk factors for
    the report of industrial back problems: a univariate analysis. Presented at the Meeting of the
    International Society for the Study of the Lumbar Spine, Miami, Florida, April 13–17.
BJELLE, A., HAGBERG, M. and MICHAELSON, G., 1979, Clinical and ergonomic factors in
    prolonged shoulder pain among industrial workers, *Scandinavian Journal of Work, Environ-
    ment and Health*, **5**, 205–210.
BJELLE, A., HAGBERG, M. and MICHAELSON, G., 1981, Occupational and individual factors in
    acute shoulder-neck disorders among industrial workers, *British Journal of Industrial Medi-
    cine*, **38**, 356–363.

BLADER, S., HOLST, B., DANIELSSON, U., FERHM, F., KALPAMAA, M., LEIJON, K., et al., 1987, Neck and shoulder complaints among sewing machine operators: frequencies and diagnoses in comparison to control population, in Buckle, P. (Ed.), *Musculoskeletal Disorders at Work*, London: Taylor & Francis, pp. 110–111.

BRINCKMANN, P., BIGGEMANN, M. and HILWEG, D., 1988, Fatigue fractures of human lumbar vertebrae, *Clinical Biomechanics*, **2**(Suppl. 1), S1–S23.

BURTON, A.K., TILLOTSON, K.M. and TROUP, J.D.G., 1989, Prediction of the low-back trouble frequency in a working population, *Spine*, **14**, 939–946.

CHAFFIN, D.B., 1974, Human strength capability and low back pain, *Journal of Occupational Medicine*, **16**, 248–254.

CHAFFIN, D.B., 1975, Ergonomic guide for the assessment of human static strength, *Annual Industrial Hygiene Association Journal*, **36**, 505–510.

CHAFFIN, D.B. and PARK, K.S., 1973, A longitudinal study of low-back pain as associated with occupational weight lifting factors, *American Industrial Hygiene Association Journal*, **34**, 513–525.

CHAFFIN, D.B., HERRIN, G.D. and KEYSERLING, W.M., 1978, Preemployment strength testing: an updated position, *Journal of Occupational Medicine*, **20**, 403.

DUNCAN, N.A. and AHMED, A.M., 1991, The role of axial rotation in the aetiology of unilateral disc prolapse, an experiment and fine element analysis, *Spine*, **16**, 1089–1098.

EHNI, G., 1969, Significance of the small lumbar spinal canal: cauda equina compression syndrome due to spondylolysis, *Journal of Neurology*, **31**, 490–494.

EVANS, F.G. and LISSNER, H.R., 1959, Biomechanical studies on the lumbar spine and pelvis, *Journal of Bone and Joint Surgery*, **41A**, 218–290.

FINE, L.J., SILVERSTEN, B., ARMSTRONG, T., JOSEPH, B. and BUCHHOLZ, B., 1986, A pilot study of postural characteristics of jobs associated with an elevated risk of rotator cuff tendinitis, in Corlett, E.N., Wilson, J. and Manenica, I. (Eds), *The Ergonomics of Working Postures*, London: Taylor & Francis, pp. 39–43.

FRYMOYER, J.W., POPE, M.H., COSTANZA, M.C., ROSEN, J.C., GOGGIN, J.E. and WILDER, D.G., 1980, Epidemiologic studies of low back pain, *Spine*, **5**, 419–423.

FRYMOYER, J., POPE, M.H., CLEMENTS, J.H., et al., 1983, Risk factors in low-back pain – an epidemiological survey, *Journal of Bone and Joint Surgery*, **65A**, 213–218.

FRYMOYER, J.W., ROSEN, J.C., CLEMENTS, J., et al., 1985, Psychologic factors in low-back pain disability, *Clinical Orthopedic Rel Research*, **195**, 178–184.

GYNTELBERG, F., 1974, One year incidence of low back pain among male residents of Copenhagen age 40–59, *Danish Medical Bulletin*, **21**, 30–36.

HAGBERG, M., 1984, Occupational musculo-skeletal stress and disorders of the neck and shoulder: a review of possible pathophysiology, *International Archives of Occupational and Environmental Health*, **53**, 269–278.

HAGBERG, M. and KVARNSTRÖM, S., 1984, Muscular endurance and electromyographic fatigue in myofascial shoulder pain, *Archives of Physical Medicine and Rehabilitation*, **65**, 522–525.

HELIOVAARA, M., 1987, Occupation and risk of herniated lumbar disc or sciatica leading to hospitalization, *Journal of Chronic Disorders*, **40**, 259.

HELIOVAARA, M., 1988, Body height, obesity, and risk of herniated lumbar intervertebral disc, *Spine*, **12**, 469–472.

HELIOVAARA, M., KNEKT, P. and AROMA, A., 1987, Incidence and risk factors of herniated lumbar disc or sciatica leading to hospitalization, *Journal of Chronic Diseases*, **3**, 251–285.

HELIOVAARA, M., VANHARANTA, H., KORPI, J., et al., 1988, Herniated lumbar disc syndrome and vertebral canals, in Heliovaara, M. (Ed.), *Epidemiology of Sciatica and Herniated Lumbar Intervertebral Disc*, Helsinki: Social Insurance Institution, pp. 433–435.

HERBERTS, P. and KADEFORS, R., 1976, A study of painful shoulder in welders, *Acta Orthopaedica Scandinavica*, **47**, 381–387.

HERBERTS, P., KADEFORS, R., HOGFORS, C. and SIGHOLM, G., 1984, Shoulder pain and heavy manual labor, *Clinical Orthopaedics and Related Research*, **191**, 166–178.

HILDEBRANDT, V.H., 1987, A review of epidemiological research on risk factors of low-back pain, in Buckle, P. (Ed.), *Musculoskeletal Disorders at Work*, London: Taylor & Francis, pp. 9–16.

HRUBEC, A. and NASHBOLD, B.S., Jr, 1975, Epidemiological of lumbar disc lesions in the military in World War II, *American Journal of Epidemiology*, **102**, 366.

HULT, L., 1954, Cervical, dorsal and lumbar spinal syndromes, *Acta Orthopaedica Scandinavica*, **17**(Suppl.), 1–102.

HULTMAN, E., BERGSTROM, J. and MCLENNAN-ANDERSON, N., 1967, Breakdown and resynthesis of phosphorycreatine and adenosine triphosphate in connection with muscular work in man, *Scandinavian Journal of Clinical Investigation*, **19**, 56–66.

HUNTING, W., LAUBLI, T. and GRANDJEAN, E., 1981, Postural and visual loads at VDT workplaces: I. Constrained postures, *Ergonomics*, **24**, 917–931.

HYMOVICH, L. and LYNDHOLM, M., 1966, Hand, wrist and forearm injuries, the result of repetitive motions, *Journal of Occupational Medicine*, **2**, 573–577.

JENSEN, R.C., 1988, Epidemiology of work-related back pain, *Topics in Acute Care and Trauma Rehabilitation*, **2**, 1–15.

KAPLAN, P.E., 1983, Carpal tunnel syndrome in typists, *Journal of the American Medical Association*, **250**, 821–822.

KEYSERLING, W.M., HERRIN, G.D., CHAFFIN, D.B., *et al.*, 1980, Establishing an industrial strength testing program, *American Industrial Hygiene Association Journal*, **41**, 730.

KUKKONEN, R., LUOPAJARVI, T. and RIIHIMAKI, V., 1983, Prevention of fatigue amongst data-entry operators, in Kvalseth, T.O. (Ed.), *Ergonomics of Workstation Design*, London: Butterworths, pp. 28–34.

KUMAR, S., 1990a, Cumulative load as a risk factor for low back pain, *Spine*, **15**, 1311–1316.

KUMAR, S., 1990b, Symmetrical and symmetrical stoop-lifting strength, *Proceedings of the 34th Annual Meeting of the Human Factors Society*, pp. 762–766.

KUMAR, S., 1991, Arm lift strength, *Applied Ergonomics*, **22**(5), 317–328.

KUMAR, S., 1994, A conceptual model of overexertion, safety and risk of injury in occupational settings, *Human Factors*, **36**, 197–209.

KUMAR, S., 1996, Isolated planar trunk strength measurement in normals: Part III – Results and database, *International Journal of Industrial Ergonomics*, **17**, 103–111.

KUMAR, S. and GARAND, D., 1992, Static and dynamic strength at different reach distances in symmetrical and asymmetrical planes, *Ergonomics*, **35**(7,8):861–880.

KUMAR, S. and MITAL, A., 1992, Margin of safety for the human back: a probable consensus based on published studies. *Ergonomics*, **35**(7,8):769–781.

KUMAR, S. and NARAYAN, Y., 1998, Spectral parameters of trunk muscles during isometric axial rotation in neutral posture, *Journal of Electromyography and Kinesiology* (in press).

KUMAR, S. and SCAIFE, W.G.S., 1979, A precision task, posture, and strain, *Journal of Safety Research*, **11**, 28–36.

KUMAR, S. and SIMMONDS, M., 1992, Effort perception as an ergonomic tool, in Kumar, S. (Ed.), *Advances in Industrial Ergonomics and Safety IV*, London: Taylor & Francis, pp. 637–643.

KUMAR, S., CHAFFIN, D.B. and REDFERN, M., 1988, Static and dynamic strength device and measurement, *Journal of Biomechanics*, **21**, 35–44.

KUMAR, S., DUFRESNE, R.M. and GARAND, D., 1991, Effect of posture on back strength. *International Journal of Industrial Ergonomics*, **7**, 53–62.

KUMAR, S., ZEDKA, M. and NARAYAN, Y., 1998, Fatigue of trunk muscles in isometric trunk rotation with flexion or extension, *European Journal of Applied Physiology* (submitted).

LAMPHIER, T., CROOKER, C. and CROOKER, J., 1965, DeQuervain's disease, *Industrial Medicine and Surgery*, **34**, 847–856.

LAWRENCE, J., 1977, *Rheumatism in Populations*, London: W. Heinemann, Medical Books Ltd.

LLOYD, G., WOLKIND, S., GREENWOOD, R. and HARRIS, D., 1979, A psychiatric study of patients with persistent low back pain, *Rheumatology Rehabilitation*, **18**, 30–34.

MAGORA, A., 1970, Investigation of the relation between low back pain and occupation, *Industrial Medicine*, **39**(11), 31–37.

MAGORA, A., 1972, Investigation of the relation between low-back pain and occupation: 3. Physical requirements: sitting, standing and weight lifting, *Industrial Medicine*, **41**(2), 5–9.

MAGORA, A., 1973, Investigation of the relation between low back pain and occupation: 4. Physical requirements: bending, rotation, reaching and sudden maximal effort, *Scandinavian Journal of Rehabilitation Medicine*, **5**, 186–190.

MANNING, D.P., MITCHELL, R.G. and BLANCHFIELD, L.P., 1984, Body movements and events contributing to accidental and non-accidental back injuries, *Spine*, **9**, 734–749.

MILLARD, V., 1988, *Report of the Task Force on the Worker's Compensation Board*, Alberta Government.

MOLBECH, S., 1963, Average percentage force at repeated maximal isometric muscle contractions at different frequencies. Communications from the Testing and Observations Institute of the Danish National Association for Infantile Paralysis, No. 16.

NIOSH (National Institute for Occupational Safety and Health), 1981, *Work Practices Guide for Manual Lifting*, DHHS [NIOSH] Publication 81–122, Cincinnati, OH: US Government Printing Office.

ONISHI, N., NOMURA, H., SAKAI, K., YAMAMOTO, T., HIRAYAMA, K. and ITANI, T., 1976, Shoulder muscle tenderness and physical fature of female industrial workers, *Journal of Human Ergology*, **5**, 87–102.

POPE, M.H., BEVINS, T., WILDER, D.G., *et al.*, 1985, The relationship between anthropometric, postural, muscular, and mobility characteristics of males aged 18–55, *Spine*, **10**, 644–648.

PORTER, R.W., 1987, Risk factors and back pain, in Buckle, P. (Ed.), *Musculoskeletal Disorders at Work*, London: Taylor & Francis, pp. 75–81.

PORTER, R.W., HIBBERT, C. and WELLMAN, P., 1980, Backache and the lumbar spinal canal, *Spine*, **5**, 99.

RALSTON, H.J., INMAN, V.T., STRAIT, L.A. and SHAFFRATH, M.D., 1974, Mechanics of human isolated voluntary muscle, *American Journal of Physiology*, **151**, 612–620.

RATHBURN, J.B. and MACNAB, I., 1970, The microvascular pattern of the rotator cuff, *Journal of Bone and Joint Surgery*, **52B**, 540–553.

ROHMERT, W., 1973, Problems in determining rest allowances. *Applied Ergonomics*, **4**, 91–95, 158–162.

ROTHMAN, R.H. and SIMONE, F.A., 1982, *The Spine*, 2nd edn, Philadelphia, London, Toronto: W.B. Sanders Co., p. 518.

ROWE, M.L., 1969, Low back pain in industry: a position paper, *Journal of Occupational Medicine*, **11**, 161–169.

SÄLLSTRÖM, J. and SCHMIDT, H., 1984, Cerviobrachial disorders in certain occupations, with special reference in the thoracic outlet, *American Journal of Industrial Medicine*, **6**, 45–52.

SCHAFFER, H., 1982, *Back Injuries Associated with Lifting*, Bulletin 2144, US Department of Labor, Bureau of Statistics, Washington, DC, pp. 1–20.

SILVERSTEIN, B.A., FINE, L.J. and ARMSTRONG, T.J., 1986, Hand, wrist cumulative trauma disorders in industry, *British Journal of Industrial Medicine*, **43**, 779–784.

SMITH, E., SONSTEGARD, D. and ANDREWS, W., 1977, Contribution of the flexor tendons to the carpal tunnel syndrome, *Archives of Physical Medicine and Rehabilitation*, **58**, 379–385.

SNOOK, S.H., 1978, The design of manual handling tasks, *Ergonomics*, **21**, 963–985.

SNOOK, S., CAMPANELLI, R.A. and HART, J.W., 1978, A study of three preventative approaches to low-back injury, *Journal of Occupational Medicine*, **20**, 478–481.

SNOOK, S.H., CAMPANELLAI, R.A. and HART, J.W., 1980, A study of back injuries at Pratt and Whitney Aircraft, Liberty Mutual Insurance Corporation, Hopkinton, MA.

SONODA, T., 1962, Studies on the compression, tension and tension strength of the human vertebral column, *Journal of the Kyoto Prefect Medical University*, **71**, 659–702.

STATISTICS CANADA, 1991, *Work Injuries, 1988–1990*, Ottawa, Ontario, Canada.

SVENSSON, H.O. and ANDERSSON, G.B.J., 1983, Low-back pain in 40- to 47-year old men: work history and work environment, *Spine*, **8**, 272.

TAUBER, J., 1970, An orthodox look at the backaches, *Journal of Occupational Medicine*, **12**, 128–130.

TICHAUER, E.R., 1973, Ergonomic aspects of biomechanics, in *Industrial Environment – Its Evaluation and Control*, Washington, DC: National Institute for Occupational Safety and Health, pp. 431–492.

VALLFORS, B., 1985, Acute, subacute and chronic low back pain: clinical symptoms, absenteeism and working environment, *Scandinavian Journal of Rehabilitation Medicine*, **11**(Suppl.), 1–98.

VARLOTTA, G.P. and BROWN, M.D., 1988, Familial predisposition for adolescent disc displacement, presentation at the Meeting of the International Society for the Study of the Lumbar Spine, Miami, Florida, April 13–17.

VERBIEST, H., 1954, A radicular syndrome from developmental narrowing of the lumbar vertebral canal, *Journal of Bone Joint Surgery*, **36B**, 230–237.

WATERS, T.R., PUTZ-ANDERSON, V., GARG, A. and FINE, L.J., 1993, Revised NIOSH equation for the design and evaluation of manual lifting tasks, *Ergonomics*, **36**, 749–776.

WEIR, B.K., 1979, Prospective study of 100 lumbosacral discectomies, *Journal of Neurosurgery*, **50**, 283–289.

WESTGAARD, R.H. and AARAS, A., 1984, Postural muscle strain as a causal factor in the development of musculoskeletal illnesses, *Applied Ergonomics*, **15**, 162–174.

WESTGAARD, R., WAERSTED, M., JANSEN, T. and AARAS, A., 1986, Muscle load and illness associated with constrained body postures, in Corlett, E.N., Wilson, J. and Manenica, I. (Eds), *The Ergonomics of Working Postures*, London: Taylor & Francis, pp. 3–18.

World Health Organisation, 1995, Global strategy on occupational health for all, WHO, Geneva.

PART ONE

Tissue Biomechanics

CHAPTER TWO

Tissue mechanics of ligaments and tendons

SAVIO L.-Y. WOO, MARIA APRELEVA AND JÜRGEN HÖHER

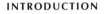

INTRODUCTION

The motion of the musculoskeletal system is stabilised and guided by ligaments and tendons, bands of tough connective tissue that traverse the joints of the body and bind the skeleton. Once thought to be relatively inert and static structures designed solely to maintain proper skeletal alignment, ligaments and tendons are now known to have many functions. The major functions of ligaments include: to *attach* articulating bones to one another across a joint; to *guide* joint movements; to maintain joint *congruency*; and to act as a *strain sensor*. In addition, laboratory experiments have shown that ligaments display complex biomechanical behaviour, providing primary stabilisation to the joints as well as maintaining normal joint kinematics. Tendons, on the other hand, attach the muscle to the bone and their major function is to *transfer* forces between muscle and bone. Tendons may be constrained as they cross joints with the purpose of maintaining their orientation during joint motion. These constraints may be formed by body prominences around or through which the tendon passes (e.g. biceptal groove in the humerus) or by specialised connective tissue sheaths. The sheaths are particularly important in the hand and feet, as tendons passing towards the fingers or toes over the numerous small joints would be susceptible to injury if displaced during finger or toe motion.

Recent advances in technology have permitted development of new methodologies which permit a careful examination of the properties of ligaments and tendons, and have identified these tissues to have viscoelastic and temperature-dependent properties. Also, the effects of freezing, strain rate, skeletal maturity, and aging on these tissues have been studied (Frank *et al.*, 1985; Woo *et al.*, 1986a, 1986b, 1987a, 1990b). This chapter briefly describes the morphological, anatomical, biochemical, and biomechanical properties of ligaments and tendons and the relationship between these properties and the stiffness and strength, function, susceptibility to injury and subsequent healing and repair.

TENDON   HIERARCHY

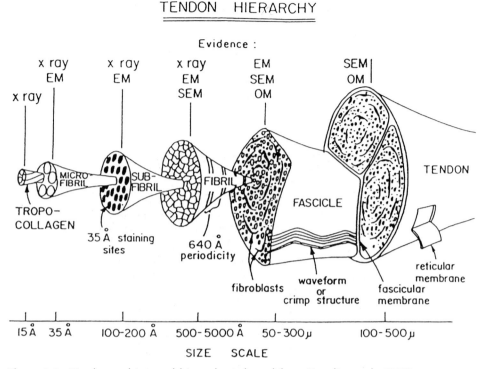

Figure 2.1   Tendon architectural hierarchy (adapted from Kastelic *et al.*, 1978).

STRUCTURE OF LIGAMENTS AND TENDONS

In ligaments, the extracellular matrix is predominant and consists of fibrillar structures that are embedded into a ground substance. The cells of ligaments and tendons are called fibrocytes. The fibrillar structures of ligaments follow a typical architectural hierarchy including tropocollagen as the basic molecular component, and a systematic arrangement in microfibrils, subfibrils, fibrils and fibres (see Figure 2.1). Type I collagen is the major component of all fibres (Frank *et al.*, 1994; Viidik, 1994). Other collagen types such as type III, V, VI, X, and XII appear only in minor amounts, and their functional role is not completely understood. Small amounts of glycoproteins (e.g. fibronectin) and proteoglycans also exist as ground substances. While fibrillar structures are responsible for the liga-ment's stiffness and strength, fibrocytes and other components are important for its *in vivo* remodelling, biological adaptation, and healing response (Frank *et al.*, 1994).

The insertions of ligaments/tendons into bone (also called osteoligamentous/tendinous junction) are of particular importance since the transfer of loads from soft to hard tissues can create large stress concentration, and therefore, make this area susceptible to injury. In those cases when the fibrous structures directly connect to bone, there are layers of uncalcified and calcified fibrocartilage in the insertion area to minimise stress concentra-tion (Woo *et al.*, 1988). In other areas such as the tibial insertion of the medial collateral ligament (MCL), the connection is complex and the surface of the ligament is connected with the periosteum, while the deeper portions of the fibres obliquely insert into the bone. In these insertions not cartilaginous layers but perpendicular oriented collagen fibres are present which connect the tendons to the periosteum of the bone (Woo *et al.*, 1988).

Table 2.1 Components of ligaments and tendons.

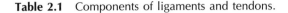

Water (up to 60%)
Collagen (70–80% of fat-free dry weight)
  Type I (predominant)
  Types III, V, VI, X, XII (minor)
Proteoglycans, glucoproteins (fibronectin), elastin
Cells (fibrocytes)

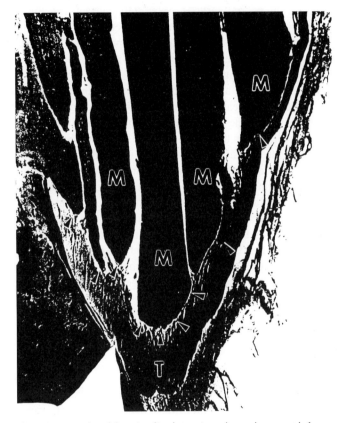

Figure 2.2 Light micrograph of longitudinal section through several frog semitendinosus muscle cells (M) attached to their tendon of insertion (T) at myotendinous junctions (arrowheads) (×250) (adapted from Woo and Buckwalter, 1998).

Tendons differ from ligaments in that they not only connect to bone but also to muscle. The musculotendinous junction is of equal importance as the tendon–bone junction since high local stress can occur and cause injury. Frequently, the tendons have an internal portion within the muscle fascia, called the aponeurosis (Zajac, 1989). The aponeurosis provides a large surface area for the load transfer from muscle to tendon and the orientation of this junction enhances its strength because cell membranes of muscle are known to be more resistant to shear stress than to tensile stress (see Figure 2.2).

A thin layer of tissue, called the epiligament or paratenon, usually covers ligaments and tendons (Frank *et al.*, 1994). This layer is abundant in cells and blood vessels and it is the major source for remodelling and healing responses. The midsubstance of ligaments and tendons usually contains small vessels mainly in the transverse orientation of the collagen fibres. However, compared to other connective tissues such as bone and skin, ligaments and tendons are poorly vascularised and have a reduced metabolism (Frank *et al.*, 1994). At locations where tendons sustain large deflections around joints (mainly at the hand and foot) they are frequently surrounded by fibrous sheaths/retinacula. An additional synovial layer can reduce friction between the tendon and the fibrous sheath and thus prevent injury (Herzog and Loitz, 1994).

Recently, free nerve endings were found in ligaments and tendons, mainly functioning by reporting tension to the central nervous system (Johannsson and Sjölander, 1993). It was found that activation of the nerves (with quick increase of tension in the structure) could lead to inhibition of muscular function, thus preventing possible injury of the musculoskeletal system. Due to these findings, tendons and ligaments are believed to play an important role in proprioception.

It is well known that tendons and ligaments have different characteristics at various age levels. Before puberty the weakest link in the bone–ligament–bone unit is the developing bone. For the MCL of the knee, we have shown that injuries occur with bony avulsions of the ligament, rather than midsubstance failures (Woo *et al.*, 1986a). Once skeletal maturity is reached, midsubstance failure is usually predominant because the strength of the insertion site is superior to that of the ligament. Studies comparing structural properties of ligament–bone complexes in the anterior cruciate ligament (ACL) of the knee between young and old donors found a substantial age related reduction in these properties. Since the cross-sectional area remained relatively constant, a large decrease in structural properties suggests that with increasing age the mechanical properties of the ACL also diminish (Noyes and Grood, 1976; Woo *et al.*, 1991). However, studies on the MCL of the knee revealed only minor changes in mechanical properties as an effect of age (Woo *et al.*, 1990a). In hamstring tendons, no age-related differences in stiffness and ultimate loads were reported (Hecker *et al.*, 1997).

STRUCTURAL AND MECHANICAL PROPERTIES

Knowledge of material and structural properties of ligaments and tendons is of clinical importance because these properties are essential to soft tissue function. The biomechanical behaviour of ligaments and tendons demonstrates that they are well suited to the physical functions they perform. The fibrillar components of ligaments and tendons are arranged in an undulating path between origin and insertion in their physiologically relaxed state. During normal movements in which tensile stretch is applied, progressive straightening and stretching of an increasing number of fibres occurs (recruitment). Different components of the tissue take up loads at different stress levels, thus contributing to a non-linear, concave, upward stress–strain curve. This mechanical behaviour is designed generally to guide the joint into appropriate motion. Due to the parallel-fibred organisation of these tissues, uniaxial tension tests are done with bone–ligament–bone or muscle–tendon–bone complexes to determine the *structural* properties represented by a non-linear load–elongation curve. This curve involves the contribution from the substance of the ligament and the bony insertion. Figure 2.3 (A) shows a typical non-linear load–elongation curve for bone–ligament–bone complex. The two regions of this curve must be distinguished. As tensile load is first applied to a ligament the relationship between load and elongation is non-linear and referred to as the 'toe' region. With increasing applied loads,

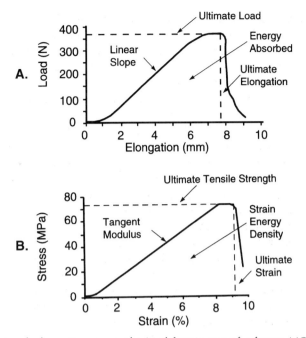

Figure 2.3 **(A)** Load–elongation curve obtained from a test of a femur–MCL–tibia complex (FMTC). **(B)** Stress–strain curve of ligament midsubstance obtained from a test of an FMTC.

increases in stiffness are seen following a more linear load–elongation relationship, referred to as the 'linear' region of the curve. Structural properties are represented by parameters such as stiffness, ultimate load, ultimate deformation, and energy absorbed to failure. The stiffness is defined as a change of load with elongation in the linear portion of the curve. This non-linear behaviour allows ligaments working at this range to guide the joint through movements with minimal resistance. At higher load, ligaments become stiffer, thus acting as a 'checkrein' to prevent excessive displacement between the two bones, and maintain joint position to accommodate for large muscle forces.

The mechanical properties of the ligament and tendon substance, on the other hand, describe the material irrespective of geometry. They should be determined from the stress–strain relationship of the midsubstance of the ligament or tendon itself to avoid the contribution from the insertion sites. These properties reflect collagen fibre organisation and orientation, as well as the microstructure. Strain, ε, can be described as the relative change in length of the tissue specimen with respect to its original length, while stress, σ, is defined as a force applied per unit area. Thus, the ultimate tensile strength or ultimate stress, for example, is the highest stress experienced by the tissue before complete failure. Mechanical properties of the ligament or tendon are represented by parameters such as the modulus, ultimate tensile strength, ultimate strain, and strain energy density. A typical stress–strain curve for a ligament midsubstance is shown in Figure 2.3 (B).

Ligaments and tendons also exhibit complex time- and history-dependent (rheological) behaviour similar to that of other viscoelastic materials. These behaviours are the consequence of complex interactions between proteoglycan molecules, water, collagen, and other structural components of soft tissues. When a ligament or tendon is pulled to a particular elongation, either once or repeatedly in cycles, the stress in the tissue decreases with time. Specifically, this means that when soft tissue is elongated to a given length,

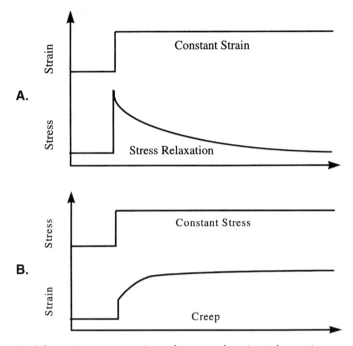

Figure 2.4 **(A)** Schematic representation of stress–relaxation (decreasing stress over time under a constant strain). **(B)** Schematic representation of creep (increasing deformation over time under a constant stress).

and remains at this same length over time, the actual load supported by the tissue progressively declines. This behaviour is referred to as *stress relaxation* (Figure 2.4 (A)). During cyclic loading, an elastic material follows the same stress–strain curve, whereas a viscoelastic material, like tendon or ligament, displays a hysteresis loop, a phenomenon in which the load–elongation curve differs during loading and unloading and results in net internal energy loss (Figure 2.5 (A)). Cyclic stress–relaxation has important implications regarding ligament and tendon behaviour during joint motion. Ligaments normally undergo cyclic loading during walking, running, and other activities. Many materials are subject to fatigue failure under these conditions – that is, repetitive stress causes failure at a much lower load than that required to cause failure from a single application of stress. As a ligament or tendon undergoes many cycles of loading and unloading *in vivo*, its relaxation behaviour results in a continuously decreasing stress, protecting the ligaments from failure by fatigue. Conversely, there is a time dependent increase in elongation when a viscoelastic material is subjected to a repetitive constant stress. This behaviour is called cyclic *creep* (Figure 2.5 (B)).

ROLE OF LIGAMENTS AND TENDONS IN HUMAN MOTION

The knee is a good example to illustrate ligament and tendon biomechanics, because, like all weight bearing joints, it needs mobility but is concerned with stability. Knee ligaments are also frequently injured during various sports activities such as football, soccer, or skiing. These injuries often result in knee instability with serious pathological sequelae. Knowledge of the properties of knee ligaments is not only important in contributing to

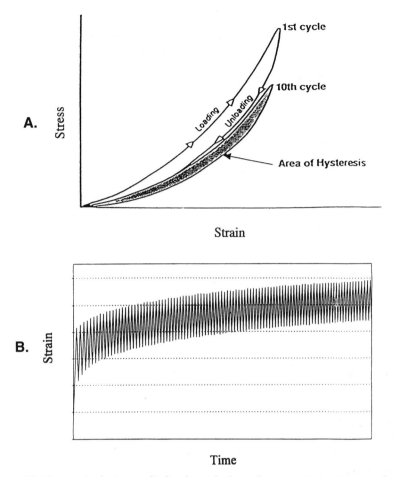

Figure 2.5   **(A)** Hysteresis during cyclic loading of a knee ligament (From Woo *et al.*, 1993).
(B) Schematic representation of cyclic creep in the MCL of the knee.

the basic understanding of the functional behaviour of these ligaments; it is also essential
for ligament repair and replacement grafts to match the properties of the graft material
with those of the native ligaments. Figure 2.6 is an anterior view of the right knee
showing the four major ligaments of the knee: anterior cruciate ligament (ACL), posterior
cruciate ligament (PCL), medial collateral ligament (MCL), and lateral collateral ligament (LCL). These ligaments act together with the joint capsule and articular surfaces of
the knee to maintain stability as well as to guide the joint through the passive range of
motion. The functional role of the ACL, for example, is mainly to limit excessive knee
motions in the anterior tibial direction, while the PCL is important to limit posterior tibial
translations (Butler *et al.*, 1980; Livesay *et al.*, 1997).

   Another example of a structure that plays major role in human motion is the calcaneal
(Achilles) tendon of the leg (Figure 2.7). It is one of the strongest tendons in the human
body and is important during running and jumping. It was estimated that the load supported by this tendon during sport activities could be as high as 1800 Newtons (400
pounds). Experimental measurements showed that failure loads for the Achilles tendon
exceed 4500 Newtons (Viidik, 1994). Injuries to this tendon are common. Tendinitis, an
injury or symptomatic degeneration of the tendon, with resultant inflammatory reaction of

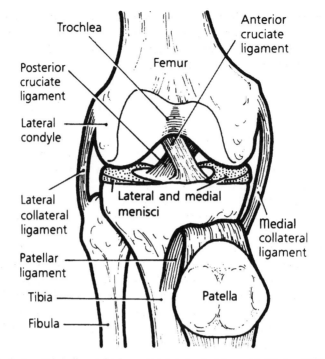

Figure 2.6   Anterior view of a right knee joint (adapted from McGinty, 1991).

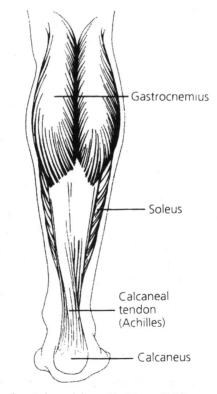

Figure 2.7   Achilles tendon (adapted from McGinty, 1991).

the surrounding structures, is frequently seen in the Achilles tendon and accounts for as much as 11 per cent of all running injuries (Friedman, 1986; James et al., 1978). It is important to understand the properties and function of the Achilles tendon in order to prescribe proper treatment and rehabilitation regimens.

RESPONSE TO IMMOBILISATION AND EXERCISE

Immobilisation of joints with casting is frequently used in clinical settings for various purposes such as fracture healing. It has been shown that immobilisation of joints leads to significant impairment of ligament properties and to stiffening of the joints (Woo et al., 1975). In rabbits and rats stiffness and ultimate load were reduced by 25–33 per cent after 4–9 weeks of immobilisation (Larson et al., 1987; Noyes, 1977; Woo et al., 1982). The reduction of structural properties appears to be a result of a combination of changes of the insertion sites and the ligament itself.

Remobilisation can reverse the effects of immobilisation on the structural properties in a bone–ligament–bone complex, but requires much longer time periods to restore the basic function of the ligaments. Experimentally, 18 weeks of remobilisation were necessary to reverse the detrimental effects of a six-week immobilisation period on the structural properties of ligaments (Laros et al., 1971). Studies from our institution on the effects of a nine-week immobilisation period of rabbit knees revealed that histologically, the tibial insertion of the MCL was not reestablished until after 52 weeks of remobilisation (Woo et al., 1987b). More importantly the failure mode was consistently shifted to the tibial insertion.

Overall the decline in structural properties of bone–ligament–bone complexes due to immobilisation is reversible, but the process is slow. Clinically, this implies that after any period of immobilisation caution is required to limit the risk of subsequent injury. Ideally, the remobilisation period would include a gradual increase in activity over a many-fold longer time period than the immobilisation to allow the tissue to restore its original function.

In recent years the awareness of health related benefits from physical activity and exercise has increased tremendously. These benefits are mainly related to the prevention and treatment of cardiovascular disease (NIH, 1996). Regarding the musculoskeletal system it should be noted that positive effects of exercise on tendons and ligaments exist, although to a much lesser degree. Experimental findings suggest that moderate exercise may enhance structural properties (stiffness and ultimate load) of ligaments by about 10–20 per cent (Tipton et al., 1975; Woo et al., 1979). Figure 2.8 represents a summary of the literature on the effects of immobilisation and exercise and their relationship to ligament mass and properties. For any ligament a physiological level of stress and strain duration exists, ensuring a certain level of mechanical properties. Any reduction in stress/strain duration, such as immobilisation, will reduce the structural properties enormously. On the other hand, an increase in stress/strain duration (or exercise) will enhance these properties, but only moderately. However, excessive increase in stress/strain as well as duration will result in structural damage and, eventually lead to failure.

RESPONSE TO INJURY (HEALING OF LIGAMENTS/TENDONS)

The term 'healing' refers to tissue repair after sustained injury. The potential of healing varies largely and depends mainly on the blood supply and the metabolic rate of the

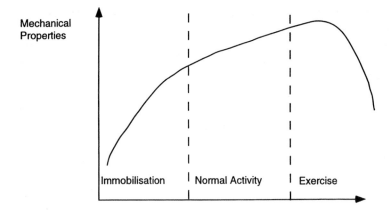

Stress and Strain Duration

Figure 2.8 Schematic diagram illustrating the effect of exercise and immobilisation on ligament properties.

involved tissue. While skin and bone, with some limitations, heal fairly quickly and predictively, ligaments and tendons are believed to have a slow and limited healing response (Frank *et al.*, 1994). Ideally, healing should lead to a complete restoration of the original tissue with identical morphological and functional characterstics (*restitutio ad integrum*). Unfortunately, ligaments are known to heal with a qualitatively inferior tissue from the original tissue.

Healing of ligaments/tendons follows phases that can be described as follows (Frank *et al.*, 1985):

(1) *Haemorrhage/inflammatory phase*: This phase is characterised by formation of a blood clot within the damaged region and the invasion of polymorphonuclear cells and monocytes/macrophages. The monocytes remove debris and attract granulation tissue-producing reparative cells.

(2) *Proliferative phase*: In this phase new blood vessels are formed while fibroblasts are recruited from the local environment or circulation to produce new matrix material (mainly collagen).

(3) *Remodeling phase*: This phase starts within weeks after the injury and can last up to several years. It is characterised by a progressive maturation of collagen fibres that align in a longitudinal orientation in response to loads experienced by the ligament.

Some ligaments/tendons can heal and their structural properties can reach normal or nearly normal stiffness and strength values, thus providing the needed function to the involved joint (Indelicato, 1995; Woo *et al.*, 1987c). Some other ligaments, such as the cruciate ligaments of the knee, heal with increased laxity and diminished strength or do not heal at all. The medial collateral ligament (MCL) of the knee has been an ideal model to study ligament healing in the laboratory due to its distinct shape and easy accessibility (Weiss *et al.*, 1991). In an isolated rupture of the MCL the ligament healed macroscopically without any treatment within six weeks (Gomez and Woo, 1989; Weiss *et al.*, 1991). The cross-sectional area of the healed ligament increases at 6–12 weeks and returns slowly back to normal with increasing time (Inoue *et al.*, 1987). While the structural properties of the femur–MCL–tibia complex may return to nearly normal, the mechanical properties of the healing MCL always remain inferior when compared to the normal tissue. This is possible because healing tissues have accumulated its mass to compensate for its inferior tissue quality. In some cases the cross-sectional area of the healed MCL was up to 2.5 times larger than that of controls after 52 weeks (Ohland et al., 1991). When severe joint laxity is associated with the ligament injury such as in a combined MCL/ACL injury of the knee, similar characteristics of healing are seen. However, the decrease in mechanical properties and increase in cross-sectional area is more pronounced (Engle et al., 1994; Ohno et al., 1995a) (see Figure 2.9).

Histologically, healed ligament tissue differs from normal tissue mainly in three regards: the collagen is more disorganised and less-oriented; there are more defects between collagen fibres; and the number of collagen fibres of larger diameter is reduced (Frank et al., 1992; Mathew et al., 1987). Additionally, there is an increased cell density and vascularity of the tissue, suggesting that metabolic rates are higher than normal (Frank, 1996). With the time of remodelling increased vascularity can diminish and the newly formed fibres become more parallel oriented in the course of its mechanical action. However, the number of large fibre diameters will remain reduced. This aspect is important since large diameter collagen fibres were shown to correlate with greater strength and stiffness of the tissue (Parry et al., 1978).

Biochemical analysis of healing tissues revealed that although the collagen content of the tissue returns to nearly normal within 14 weeks collagen crosslinks remain below 50 per cent of normal up to one year after injury (Inoue et al., 1987; Weiss et al., 1991; Woo et al., 1997). Further, the amount of type I collagen is reduced in favour of minor collagen types, and the size of proteoglycans is increased (Frank, 1996).

In summary, experimental data indicate that ligaments and tendons heal with the formation of new tissue of inferior quality following sequential and time-dependent phases and, even under optimal conditions, the quality of normal ligament tissue will not be matched for up to two years.

EFFECTS OF VARIOUS TREATMENTS ON THE HEALING RESPONSE OF LIGAMENTS AND TENDONS

The clinical literature has provided numerous studies focusing on treatment regimens for ligament and tendon injuries. However, it has to be kept in mind that several ligament/tendon injuries heal without any specific treatment and that a number of injuries do not lead to any functional impairment, even without any evidence of efficient healing response. Valuable information on the effect of various treatment regimens for ligament and tendon injuries can be derived from experimental studies where variables can more easily be controlled than in clinical settings. There are three major variables that affect the healing response of ligaments and tendons: non-repair versus surgical repair; immobilisation versus early motion; and biological manipulations such as the use of growth factors.

Using the rabbit MCL as a model, the effect of surgical repair of ligaments was compared to conservative treatment. A long-term study failed to demonstrate a benefit from suture repair when compared to conservative treatment (Inoue et al., 1987; Weiss et al., 1991). In both groups ligaments were macroscopically well healed after 12 weeks, ligament laxity was slightly increased initially and returned to normal at one year, and structural properties such as stiffness and ultimate load were slightly diminished even at one year. Mechanical properties remained about 50 per cent of normal, indicating the

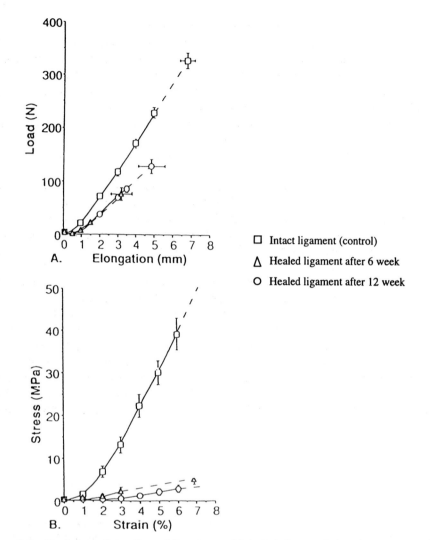

Figure 2.9 Healed medial collateral ligament exhibits inferior mechanical properties when compared to the intact state. **(A)** Load–elongation curve for MCL. **(B)** Stress–strain curve for femur–MCL–tibia complex.

decreased tissue quality (Weiss *et al.*, 1991). On the other hand, in a combined injury model (MCL and ACL combined) surgical repair of the MCL improved structural properties in the early phase (Ohno *et al.*, 1995b; Yamaji *et al.*, 1996). Other ligaments such as the cruciate ligaments of the knee, do not heal sufficiently with or without surgical repair (Feagin and Curl, 1976; Sommerlath *et al.*, 1991). In these cases reconstructive procedures are necessary in an attempt to restore normal ligament function.

Tendons are more frequently repaired surgically since it is believed that muscle pull can increase the gap between rupture ends and thus prevent healing. However, recent results show that in partial flexor tendon ruptures up to 60 per cent can heal sufficiently without surgery (Morifusa *et al.*, 1995) and that complete Achilles tendon ruptures do not necessarily benefit from surgical repair (Thermann *et al.*, 1995).

As described earlier, mechanical stimuli as well as stress deprivation in the form of immobilisation have a profound effect on intact tendons and ligaments. For the healing tissue mechanical stimuli appear to be equally important. Studies from our research centre as well as others revealed that tendons and ligaments regain a higher strength after sustained rupture when treated with passive motion compared to immobilisation (Gelberman and Woo, 1989; Woo *et al.*, 1981, 1990c). Clinical studies also suggested that early mobilisation and aggressive rehabilitation protocols may be effective in restoring joint motion without compromising stability (Kannus, 1988; Shelbourne and Nitz, 1990). However, in severely unstable joints early motion may be not beneficial to the healing tissue (Woo *et al.*, 1990c).

Since restoration of normal tissue quality in ligament healing has yet to be accomplished under normal circumstances, different biological approaches, such as cell manipulations by cytokines to enhance the quality of the healing tissue have recently been discussed. Cell migration and proliferation, as well as protein and collagen synthesis, are essential characteristics of the tissue's healing response. Endogenous growth factors that are released by inflammatory cells can act as mediators of the healing response. In the past many growth factors have been evaluated both *in vitro* and *in vivo* on their effect of ligament healing with variable results (Batten *et al.*, 1996; Letson and Dahners, 1994; Scherping *et al.*, 1997; Schmidt *et al.*, 1995; Weiss *et al.*, 1995). In our laboratory, we have found that epidermal growth factor (EGF) and platelet derived growth factor (PDGF) increase fibroblast proliferation *in vitro*, while transforming growth factor-beta 1 (TGF-β1) increases protein synthesis (Hildebrand and Frank, 1997). When these growth factors are combined and tested in an *in-vivo* model, the structural properties of the healing rabbit bone–MCL–bone complex and the mechanical properties of the healing MCL appeared to be enhanced (Hildebrand and Frank, 1997). Longer-term results are needed to put this concept on a more definitive basis.

CLINICAL SIGNIFICANCE AND FUTURE DIRECTIONS

In this chapter we have given an overview of structural and functional characteristics of ligaments and tendons and their response to injury. In the future the effects of biological stimulation of ligament healing using various cytokines needs to be further evaluated. Although little is known about the tissue's sensitivity to growth factors over time within the healing period, it is currently believed that application at an early stage is better than at a later stage of healing (Batten *et al.*, 1996). Further, since the half-life of growth factors is only minutes to hours, there is a debate about whether or not continuous or intermittent application of growth factors is better than single shot application. As a delivery vehicle fibrin sealant can be used for single shot application with a short-term effect, whereas gene therapy might be a vehicle for long-term delivery of growth factors to the tissue in the future.

In this chapter we have mainly focused on complete injuries of tendon and ligaments. However, it is known that at 50–70 per cent of the ultimate load of tendons and ligaments partial failure may occur (single fibril tears). This includes fragmentation, thinning and separation of collagen. As a biological response, oedema, proliferation of capillaries and finally calcification of the tendon may occur. Frequently, this is associated with pain experienced during activity of the tendon or ligament. Since the chronic biological changes seen in tendon/ligament tissue do not meet the criteria of a true inflammation, they are referred to as tendinosis, rather than tendinitis. An example for this is the patellar tendinosis, also called jumper's knee, which consists of chronic intratendinous changes at the tendon–bone junction at the tip of the patella. On the other hand, peritendinosus tissue such as tendon sheath may develop an acute inflammation, as a response to acute overuse. This is accompanied by pain and swelling and is referred to as peritendinitis. Examples of possible areas affected by peritendinitis include the flexor tendon sheath of the forearm and the Achilles tendon. In addition to partial failures microscopic changes such as loss of physiological crimp pattern may be seen under loads as low as one third of the maximum load. Overall, workplace related injuries of the musculoskeletal system might more frequently include prefailure injuries, presented as overuse syndromes with acute or chronic onset. Although basic science has characterised the morphological changes of these injuries well, future research should focus on the prevention and treatment of these injuries.

References

BATTEN, M.L., HANSEN, J.C. and DAHNERS, L.E., 1996, Influence of dosage and timing of application of platelet-derived growth factor on early healing of the rat medial collateral ligament, *J Orthop Res*, **14**, 736–741.

BUTLER, D.L., NOYES, F.R. and GROOD, E.S., 1980, Ligamentous restraints to anterior–posterior drawer in the human knee: a biomechanical study, *J Bone Joint Surg*, **62A**(2), 259–270.

ENGLE, C.P., NOGUCHI, M., OHLAND, K.J., SHELLEY, F.J. and WOO, S.L.-Y., 1994, Healing of the rabbit medial collateral ligament following an O'Donoghue triad injury: the effects of anterior cruciate ligament reconstruction, *J Orthop Res*, **12**, 357–364.

FEAGIN, J.A. and CURL, W.W., 1976, Isolated tear of the anterior cruciate ligament: 5 year follow-up study, *Am J Sports Med*, **4**, 95.

FRANK, C.B., 1996, Ligament healing: current knowledge and clinical applications, *J Am Acad Orthop Surg*, **4**, 74–83.

FRANK, C.B., AMIEL, D., WOO, S.L.-Y. and AKESON, W.H., 1985, Normal ligament properties and ligament healing, *Clin Orthop*, **196**, 15–25.

FRANK, C.B., MacDONALD, D., BRAY, D.F., RANGAYYAN, R.M., CHIMICH, D.D. and SHRIVE, N.G., 1992, Collagen fibril diameters in the healing rabbit medial collateral ligament, *Connect Tiss Res*, **27**(4), 251–263.

FRANK, C.B., BRAY, R.C., HART, D.A., SHRIVE, N.G., LOITZ, B.J., MAYTAS, J.R. and WILSON, J.E., 1994, Soft tissue healing, in Fu, F.H., Harner, C.D. and Vince, K.G. (Eds), *Knee Surgery*, Baltimore, MD: Williams and Wilkins, pp. 189–229.

FRIEDMAN, M.J., 1986, Injuries to the leg in athletes, in Nicholas, J.A. and Hershman, E.B. (Eds), *The Lower Extremity and Spine in Sports Medicine*, St Louis: Mosby, pp. 601–655.

GELBERMAN, R.H. and WOO, S.L.-Y., 1989, The physiological basis for application of controlled stress in the rehabilitation of flexor tendon injuries, *J Hand Ther*, **14**, 66–70.

GOMEZ, M.A. and WOO, S.L.-Y., 1989, The advantages of applied tension on healing medial collateral ligament, *Trans ORS*, **14**, 184.

HECKER, A.T., BROWN, C.H., DEFFNER, K.T. and ROSENBERG, T.D., 1997, Tensile properties of young multiple stranded hamstring grafts, in *AOSSM Specialty Day*, San Francisco: AAOS.

HERZOG, W. and LOITZ, B., 1994, Tendon, in Nigg, B.M. and Herzog, W. (Eds), *Biomechanics of the Musculo-skeletal System*, Chichester: Wiley, pp. 133–153.

HILDEBRAND, K.A. and FRANK, C.B., 1997, The normal structure and function of the ligaments and their responses to injury and repair, in Dee, R.M. *et al.*, (Eds), *Principles of Orthopaedic Practice*, New York: McGraw-Hill, pp. 109–117.

INDELICATO, P.A. 1995, Isolated medial collateral ligament injuries in the knee, *J Am Acad Orthop Surg*, **3**(1), 9–14.

INOUE, M., McGURK-BURLESON, E., HOLLIS, J.M. and WOO, S.L., 1987, Treatment of the medial collateral injury. I: The importance of anterior cruciate ligament on the varus-valgus knee laxity, *Am J Sports Med*, **15**(1), 15–21.

JAMES, S.L., BATES, B.T. and OSTERNIG, L.R., 1978, Injuries to runners, *Am J Sports Med*, **6**, 40.

JOHANNSSON, H. and SJÖLANDER, P., 1993, Neurophysiology of joints, in Wright, V. and Radin, E.L. (Eds), *Mechanics of Human Joints: Physiology, Pathophysiology, and Treatment*, New York: Marcel Dekker, pp. 243–290.

KANNUS, P., 1988, Long-term results of conservatively treated medial collateral ligament injuries of the knee joint, *Clin Orthop*, **226**, 103–112.

KASTELIC, J., GALESKI, A. and BAER, E., 1978, The multicomposite structure of tendon, *Conn Tiss Res*, **6**, 11–23.

LAROS, G.S., TIPTON, C.M. and COOPER, R.R., 1971, Influence of physical activity of ligament insertions in the knees of dogs, *J Bone Joint Surg*, **53-A**, 275–286.

LARSON, N.P., FORWOD, M.R. and PARKER, A.W., 1987, Immobilization and re-training of cruciate ligaments in the rat, *Acta Orthop Scand*, **58**, 260–264.

LETSON, A.K. and DAHNERS, L.E., 1994, The effect of combinations of growth factors on ligament healing, *Clin Orthop*, **308**, 207–212.

LIVESAY, G.A., RUDY, T.W., WOO, S.L.-Y., RUNCO, T.J., SAKANE, M., LI, G. and FU, F.H., 1997, Evaluation of the effect of joint constraints on the in-situ force distribution within the anterior cruciate ligament, *J Orthop Res*, **15**(2), 278–284.

MATHEW, C., MOORE, M.J. and CAMPBELL, L., 1987, A quantitative ultrastructural study of collagen fibril formation in the healing extensor digitorum longus tendon of the rat, *J Hand Surg*, **12-B**(3), 313–320.

McGINTY, J.B., 1991, *Athletic Training and Sports Medicine*, Park Ridge, IL: Am Acad Orthop Surg.

MORIFUSA, S., CHAN, S.S., BOARDMAN, N.D., TRAMAGLINI, D.M., PFAEFFLE, H.J., SOTEREANOS, D.G. and HERNDON, J.H., 1995, Effect of partial laceration on the gliding function and structural properties of the canine flexor digitorum profundus tendon, *Trans Orth Res Soc*, **137**, 23.

NIH, 1996, CONSENSUS CONFERENCE: Physical activity and cardiovascular health, *JAMA*, **276**(3), 241–246.

NOYES, F.R., 1977, Functional properties of knee ligaments and alterations induced by immobilization: a correlative biomechanical and histological study in primates, *Clin Orthop*, **123**, 210–242.

NOYES, F.R. and GROOD, E.S., 1976, The strength of the anterior cruciate ligaments in humans and rhesus monkeys. Age-related and species-related changes, *J Bone Joint Surg*, **58A**, 1074–1082.

OHLAND, K.J., WEISS, J.A., ANDERSON, D.R. and WOO, S.L.-Y., 1991, Long-term healing of the medial collateral ligament (MCL) and its insertion sites, *Trans Orth Res Soc*, **16**, 158.

OHNO, K., POMAYBO, A.S., SCHMIDT, C.C., LEVINE, R.E., OHLAND, K.J. and WOO, S.L.-Y., 1995a, Healing of the MCL after a combined MCL and ACL injury and reconstruction of the ACL: comparison of repair and nonrepair of MCL tears in rabbits, *J Orthop Res*, **13**, 442–449.

OHNO, K., POMAYBO, A.S., SCHMIDT, C.C., LEVINE, R.E., OHLAND, K.J. and WOO, S.L.-Y., 1995b, Healing of the medial collateral ligament after a combined medial collateral and anterior cruciate ligament injury and reconstruction of the anterior cruciate ligament: comparison of repair and nonrepair of medial collateral ligament tears in rabbits, *J Orthop Res*, **13**, 442–449.

PARRY, D.A., BARNES, G.R. and CRAIG, A.S., 1978, A comparison of the size distribution of collagen fibrils in connective tissues as a function of age and a possible relation between fibril size distribution and mechanical properties, *Proc Royal Soc London – Series B: Biological Sciences*, **203**(1152), 293–303.

SCHERPING, S.C., SCHMIDT, C.C., GEORGESCU, H.I., KWOH, C.K., EVANS, C.H. and WOO, S.L.-Y., 1997, Effects of growth factors on the proliferation of ligament fibroblasts from skeletally mature rabbits, *Conn. Tiss Res*, **36**, 1–8.

SCHMIDT, C.C., GEORGESCU, H.I., KWOH, C.K., BLOMSTROM, G.L., ENGLE, C.P., LARKIN, L.A., *et al.*, 1995, Effect of growth factors on the proliferation of fibroblasts from the medial collateral and anterior cruciate ligaments, *J Orthop Res*, **13**, 184–190.

SHELBOURNE, K.D. and NITZ, P., 1990, Accelerated rehabilitation after anterior cruciate ligament reconstruction, *Am J Sports Med*, **18**(3), 292–299.

SOMMERLATH, K., LYSHOLM, J. and GILLQUIST, J., 1991, The long-term course after treatment of acute anterior cruciate ligament ruptures. A 9 to 16 year followup, *Am J Sports Med*, **19**(2), 156–162.

THERMANN, H., FRERICHS, O., BIEWENER, A., KRETTEK, C. and SCHANDELMEIER, P., 1995, Functional treatment of acute rupture of the Achilles tendon. An experimental biomechanical study, *Unfallchirurg*, **98**(10), 507–513.

TIPTON, C.M., MATHES, R.D., MAYNARD, J.A. and CAREY, R.A., 1975, The influence of physical activity on ligaments and tendons, *Med Sci Sports*, **7**, 165–175.

VIIDIK, A., 1994, Structure and function of normal and healing tendons and ligaments, in Leadbetter, W.B. Buckwalter, J.A. and Gordon, S.L. (Eds), *Sports-induced Inflammation*, Am. Acad. Orthop. Surg. pp. 3–37.

WEISS, J.A., WOO, S.L.-Y., OHLAND, K.J., HORIBE, S. and NEWTON, P.O., 1991, Evaluation of a new injury model to study medial collateral ligament healing: primary repair versus nonoperative treatment, *J Orthop Res*, **9**, 516–528.

WEISS, J.A., BECK, C.L., LEVINE, R.E. and GREENWALD, R.M., 1995, Effects of platelet-derived growth factor on early medial collateral ligament healing, *Trans Orthop Res Soc*, **20**, 159.

WOO, S.L.-Y. and BUCKWALTER, J.A., 1998, *Injury and Repair of the Musculoskeletal Soft Tissues*, Park Ridge, IL: Am Ac Orthop Surg.

WOO, S.L.-Y., MATTHEWS, J.V., AKESON, W.H., AMIEL, D. and CONVERY, F.R., 1975, Connective tissue response to immobility: a correlative study of biomechanical measurements of normal and immobilised rabbit knees, *Arthritis Rheum*, **18**, 257–264.

WOO, S.L.-Y., KUEI, S.C., GOMEZ, M.A., WINTERS, J.M. and AMIEL, D., 1979, The effect of immobilisation and exercise on the strength characteristics of bone-medal collateral ligament-bone complex, in *ASME Bimech Symp AMD*.

WOO, S.L.-Y., GELBERMAN, R.H., COBB, N.G., AMIEL, D., LOTHRINGER, K. and AKESON, W.H., 1981, The importance of controlled passive mobilization on flexor tendon healing, *A Orthop Scand*, **52**, 615–622.

WOO, S.L.-Y., GOMEZ, M.A., WOO, Y.-K. and AKESON, W.H., 1982, Mechanical properties of tendons and ligaments II: The relationships of immobilization and exercise on tissue remodeling, *Biorheology*, **19**, 397–408.

WOO, S.L.-Y., ORLANDO, C.A., GOPMEZ, M.A., FRANK, C.B. and AKESON, W.H., 1986a, Tensile properties of the medial collateral ligament as a function of age, *J Orthop Res*, **4**, 133–141.

WOO, S.L.-Y., ORLANDO, C.O., CAMP, J.F. and AKESON, W.H., 1986b, Effects of postmortem storage by freezing on ligament tensile behavior, *J Biomech*, **19**, 399–404.

WOO, S.L.-Y., LEE, T.Q., GOMEZ, M.A., SATO, S. and FIELD, F.P., 1987a, Temperature dependent behavior of the canine medial collateral ligament, *J Biomech Eng*, **109**, 68–71.

WOO, S.L.-Y., GOMEZ, M.A., SITES, T.J., NEWTON, P.P., ORLANDO, C.A. and AKESON, W.H., 1987b, The biomechanical and morphological changes in the medial collateral ligament of rabbit after immobilisation and remobilisation, *J Bone Joint Surg*, **69-A**, 1200–1211.

WOO, S.L.-Y., INOUE, M. and McGURK-BURLESON, E., 1987c, Treatment of the medial collateral ligament injury: structure and function of canine knees in response to differing treatment regimens, *Am J Sports Med*, **15**, 22–29.

WOO, S.L.-Y., MAYNARD, J., BUTLER, D.L., LYON, R., TORZILLI, P.A., AKESON, W.H., *et al.*, 1988, Ligament, tendon and joint capsule insertions into bone, in Woo, S.L.-Y. and Buckwalter, J.A. (Eds), *Injury and Repair of the Musculoskeletal Soft Tissues*, Park Ridge, IL: Am Acad Orthop Surg, pp. 133–166.

WOO, S.L.-Y., OHLAND, K.J. and WEISS, J.A., 1990a, Aging and sex-related changes in the biomechanical properties of the rabbit MCL, *Mech Age Develop*, **56**, 129–142.

WOO, S.L.-Y., WEISS, J.A., GOMEZ, M.A. and HAWKINS, D.A., 1990b, Measurement of changes in ligament tension with knee motion and skeletal maturation, *J Biomech Eng*, **112**(1), 46–51.

WOO, S.L.-Y., YOUNG, E.P., OHLAND, K.J., MARCIN, J.P., HORIBE, S. and LIN, H.C., 1990c, The effects of transection of the anterior cruciate ligament on healing of the medial collateral ligament: a biomechanical and histological study in dogs, *J Bone Joint Surg*, **72-A**(3), 382–392.

WOO, S.L.-Y., HOLLIS, J.M., ADAMS, D.J., LYON, R.M. and TAKAI, S., 1991, Tensile properties of the human femur–anterior cruciate ligament-tibia complex: the effect of specimen age and orientation, *Am J Sports Med*, **19**, 217–225.

WOO, S.L.-Y., SMITH, B.A., LIVESAY, G.A. and BLOMSTROM, G.L., 1993, Why do ligaments fail? *Curr Orthop*, **7**, 73–84.

WOO, S.L.-Y., NIYIBIZI, C., MATYAS, J., KAVALKOVICH, K.W., WEAVER-GREEN, C.M. and FOX, R.J., 1997, A histologic and biochemical evaluation of MCL healing after a concurrent MCL and ACL injury in the rabbit knee, *Acta Orthop Scand*, **68**, 142–148.

YAMAJI, T., LEVINE, R.E., WOO, S.L.-Y., NIYIBIZI, C., KAVALKOVICH, K.W. and WEAVER-GREEN, C.M., 1996, Medial collateral ligament healing one year after a concurrent medial collateral ligament and anterior cruciate ligament injury: an interdisciplinary study in rabbits, *J Orthop Res*, **14**, 223–227.

ZAJAC, F.E., 1989, Muscle and tendon: properties, models, scaling, and application to biomechanics and motor control, *Crit Rev Biomed Eng*, **17**(4), 359–411.

CHAPTER THREE

Ligament sprains

S.A. TIMMERMANN, S.P. TIMMERMANN,
R. BOORMAN AND C.B. FRANK

NORMAL LIGAMENT STRUCTURE AND FUNCTION

Definition

The term ligament is derived from the Latin term '*ligare*', meaning 'to bind' or 'to tie' (Webster, 1970). Skeletal ligaments have since been defined as dense bands of connective tissue that function not only to guide joint motion (Bray *et al.*, 1991), but also act as joint stabilisers (Solomonow *et al.*, 1987) and as proprioceptive monitors of joint kinematics (Abbott *et al.*, 1944; Barrach and Skinner, 1990; Schultz *et al.*, 1984; Zimney *et al.*, 1986).

There are several hundred skeletal ligaments in the human body which are named by a variety of gross, structural, and functional features (Basmajian and Slonecher, 1989). Most commonly, these ligaments are named by their points of bony attachment (i.e. glenohumeral, scapholunate); however, other anatomic adjectives such as shape (i.e. deltoid), function (i.e. capsular), relation to a joint (i.e. collateral), relation to a surface (i.e. superficial or deep) or simply their relation to one another (i.e. cruciates) can also be used to describe them. Yet as simple and similar as ligaments appear grossly, they are very complex heterogeneous structures that differ in many respects, including their response to injury.

Gross appearance

Skeletal ligaments have a wide variety of gross appearances and locations. The majority of them are anatomically distinct, homogeneous-appearing, dense, white structures that appear to be stretched between their points of bony attachment (Figure 3.1). Next in the spectrum of ligament forms are the somewhat less distinct sheetlike ligaments which are, nonetheless, still fairly discrete and well oriented for their functions. The last type of ligament, termed 'capsular ligaments', is nearly impossible to distinguish without delicate dissection. These broad complex fibrous forms have been the last to be defined as discrete anatomic entites because of their deep periarticular location and interdigitation with other structures (Loitz and Frank, 1993).

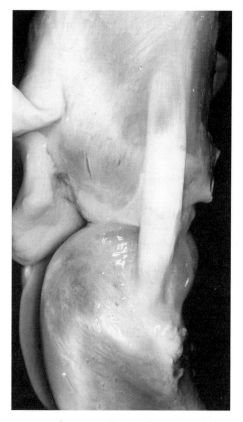

Figure 3.1 Gross appearance of a very distinct ligament – the rabbit medial collateral ligament (MCL).

Upon closer inspection, even with the naked eye, all ligaments can be seen to be composed of roughly parallel fibres that tighten or loosen in different joint positions as different forces are applied across a joint. In some cases fibres appear bundled or grouped, suggestive of subtle functional differences in fibres within the same structure (Frank *et al.*, 1985). In others, fibres remain separate and distinct.

Ultrastructure/histological appearance

At a microscopic level all ligaments have been shown to be made up of multiple parallel collagen fibres spanning between two bony insertions. Collagen appears to be oriented roughly in line to the long axis of the ligament, providing maximum resistance to tensile loads in that direction. Specific ultrastructural organisation, however, differs within and among ligaments, and distinguishes ligaments from tendons (Amiel *et al.*, 1983; Kennedy *et al.*, 1974; Yahia and Drovin, 1989).

Using polarised light, another subtlety of ligament substance can be observed. A regular wavy undulation of cells and matrix can be seen, known as collagen 'crimp' (Figure 3.2) (Diamant *et al.*, 1972; Frank *et al.*, 1988; Viidik, 1972). Although its functional significance continues to be investigated, it appears that this accordion-like pattern

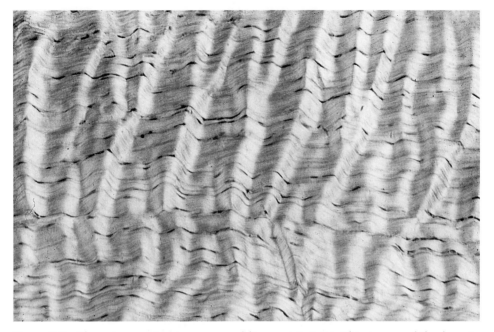

Figure 3.2 The microscopic appearance of ligament 'crimp'. This is one of the keys to normal fibre recruitment (H&E, × 60).

of crimp creates a loading 'buffer' or 'shock absorbing' phenomenon that plays a protective role during rapid loading (Amiel *et al.*, 1990).

Ligament insertions are even more complex, heterogeneous and dynamic than ligament substance (Woo *et al.*, 1988). Contrary to popular belief, ligaments are not simply riveted to their bony insertions by Sharpey's fibres. These fibres do act as anchors but only as part of a transition continuum of collagen fibres and cells from ligament substance into bone. The transition of midsubstance cells from fibroblasts through to fibrochondrocytes very near the insertion, into mineralised fibrocartilage and finally into bone creates a progressive stiffening of matrix at the normal ligament insertion, thus normally preventing the presence of a sharp stress interface between the ligament and the bone. This is a clever means by which nature has likely created a configuration and a transition of tissue properties which can help minimise injuries at insertion sites.

Biochemical composition

Normal skeletal ligaments are composed of a number of substances that can be chemically isolated and characterised (Amiel *et al.*, 1990). In general, ligaments consist of several biochemical parts (Figure 3.3). Most contain approximately two-thirds water by weight, while roughly three-quarters of their dry mass is made up of collagen. More than 90 per cent of this collagen is type I, with a few percent being made up of type III plus other minor collagens. Smaller proportions of the normal ligament matrix are composed of elastin, glycosaminoglycans (GAGs), and other substances.

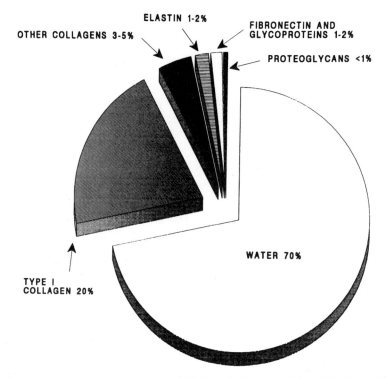

Figure 3.3   Pie graph showing the normal biochemical composition of a typical ligament (used with permission from Frank *et al.*, 1994).

Biomechanical properties

Ligament properties in response to loads can be described in three different ways: structural behaviour (load–deformation), material behaviour (stress–strain), and viscoelastic behaviour (relaxation and creep) (Butler *et al.*, 1978; Frank, 1996; Woo and Adams, 1990; Woo and Young, 1991; Woo *et al.*, 1982).

Structural behaviour refers to a ligament's response to a mechanical load regardless of its size or shape. Under load, ligaments resist displacement with increasing stiffness until eventually some part of the bone–ligament–bone complex fails. This increasing tensile resistance of ligaments as they are distracted has been characterised and described as non-linear (Figure 3.4).

The reasons for this non-linear behaviour are multifactorial. During the stretching of a complex, an increasing number of ligament fibres are recruited under tension. Under relatively small tensile loads, crimped fibrils begin to straighten. Initially, there is little resistance to tension as the fibres lengthen, but as elongation progresses, an increasing number of fibrils become taut and carry load. This process of straightening and fibre recruitment results in the non-linear characteristic of the load–deformation curve of a ligament referred to as its 'toe' region. As elongation continues at higher loads, all remaining fibrils become taut, and ligaments display a more linear 'stiffer' response. Ultimately, as elongation exceeds the capacity of the fibres, yield and failure of the ligament then results from progressive fibril failure.

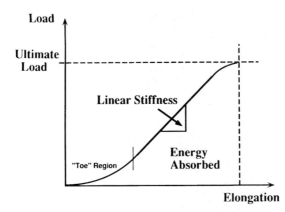

Figure 3.4 Schematic representation of a typical ligament load–elongation curve as the ligament is loaded in tension (used with permission from Woo *et al.*, 1994b).

In order to compare properties between ligaments of different size, the concept of material properties is used. Normalising load with respect to tissue cross-sectional area (stress) and elongation relative to initial tissue length (strain) eliminates some of the influences of tissue geometry, thus expressing the behaviour of the tissue in terms of a standard amount of tissue itself. Material properties thus allow all ligament tissues to be compared with each other and with many other materials as well (tendons, etc.). This comparison shows that ligaments, like tendons, are highly adapted to resist tensile stress and strain.

The third behaviour which is important to recognise is referred to as ligament viscoelasticity. Viscoelasticity refers to the ability of tissues to adapt or adjust to repetitive loading by altering either their length or their load over time. In a tissue which is viscous, sustained load, for example, results in tissue 'flow', known as creep (deformation that changes with time). A more elastic tissue would return to its original shape or length after load is removed and its stress–strain behaviour would remain unchanged with repeated or cycled loads. Interestingly, ligaments normally maintain the capacity for both viscous and elastic responses: at low loads viscous behaviours dominate, whereas at higher loads, elastic behaviours dominate. This balance likely allows normal ligaments to function within a fairly wide range of loads without their fibres or other components being damaged. The mechanisms of these behaviours are currently being investigated, but clearly involve a dynamic reorganisation of several tissue components during loading (water, collagen, etc.).

LIGAMENT INJURY AND HEALING

Mechanisms of injury

Based on these biomechanical properties of normal ligaments, an understanding of the mechanisms of ligament injury can be gained. However, it must again be emphasised that all ligaments are not identical, and various ligaments are biomechanically adapted to their own unique environment. For instance, the ligamentum nuchae of the neck must be able to allow repetitive cycles of elongation, but still be able to return to its original length (Davidson *et al.*, 1992) This ligament has much greater quantities of elastic fibres than most skeletal ligaments, which are apparently able to protect it against permanent elongation.

On the other hand, as noted in the previous section, many ligaments, if loaded repetitively will either deform permanently or fail. At higher loads, all ligaments will either partially or completely fail. Interestingly, it has been shown that the failure strength of ligaments increases slightly with exercise and decreases quite dramatically with immobilisation (Cabaud et al., 1980; Woo et al., 1982).

Ligament injuries can be classified into two main categories: the first is 'repetitive micro-trauma' and the second can be called 'macro-trauma'. Repetitive micro-trauma causes the failure of a soft-tissue structure secondary to multiple exposures to forces which are actually well below the normal ultimate tensile strength of that structure when exposed to a single load. Wilson (1996) for example, has suggested that the ultimate tensile stress of the rabbit patellar tendon decreases with increasing cycle number in vitro, supporting the concept that fatigue failures of these structures can occur. Fatigue failure has been shown to result from the propagation of micro-tears in materials, causing this type of structural failure at a lower than normal load. Importantly, a chronic state of inflammation and repair may be established in an attempt to heal micro-tears in living tissues, potentially leading to pain and disability for the patient (Safran, 1995). It has been hypothesised that if the rate of micro-tear production and propagation is more rapid than the rate of repair in vivo, then persisting symptoms and signs of an injury will be manifested. This type of injury is common and well documented in tendons, since these structures tend to carry higher loads in vivo than ligaments (Beynnon et al., 1995; Safran, 1995; Woo et al., 1994a). However, it has also been speculated that ligaments can also be injured by this mechanism. For instance, the medial collateral ligament of the elbow has been diagnosed as one structure which may be damaged as a result of repetitive loading in throwing athletes (Safran, 1995).

By far the most clinically recognisable ligament injuries result from acute macro-trauma, in which forces are sufficient within a ligament to cause partial or complete rupture of its fibres. These injuries, which are generally known as 'ligament sprains', tend to occur in skeletally mature individuals with strong bone (Hurov, 1986; Lam, 1988; Matyas et al., 1990). Most tend to have well documented mechanisms of injury and each is based on loads which must be resisted by a specific ligament. For instance the lateral collateral ligament of any joint is injured through a varus producing force, while the medial collateral ligament will be injured through a valgus producing force. The anterior cruciate ligament of the knee is torn commonly during a quick, turning (twisting) deceleration, producing anterior tibial translation and tibial external rotation (Dehaven, 1986).

Ligament sprains have historically been graded according to the severity of a tear: grade 1 is an incomplete tear with no, or minimal clinical laxity; grade 2 is an incomplete tear with obvious joint laxity, but an attainable 'end-point' on physical examination; and grade 3 is a complete ligament tear resulting in significant joint laxity. Grade 2, and especially grade 3 tears, often involve more than one ligamentous structure, since the forces often progress through other ligamentous restraints. Ligaments normally work in concert with each other and with other joint stabilisers to maintain stability throughout the range of motion of a joint. Therefore, after a particular ligament is injured, other joint stabilisers must adapt and assume the increased load (Frank et al., 1985).

Healing response

Just as the morphology and biomechanical properties of skeletal ligaments differ significantly, so do their responses to injury (Frank et al., 1983). The ligaments of the knee have been studied most extensively, and it has been well documented that the functional healing potential of the medial collateral ligament exceeds that of the anterior cruciate ligament (Frank *et al.*, 1983; Inoue *et al.*, 1987; O'Donoghue *et al.*, 1971). Many hypotheses have been postulated to explain these different healing potentials. These include differences in: intrinsic ligament fibroblastic response to injury, mechanical environment, intra-articular versus extra-articular environment (synovial fluid effects), blood supply, and inflammatory response.

The actual phases of ligament healing are analogous to healing in other connective tissues, such as the skin (Frank *et al.*, 1983). Specifically, ligaments generally appear to attempt to heal through scar tissue production; scar formation is best explained by examining it in three specific phases: bleeding and inflammation, proliferation, and remodelling.

Bleeding and inflammation

When ligaments tear, there is immediate local pain (due to pain fibres within the ligament) and bleeding (due to tearing blood vessels in and around the ligament). As with bleeding in any other injured structure, a rapid inflammatory response is initiated. A platelet and fibrin clot is produced, and a complex cascade of cytokines and growth factors are released which promote and direct the inflammatory response. Local blood vessels dilate, acute inflammatory cells infiltrate, and fibroblastic scar cells begin to appear. This first phase of ligament healing lasts for hours to a few days.

Scar proliferation

The second phase of ligament healing involves the production of scar matrix by proliferating scar fibroblasts (Akeson *et al.*, 1984). The source of these cells is controversial; however, they are likely to be a combination of local fibroblasts and differentiating mesenchymal cells from the vasculature. Macrophages and other inflammatory cells simultaneously remove damaged ligament, clot, and other cellular debris in an attempt to leave only the dense scar matrix. While gaps may not be filled by scar in some cases (e.g. anterior cruciate ligament (ACL) of knee) the gap injury in most extra-articular ligaments probably does become filled with a disorganised scar matrix within days (Figure 3.5). Neovascular in-growth is then seen. This new matrix then increases in mass, and becomes less viscous and more elastic as the inflammation decreases over the next few weeks of healing.

Scar remodelling

The third and final phase of ligament healing is matrix remodelling. Once bridging has occurred, the scar matrix begins to contract, becomes less viscous, and becomes both more dense and better organised. Electron microscopic evidence reveals that biomechanical flaws within the scar matrix (debris, fat cells, loose matrix, hypercellular areas, and areas without matrix) are gradually filled in with collagenous matrix. This has been shown to correlate with increased biomechanical strength (Shrive *et al.*, 1995). Collagen fibres are also reorganised to become less random, and more aligned to resist tensile forces (Figure 3.6). Interestingly, however, normal crimp is never restored. In fact, it has also been shown that even after years of remodelling, ligament scar matrix remains different to normal ligament. The specifics of these differences have been well documented elsewhere (Chimich *et al.*, 1991; Frank *et al.*, 1983). Importantly, it has been shown in animal models of collateral ligament injury that even after one year of healing, the

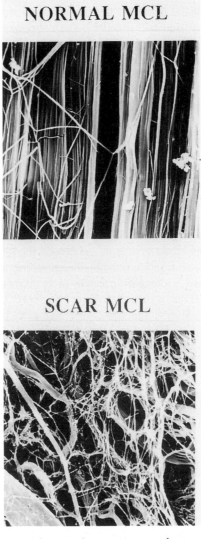

Figure 3.5 Scanning electron microscopic appearance of a normal medial collateral ligament (MCL) versus a disorganised three-week MCL scar.

ligament is not normal histologically, biochemically, or mechanically (Frank *et al.*, 1983). The ultimate tensile strength of a rabbit or canine medial collateral ligament (MCL) at one year, for example, is only about 50–70 per cent of that of a normal ligament (Chimich *et al.*, 1991; Woo *et al.*, 1987).

TREATMENT OPTIONS

Goals of treatment for ligament injuries include eliminating symptoms and impairments with the aim of returning the employee to work in a safe and healthy work environment. Initial treatment of an acute injury involves providing possible anti-inflammatory medication, rest, patient education, and therapeutic modalities.

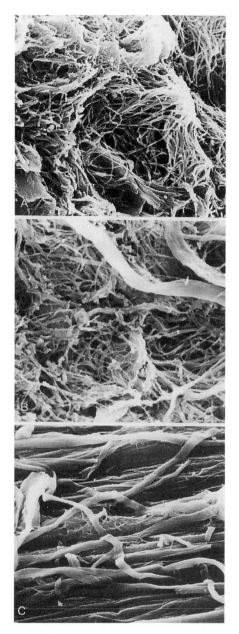

Figure 3.6 A composite of scanning electron micrographs of ligament scars at 00 weeks (A), 6 weeks (B) and 14 weeks (C) of healing showing reorganisation and realignment of matrix along the axis of the ligament (the ligament is horizontal in each case) (used with permission from Frank *et al.*, 1994).

Mobilisation versus immobilisation

Controlled movement of a joint in which stresses on injured ligaments are low appears to have several beneficial effects on healing. Controlled motion may provide improved scar strength and stiffness without compromising scar length (Frank *et al.*, 1984; Gomez

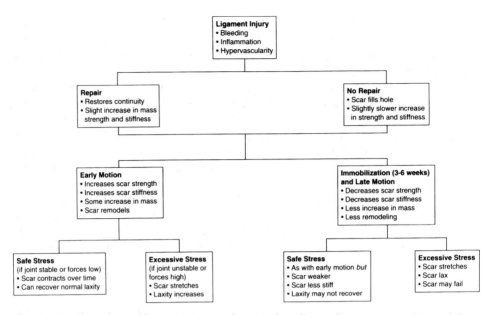

Figure 3.7   Flow chart of ligament injury, showing the effects of movement and immobilisation on ligament healing (used with permission from Frank, 1996).

et al., 1989; Hart and Dahners, 1987). Mobilisation of a joint stimulates fibroblast synthesis of collagen and proteoglycans within the sprained ligament. In addition, motion may promote return of proper collagen fibre orientation (Muneta *et al.*, 1993). Collectively, a stronger scar is produced. On the other hand, excessive motion or high loading of ligament scar may cause ligament stretching or creep. What load or amount of motion that are too great, however, are unknown at present (Figure 3.7).

Contrary to motion, immobilisation of ligament scar tissue appears to inhibit its mass and decrease its mechanical quality (Bray *et al.*, 1992; Gomez *et al.*, 1989; Newton *et al.*, 1995; Padgett and Dahners, 1992). Immobilised ligament scars are smaller, weaker and less viscous than non-immobilised scars. However, immobilisation also causes changes to the whole joint, including: fibro-fatty connective tissue proliferation, increased collagen cross links, loss of water and GAGs, articular cartilage degeneration and the development of a haphazard arrangement of collagen fibres (Enneking, 1972), making the joint stiffer than normal.

Therapeutic modalities

A plethora of therapeutic modalities have been advocated for use in the attempt to improve joint function after ligament sprains. These include: ice, heat, electromodalities, proprioception, and bracing. While these treatments are based on sound scientific principles, their actual efficacy has yet to be documented. The current understanding of some commonly used clinical modalities will be discussed briefly below.

The use of ice during the inflammatory stage of ligament healing is thought to: reduce bleeding by arteriolar vasoconstriction, reduce inflammation and swelling by decreasing metabolism and inflammatory mediators, and decrease sensory nerve conduction thereby reducing pain sensation (Michlovitz, 1990). On the other hand, the application of heat to an injured joint theoretically increases blood flow by arterial vasodilatation while reducing the viscosity of connective tissue. Collectively these effects have the potential of reducing pain and stiffness; however, their actual effects on ligament healing have not been documented specifically.

Many studies in the literature have attempted to determine the effectiveness of therapeutic ultrasound in soft tissue healing. While ultrasound can elevate tissue temperature to depths of 5 cm or more (Michlovitz, 1990), thus theoretically increasing collagen extensibility, increasing blood flow, altering nerve conduction velocity with increasing pain thresholds, and changing contractile activity of muscle tissue and permeability along cell membranes, the speculation that ultrasound may increase ligament scar tissue synthesis still requires proof.

Transverse friction massage is a type of deep massage used on tendons and ligaments for the purpose of facilitating their healing. Potential effects of transverse frictions include hyperaemia, stimulation of type I and II mechanoreceptors to reduce pain perception, and prevention of adhesion formation between neighbouring tissues. In addition, it is postulated that deep friction massage may assist orientation of collagen along the appropriate lines of stress and also help synthesise new collagen (Cyriax, 1982). As with other modalities, this speculation requires validation.

Prophylactic use of bracing and taping for ligamentous injury also remains controversial. Recent biomechanical studies indicate that although braces may provide protection to the knee during low loads, they probably do not have as great an effect during high loads (Beynnon and Johnson, 1996). In another recent study, ankle lace up stabilisers were found to be effective in preventing ankle injury and reinjury (Rovere et al., 1988). Further work in this area is required.

ERGONOMIC CONSIDERATIONS

As noted above, the knowledge of ligament structure, function, injury and rehabilitation can be used in ergonomic planning. Specifically, measures can be taken which will help prevent ligamentous injuries and aid in the recovery of workers who have already suffered a sprain. This may entail a job analysis and work place revisions in order to identify hazardous exposures and to eliminate excessive biomechanical stresses associated with the job. Ergonomic factors such as constrained or static postures, repetitive motions, and poor ergonomic or equipment design can be found to be responsible for ligamentous injuries. With the aim of minimising ligamentous overload and subsequent reinjury, ergonomic assessment must address both the high load stress and the low load repetitive mechanisms in the workplace.

The key to both the prevention and treatment of ligament injuries is the minimisation of excessive forces on the joint(s) in question. Prevention and treatment of ligament macrotrauma involve attention to the details of a person's job description and to the workplace in an effort to minimise the chances that the worker may suffer a sudden, forceful loading of any joint. Uneven surfaces, wet or slippery surfaces, and stairs/ladders are the most common sites of a sudden load on the lower extremities. Falls, due to any cause, are the reasons for most upper limb ligament sprains. Attention to the details of the work environment, in an effort to prevent such falls or slips, is obviously critical. Also as noted above, ligament microtrauma is caused by joint overloading; but in the case of these injuries, the cause is most commonly 'repetitive joint overloading' at sub-failure stresses. Ergonomic measures which can either modify the task to decrease the joint stresses, or alternatively, decrease the number of repetitions that must be performed sequentially can keep a ligament within its viscoelastic adaptive range, and prevent its injury. Similarly, once injured, the same stress-minimisation measures need to be considered in order to optimise ligament healing. The design of the workplace is central to keeping all joints within their physiological, comfortable 'safety limits'.

As with all areas of medicine, attention to prevention of ligament injuries by paying attention to measures which can be taken to prevent them is preferable to trying to implement these measures after an injury has occurred. A ligament sprain, if serious, can have permanent consequences to the worker. Ligament injuries, ideally, therefore should be prevented if at all possible.

References

ABBOTT, L., SANDERS, J., BOST, F. and ANDERSON, C., 1944, Injuries to the ligaments of the knee joint, *Journal of Bone and Joint Surgery*, **26**, 503–521.

AKESON, W.H., WOO, S.L.-Y., AMIEL, D. and FRANK, C.B., 1984, The chemical basis of tissue repair. The biology of ligaments, in Hunter, L.Y. and Funk, F.J. (Eds), *Rehabilitation of the Injured Knee*, St Louis: Mosby, C.V., pp. 93–148.

AMIEL, D., FRANK, C. and HARWOOD, F., 1983, Tendons and ligaments – a morphological and biochemical comparison, *Journal of Orthopaedic Research*, **1**, 257–265.

AMIEL, D., BILLINGS, E. and AKESON, W., 1990, Ligament structure, chemistry, and physiology, in Daniel, D.D., Akeson, W.H. and O'Conner, J.J. (Eds), *Knee Ligaments: Structure, Function, Injury, and Repair*, New York: Raven Press, pp. 77–91.

BARRACH, R. and SKINNER, H., 1990, The sensory function of knee ligaments, in Daniel, D.D., Akeson, W.H. and O'Conner, J.J. (Eds), *Knee Ligaments: Structure, Function, Injury, and Repair*, New York: Raven Press, pp. 95–114.

BASMAJIAN, J. and SLONECHER, C., 1989, *Grants Method of Anatomy. A Clinical Problem Solving Approach*, 11th edn., Baltimore: Williams & Wilkens.

BEYNNON, B.D. and JOHNSON, R.J., 1996, Anterior cruciate ligament injury rehabilitation in athletes. Biomechanical considerations, *Sports Medicine*, **22**, 54–64.

BEYNNON, B.D., FLEMING, B.C., JOHNSON, R.J., NICHOLS, C.E., RENSTROM, P.A. and POPER, M.H., 1995, Anterior cruciate ligament strain behavior during rehabilitation exercises in vivo, *American Journal of Sports Medicine*, **23**(1), 24–34.

BRAY, R.C., FRANK, C. and MINIACI, A., 1991, Structure and function of diathrodial joints, in McGinty, J.B. (Ed.), *Operative Arthroscopy*, New York: Raven Press, pp. 79–123.

BRAY, R.C., SHRIVE, N.G., FRANK, C.B. and CHIMICH, D.D., 1992, The early effects of joint immobilization on medial collateral ligament healing in an ACL deficient knee: a gross anatomic and biomechanical investigation in the adult rabbit model, *Journal of Orthopaedic Research*, **10**, 157–160.

BUTLER, D., GROOD, E., NOYES, F. and ZERNICKE, R., 1978, Biomechanics of ligaments and tendons, in *Exercise and Sport Sciences Reviews*, Baltimore: Williams & Wilkens.

CABAUD, H.E., CHATTY, A., GILDENGORIN, V. and FELTMAN, R.J., 1980, Exercise effects on the strength of the rat anterior cruciate ligament, *American Journal of Sports Medicine*, **8**(2), 79–86.

CHIMICH, D., FRANK, C., SHRIVE, N., DOUGALL, H. and BRAY, R., 1991, The effects of initial end contact on medial collateral ligament healing: a morphological and biomechanical study in a rabbit model, *Journal of Orthopaedic Research*, **9**, 37–47.

CYRIAX, J., 1982, Textbook of Orthopaedic Medicine, in Vol. 1., *Diagnosis of Soft Tissue Injuries*, London: Bailliere and Tindall.

DAVIDSON, J.M., QUAGLINO, J.D. and GIRO, M.G., 1992, Elastin repair, in Cohen, I.K., Diegelmann, R.E. and Lindblad, W.J. (Eds), *Wound Healing; Biochemical and Clinical Aspects*, Philadelphia, PA: W.B. Saunders, pp. 223–236.

DEHAVEN, K.E., 1990, Acute ligament injuries and dislocations, in Evarts, C.M. (Ed.), *Surgery of the Musculoskeletal System*, 2nd edn, Vol. 4, New York: Churchill Livingstone, pp. 3255–3282.

DIAMANT, J., KELLER, A., BAER, E., LITT, M. and ARRIDGE, R., 1972, Collagen: ultrastructure and its relation to mechanical properties as a function of aging, *Proceedings of the Royal Society of London: Series B – Biological Sciences*, **180**(60), 293–315.

ENNEKING, W.F. and HOROWITZ, M., 1972, The intra articular effects of immobilization on the human knee, *Journal of Bone and Joint Surgery*, **54A**, 973–985.

FRANK, C., 1996, Ligament healing: current knowledge and clinical applications. A comprehensive review, *Journal of the American Academy of Orthopaedic Surgeons*, **4**(2), 74–83.

FRANK, C., WOO, S.L.-Y., AMIEL, D., HARWOOD, T., GOMEZ, M. and AKESON, W., 1983, Medial collateral ligament healing. A multidisciplinary assessment in rabbits, *Americal Journal of Sports Medicine*, **11**(6), 379–389.

FRANK, C., AKESON, W.H., WOO, S.L.-Y., AMIEL, D. and COUTTS, R.D., 1984, Physiology and therapeutic value of passive joint motion, *Clinical Orthopaedics and Related Research*, **185**, 113–125.

FRANK, C., AMIEL, D., WOO, S.L.-Y. and AKESONW, W., 1985, Normal ligament properties and ligament healing, *Clinical Orthopaedics and Related Research*, **196**, 15–25.

FRANK, C., WOO, S.L.-Y., ANDRIACCHI, T., BRAND, R., OAKES, B., DAHNERS, L., *et al.*, 1988, Normal ligament: structure, function, and composition, in Woo, S.L.-Y. and Buckwalter, J.A. (Eds), *Injury and Repair of the Musculoskeletal Soft Tissues*, Park Ridge, IL: American Academy of Orthopaedic Surgeons, pp. 45–101.

FRANK, C.B., BRAY, R.C., HART, D.A., SHRIVE, N.G., LOITZ, B.J., MATYAS, J.R. and WILSON, J.E., 1994, Soft tissue healing, in Fu, F.H., Harner, C.D. and Vince, K.G. (Eds), *Knee Surgery*, Baltimore, MD: Williams and Wilkins, pp. 189–229.

GOMEZ, M.A., WOO, S.L.-Y., INOUE, M., AMIEL, D., HARWOOD, F.L. and KITZBAYASHI, L., 1989, Medial collateral ligament healing subsequent to different treatment regimens, *Journal of Applied Physiology*, **66**, 245–252.

HART, D.P. and DAHNERS, L.E., 1987, Healing of the medial collateral ligament in rats: the effects of repair, motion, and secondary stabilizing ligament, *Journal of Bone and Joint Surgery*, **69(A)**, 1194–1199.

HUROV, J.R., 1986, Soft tissue interface: how do attachments of muscles, tendons, and ligaments change during growth. A light microscopic study, *Journal of Morphology*, **189**, 313–325.

INOUE, M., McGURK-BURLESON, E., HOLLIS, J.M. and WOO, S.L.-Y., 1987, Treatment of the medial collateral ligament injury. I. The importance of anterior cruciate ligament on the varus-valgus knee laxity, *Americal Journal of Sports Medicine*, **15**, 15–21.

KENNEDY, J., WEINBERG, H. and WILSON, A., 1974, Anatomy and function of the anterior cruciate ligament – as determined by clinical and morphologic studies, *Journal of Bone and Joint Surgery*, **56(A)**, 223–235.

LAM, T.C., 1988, The Mechanical Properties of the Maturing Medial Collateral Ligament, University of Calgary, PhD Thesis.

LOITZ, B. and FRANK, C., 1993, Biology and mechanics of ligament and ligament healing, in Holloszy, J. (Ed.), *Exercise and Sport Sciences Reviews*, Baltimore, MD: Williams & Wilkens.

MATYAS, J.R., BODIE, D., ANDERSEN, M. and FRANK, C.B., 1990, The developmental morphology of a 'periosteal' ligament insertion: growth and maturation of the tibial insertion of the rabbit medial collateral ligament, *Journal of Orthopaedic Research*, **8**(3), 412–424.

MICHLOVITZ, S.L., 1990, *Thermal Agents in Rehabilitation*, Philadelphia: F.A. Davis Company.

MUNETA, T., YAMAMOTO, H., TAKAKUDA, K., SAKAI, H. and FURUYA, K., 1993, Effects of postoperative immobilization, *American Journal of Sports Medicine*, **21**, 305–313.

NEWTON, P.O., WOO, S.L.-Y., MacKENNA, D.A. and AKESON, W.H., 1995, Immobilization of the knee joint alters the mechanical and ultrastructural properties of the rabbit anterior cruciate ligament, *Journal of Orthopaedic Research* **13**, 191–200.

O'DONOGHUE, D.H., FRANK, G.R., JETER, G.L., *et al.*, 1971, Repair and reconstruction of the anterior cruciate ligament in dogs: factors influencing long-term results, *Journal of Bone Joint Surgery*, **53A**, 710–718.

PADGETT, L.R. and DAHNERS, L.E., 1992, Rigid immobilization alters matrix organization in the injured rat medial collateral ligament, *Journal of Orthopaedic Research*, **10**, 895–900.

PEATE, W.F., 1994, Occupational musculoskeletal disorders, primary care, *Clinics in Office Practice*, **21**, 313–327.

PRAEMER, A., *et al.*, 1992, *Musculoskeletal Conditions in the United States*, Rosemont, IL: American Academy of Orthopaedic Surgeons.

ROVERE, G.D., CLARKE, T.J., YATES, C.S. and BURLEY, K., 1988, Retrospective comparison of taping and ankle stabilisers in preventing ankle injuries, *American Journal of Sports Medicine*, **16**, 228–233.

SAFRAN, M.R., 1985, Elbow injuries in athletes: a review, *Clinical Orthopaedics and Related Research*, **310**, 257–277.

SCHULTZ, R., MILLER, D., KERR, C. and MICHELI, L., 1984, Mechanoreceptors in the human cruciate ligaments, *Journal of Bone and Joint Surgery*, **66A**, 1072–1076.

SHRIVE, N.G., CHIMICH, D., MARCHUK, L., WILSON, J., BRANT, R. and FRANK, C., 1995, Soft tissue 'flaws' are associated with the material properties of the healing rabbit medial collateral ligament, *Journal of Orthopaedic Research*, **13**, 923–929.

SOLOMONOW, M., BARATTA, B., ZHOU, H., SHOJI, W., BOSE, W., BECK, C. and D'AMBROSIA, R., 1987, The synergistic action of the anterior cruciate ligament and thigh muscles in maintaining joint stability, *American Journal of Sports Medicine*, **15**, 207–213.

VIIDIK, A., 1972, Simultaneous mechanical and microscopic studies of collagen fibres, *Zeitschrift fur Anatomie and Entwicklungegeschichte*, **136**(2), 204–212.

WEBSTER, A.M., 1970, *Webster's Seventh New Collegiate Dictionary*, Springfield, MA: G&C Merriam Company.

WILSON, A., 1996, Characterization of the fatigue behavior of the patellar tendon. Unpublished data.

WOO, S. and ADAMS, D.J., 1990, Tensile properties of human anterior cruciate ligaments and ACL graft tissues, in Daniel, D.D., Akeson, W.H. and O'Conner, J.J. (Eds), *Knee Ligaments: Structure, Function, Injury, and Repair*, New York: Raven Press, pp. 279–289.

WOO, S. and YOUNG, E., 1991, Structure and function of tendons and ligaments, in Hayes, W.C. (Ed.), *Basic Orthopaedic Biomechanics*, New York: Raven Press.

WOO, S.L.-Y., GOMEZ, M.A., WOO, Y.K. and AKESON, W.H., 1982, Mechanical properties of tendons and ligaments. The relationships of exercise in tissue remodeling, *Biorheology*, **19**, 379–408.

WOO, S.L.-Y., INOUE, M., McGURK-BURLESON, E. and GOMEZ, M.A., 1987, Treatment of the medial collateral ligament injury. II. Structure and function of canine knees in response to different treatment regimens, *American Journal of Sports Medicine*, **15**, 22–29.

WOO, S.L.-Y., MAYNARD, J., BUTLER, D., LYON, R., TORZILLI, P., AKESON, W.H., *et al.*, 1988, Ligament, tendon, and joint capsule insertions to bone, in Woo, S.L.-Y. and Buckwalter, J.A. (Eds), *Injury and Repair of the Musculoskeletal Soft Tissues*, Park Ridge, IL: American Academy of Orthopaedic Surgeons, pp. 133–166.

WOO, S.L.-Y., AN, K.-N., ARNOCZKY, S.P., WAYNE, J.S., FITHIAN, D.C. and MYERS, B.C., 1994a, Anatomy, biology and biomechanics of tendon, ligament, and meniscus, in Simon, S.R. (Ed.), *Orthopaedic Basic Science*, Rosemont, IL: American Academy of Orthopaedic Surgeons, pp. 45–87.

WOO, S.L.-Y., SMITH, B.A. and JOHNSON, G.A., 1994b, Biomechanics of knee ligaments, in Fu, F.H., Harner, C.D. and Vince, K.G. (Eds), *Knee Surgery*, Baltimore, MD: Williams and Wilkins, pp. 155–172.

YAHIA, L. and DROVIN, G., 1989, Microscopical investigation of canine anterior cruciate ligament and patellar tendon: collagen fascicle morphology and architecture, *Journal of Orthopaedic Research*, **7**, 243–251.

ZIMNEY, M., SCHUTTE, M. and DABEZIES, E., 1986, Mechanoreceptors in the human anterior cruciate ligament, *Anatomical Record*, **214**, 204–209.

CHAPTER FOUR

Bone biomechanics and fractures

STEFAN JUDEX, WILLIAM WHITING AND RONALD ZERNICKE

COMPOSITION AND FUNCTION OF BONE

Bone is a specialised connective tissue and one of the hardest and strongest tissues in the human body. Although, macroscopically, it appears to be inert, it is a dynamic structure undergoing continuous remodelling throughout life. These dynamics are highlighted by bone's ability to adjust its mass and morphology in response to changes in endogenous (e.g. hormones) or exogenous (e.g. mechanical loading) factors.

The function of bone is multifaceted, including serving as levers to facilitate muscle controlled movements, protection of vital organs, storehouse of minerals, and production of hematopoietic cells. These factors are synergistically interrelated and, on a larger scale, may represent mutually antagonistic objectives. For instance, bones have to be strong enough to withstand forces generated during daily activities but, at the same time, should minimise their mass as maintaining bone tissue is metabolically very costly.

Grossly, bone tissue can be classified as cortical (also called compact) or trabecular (spongy or cancellous) (Figure 4.1). The middiaphysis of long bones typically consists of cortical bone whereas vertebrae comprise trabecular bone covered with a cortical shell. The distinct morphology of trabecular bone can be attributed to the arrangement of interconnecting trabeculae which may be of rod-to-rod, rod-to-plate, or plate-to-plate structure. The lattice-work organisation of trabecular bone can vary substantially among bones and among individuals. With its high surface-to-volume ratio, trabecular bone plays a central role in mineral homoeostasis as calcium stores can be mobilised quickly in response to decreased serum calcium levels.

At the tissue level, bone can be divided into woven, primary, and secondary bone. Woven bone can be deposited *de novo* (without a pre-existing bony or cartilaginous model). It is laid down as a disorganised structure of collagen fibres and osteocytes in situations in which temporary, rapid mechanical support is required, such as after traumatic injuries. Primary bone comprises several types of bone tissue, each with unique morphology and function. For instance, trabecular bone of vertebral bodies and in epiphyses of long bones consists mostly of primary lamellar bone. Other types of primary bone are plexiform bone, as found in rapidly growing animals, and primary osteons that are formed during growth. Secondary bone is generated when pre-existing primary (or secondary) bone is replaced during remodelling.

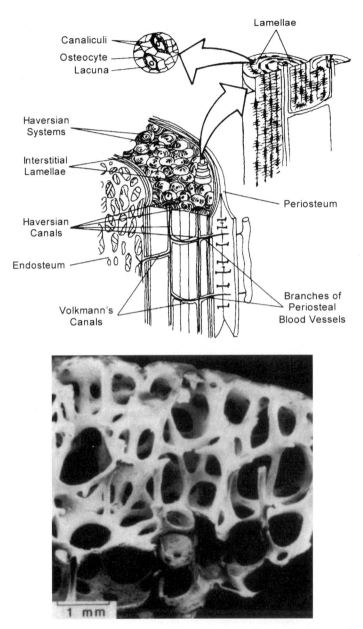

(a)

(b)

Figure 4.1 **(a)** Organisation of Haversian cortical bone in the middiaphysis of a long bone (from Nordin and Frankel, 1989 with permission). **(b)** Micro-photograph of the rod-to-rod lattice arrangement of human trabecular bone in the femoral head (from Gibson, 1985 with permission).

Bone is richly innervated and vascularised. An estimated 11 per cent of the cardiac output is sent to the skeleton (Gross *et al.*, 1979). Within cortical bone, primary arteries and veins travel within the Haversian canals that are aligned with bone's longitudinal axis (Figure 4.1a). Volkman canals interconnect Haversian canals and are oriented transversely to them. Trabecular bone is void of Haversian and Volkman canals, however, individual trabeculae are in intimate contact with a rich vascular supply via bone marrow. Osteocytes are the housekeeping cells in bone and are located in small caves, called lacunae. Small bone canals (cannaliculi) connect the lacunae. An osteocytic cellular net-work exists within the lacunae–cannaliculi system, creating the potential for communica-tion among osteocytes via gap junctions. Other major bone cell populations are osteoblasts (bone forming cells) and osteoclasts (bone resorbing cells). Despite obvious structural differences between cortical and trabecular bone, they share the same types of cells.

The extracellular matrix of bone comprises inorganic, organic, and fluid components. Calcium hydroxyapatite crystals (inorganic) constitute about half of total bone volume and account for 99 per cent of total body calcium. Another 39 per cent of bone volume consists of organic components, primarily type I collagen (95 per cent) and proteoglycans (5 per cent). The remaining volume is taken up by fluid in lacunea and cannaliculi, within the hydroxyapatite matrix, and in vascular channels.

MECHANICAL PROPERTIES OF BONE

Stress and strain

The concepts of stress and strain are central to bone biomechanics. Mechanical stress (σ) in a structure can be considered as the internal resistance developed in response to an externally applied load. Stress is defined as a force (F) per unit area (A), ($\sigma = F \cdot A^{-1}$), and is expressed in Pascals (1 Pa = 1 N $\cdot$ m^{-2}). Mechanical strain (ε) is a change in length (ΔL) normalised to the original length (L) of any given specimen ($\varepsilon = \Delta L \cdot L^{-1}$). Thus, strain is a dimensionless measure and is commonly expressed in microstrain (10^{-6} strain); 1 per cent deformation = 0.01 ε (or strain) = 10 000 $\mu\varepsilon$ (or μstrain). Strains are closely related to stress through material properties. In its simplest form, $\varepsilon = \sigma \cdot E^{-1}$, where E is a material constant (elastic modulus).

Mechanical testing of bone tissue

Material testing of tissue is essential in order to understand both its function and its response to mechanical load. The mechanical properties of cortical bone can be investig-ated with a variety of methods such as testing in uniaxial compression/tension, in three-point or four-point bending, in torsion, by accoustic microscopy, or non-invasively by ultrasound. Mechanical tests generate simplified stress configurations as bones are loaded multiaxially during functional activities. Consequently, each test reveals different details about bone's mechanical behaviour, and different tests are necessary for a complete description of bone's mechanical response.

The basic output from a mechanical test is a load–deformation curve (Figure 4.2). Initially, the load–deformation curve increases in a relatively linear fashion with increas-ing loads (Hooke's Law). The slope of this linear region is related to bone's structural stiffness or rigidity which is refered to as flexural rigidity in bending tests or as torsional rigidity in torsional tests. The yield region marks the transition from the elastic to the plastic region. Once the yield point (region) is passed, the bone sample does not return to its original configuration after load release. In the plastic region, further load increments produce over-proportional increases in deformation. Catastrophic failure occurs at the failure point. The area under the load deformation curve is the amount of energy that the specimen has absorbed at a given load or deformation. Load behaviour, stiffness, and energy absorbed are *structural properties* of a tested bone sample as they provide infor-mation on bone as a structural element within the body. Thus, parameters obtained from the load deformation curve depend highly on geometry and bone quantity of the sample.

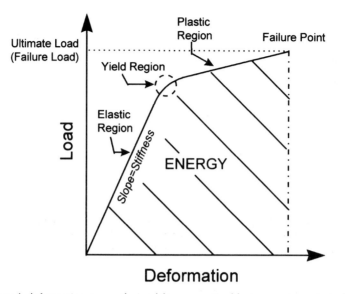

Deformation

Figure 4.2 Load–deformation curve derived from a cortical bone specimen tested in uniaxial tension. The ultimate and failure load are typically similar for cortical bone.

If the geometry (shape) of the sample is known, the *material properties* of the bone can be determined to provide information on the mechanical quality of bone. For this purpose, the applied force is normalised to unit area (stress), and deformation is transformed into strain. In the resulting stress–strain diagram, the slope of the linear portion of the curve refers to the elastic modulus (also called Young's modulus) of the material. The elastic modulus is a measure of the stiffness of the *material*. The strength of the material can be referred to as the stress at yield (yield strength) or as the maximum stress sustained (ultimate strength). The area under the stress–strain curve is a measure of toughness of the material.

Bone stress cannot be measured directly but can be calculated indirectly. For instance in a uniaxial test, the generated axial stress (sufficiently far away from the clamps) is equal to the applied force divided by the cross-sectional area of the specimen. Bone strain, on the other hand, can be measured directly by using a clip-on extensometer or by bonding strain gauges onto the surface of the bone. Strain values can also be derived from the machine displacement and the measured length of the sample, however, this method may be inaccurate due to inhomogeneous strain fields.

Mechanical behaviour of bone tissue

The mechanical behaviour of bone often is compared to steel-reinforced concrete, with the collagen fibres of bone providing tensile strength (analogous to steel rods) and the mineral phase (concrete) contributing stiffness. This composite material analogy, however, does not account for the fluid phase of bone that, largely, is responsible for bone's viscoelastic behaviour.

Viscoelastic materials are sensitive to the applied strain rate. Strain rate is defined as change in strain (deformation) per unit time. Many mechanical properties of bone are highly strain rate dependent. Ultimate strength, for instance, increases significantly when

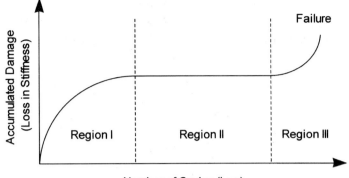

Figure 4.3 Fatigue plotted as a function of loading cycles. Microcracks have been associated with decreased strength and stiffness of the bone matrix. These microcracks are initiated in region I, then accumulate and grow until failure (adapted from Martin and Burr, 1989).

a bone is loaded more rapidly. For instance, the ultimate compressive strength of a bovine bone sample at a strain rate of 0.001 sec^{-1} is 176 MPa compared to 365 MPa at a strain rate of 1500 sec^{-1} (McElhaney, 1966).

Most materials can be characterised as brittle (e.g. glass) or ductile (e.g. gold). Bone is relatively ductile. Although bone is not as strong as most engineering materials, it is very tough (i.e., a great deal of energy can be absorbed before it fractures or yields). With increasing age, bone becomes more brittle and its toughness decreases significantly.

Fatigue in bone is characterised by a loss of strength and stiffness when subjected to cyclic loading and is associated with microcracks in the bone matrix. In general, fatigue life of a material is dependent on its ability to prevent microcrack initiation and to resist subsequent crack propagation. The latter quality is more important for a fatigue resistant material, and bone displays this characteristic (Martin and Burr, 1989). The fatigue behaviour of bone (and many other composite materials) can be subdivided into three regions (Figure 4.3). The first region is associated with the initiation of microcracks and a rapid loss of stiffness. Stiffness is stabilised in the second region. In the third region, stiffness decreases rapidly and leads to catastrophic failure of the bone that is related to the accumulation and growth of microcracks (Martin and Burr, 1989).

Bone is an anisotropic material, and as such, its mechanical properties depend on the loading direction. Bone is much stiffer longitudinally (along a bone's long axis) than it is in any other direction. In human femoral bone, the modulus of elasticity may vary from about 17 GPa in the longitudinal direction to about 12 GPa in a circumferential direction (Reilly and Burstein, 1975). Nonetheless, in simplified models, Haversian bone can be considered an orthotropic material possessing three axes of material symmetry. This model is analogous to wood which exhibits material symmetry longitudinally along the stem, radially from the centre, and circumferentially along the rings formed during growth. In extensively remodelled bone, there is no significant difference between material properties in the radial and circumferential direction and, hence, older secondary Haversian bone can be modelled as transversely isotropic (Katz et al., 1984).

Mechanical properties of bone are also affected by the applied strain mode. Bone is the strongest in compression, moderately strong in tension, and weakest in shear. For human femora (19–80 years old) tested longitudinally, the ultimate compressive stress is about 193 MPa, the ultimate tensile stress is about 133 MPa, while the ultimate shear strength is less than 30 per cent of the ultimate compressive strength (68 MPa) (Reilly and Burstein, 1975). Relatively low ultimate shear stresses are typical of ductile materials.

While mechanical properties of bones across a variety of species are similar for functionally equivalent bones, they may differ dramatically for bones with different functions (Currey, 1979). Comparative osteological studies reveal that calcium content and porosity in the bone matrix accounts for approximately 80 per cent of the variation seen in a bone's elastic modulus (Currey, 1988). The reader is referred to Keaveny and Hayes (1993) or Martin and Burr (1989) for excellent and more comprehensive reviews of the mechanical properties and mechanical behaviour of cortical and trabecular bone.

Influence of structural and material properties on bone strength

Structural and material properties of bone both can be affected significantly by age, hormonal variations (e.g. oestrogen), diet (e.g. high fat), diseases (e.g. diabetes), drugs (e.g. corticosteroids), genetics (e.g. osteogenesis imperfecta), or its physical environment (e.g. exercise). While changes in structural properties (e.g. increased cross-sectional area) may lead to a stronger bone, the positive effect may be offset by concomitant changes in material properties. For instance, fluoride treatment may induce new bone formation leading to increases in bone mass. However, biomechanical studies have demonstrated that, depending on fluoride dosage, this structural enhancement may be accompanied by a deterioration of bone quality, possibly leading to a bone that is more prone to fracture. (Riggs *et al.*, 1990; Sogaard *et al.*, 1995; Turner *et al.*, 1992).

True bone mineral density is commonly considered as a good measure of bone quality (material property). In general, factors that increase bone mineral density, also enhance the strength of the tissue and, consequently, decrease the risk of bone fracture. Osteomalacia, which may be caused by diets insufficient in calcium and phosphorus, represents a condition in which a poorly mineralised matrix dramatically increases fracture risk. Extremely high bone mineral densities, however, are not desirable as the bone becomes increasingly brittle and susceptible to fracture at higher loading rates. Theoretically, the optimum percentage of mineral (by weight) in the bone matrix is around 67 per cent (Currey, 1969). Interestingly, bones from people afflicted with osteoporosis are often referred to as brittle although there is little evidence that osteoporotic bones are more highly mineralised than normal bones. In fact, osteoporosis is a clinical condition commonly defined as a bone fracture subsequent to a loss in bone mass. The decline in mechanical integrity may be attributed to a deterioration in structural and/or material properties.

Particular considerations for trabecular bone

Trabecular bone can be tested either as an isolated structure or in whole bone preparation, such as with a femoral neck or a vertebra. While the first approach is necessary to determine the mechanical behaviour of trabecular bone, the latter approach is ergonomically (clinically) relevant because the integrated behaviour of the composite structure can be determined.

Most studies on mechanical properties of trabecular bone focus on its structural properties, because the material properties of separate trabeculae are difficult to measure. Even when measuring structural properties, results have to be interpreted with great care due to the following reasons. Firstly, mechanical properties of trabecular bone are highly dependent on its apparent density. Apparent density is the ratio of mineral mass of a given bone specimen to its total volume (trabeculae and spaces between trabeculae). The typical apparent density of tibial trabecular bone is about 0.3 gm · cc^{-1} (Carter and Hayes, 1977) compared to 1.9 gm · cc^{-1} in femoral cortical bone (Snyder and Schneider, 1991). However, variations in apparent density are very large for trabecular bone, and local changes in apparent density within the human proximal tibia can influence mechanical trabecular bone properties by up to two orders of magnitude (Goldstein *et al.*, 1983). Secondly, the architecture of trabecular bone dictates potent non-linear effects. The orientations of trabeculae appear to be aligned with principal stresses generated during loading. These trabecular patterns add a layer of structural anisotropy to bone tissue's intrinsic anisotropy, and together make mechanical testing of trabecular bone specimens dependent on the direction of load application. Finally, spaces between trabeculae are typically filled with marrow which can contribute significantly to the mechanical behaviour of trabecular bone when tested under high-speed impact (Carter and Hayes, 1977). These factors demonstrate that it is difficult to make general statements about values for mechanical properties of trabecular bone but, typically, the strength of trabecular bone is less than 10 per cent of the strength of cortical bone (Keaveny and Hayes, 1993).

IN VIVO MECHANICAL LOADING OF BONES

The mechanical environment of bone

Unlike *in vitro* mechanical tests (e.g. uniaxial tensile test), daily activities generate a very complex *in vivo* mechanical environment in bones. During functional loading, bone tissue is subjected to a combination of bending moments, torsional moments, axial loads, and shear loads (Figure 4.4a). The relative composition of moments and forces acting on a cross-section depends on the kind of activity, the specific bone, the location of the section, the degree of eccentric loading, the amount of diaphyseal curvature of the bone, and the existence of diaphyseal muscular attachments.

This already complex loading environment is further complicated in injury situations when large additional forces act on the bone. These forces may be created directly (e.g. by an opponent's foot during a soccer match) or indirectly by load transfer through adjacent tissues (i.e., bones, ligaments, and tendons). At the tissue level, any loading environment generates normal stresses and shearing stresses in a given volume of bone. Consider a cube of unit length at an arbitrary position (Figure 4.4b). Normal stresses (σ) act perpendicular to the faces of the cube and can be classified as tensile or compressive. Thus, normal stresses either elongate or compress the cube, but leave the angles of the cube intact. Shearing stresses (τ) act tangential to the faces and alter the angles of the cube.

Stresses produced in the cube depend not only on the location of the cube within the bone but to a large extent on the orientation of the cube. In fact, normal and shear stresses in the cube change their magnitude with a rotation of the cube about any of the three orthogonal axes. If the cube is rotated so that all shear stresses become zero, then the normal stresses are called principal stresses, and the directions of these stresses are defined as principal stress directions. Principal stresses represent the maximal or minimal values of normal stresses that can be generated in the cube for the given loading configuration. As noted earlier, stress and strain are closely interrelated, but because bone is an anisotropic material, the principal directions for stress and strain do not coincide.

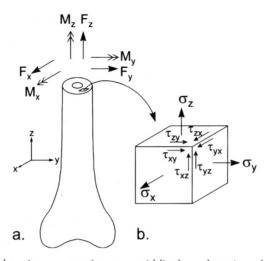

Figure 4.4 **(a)** Load environment acting on a middiaphyseal section of a long bone consisting of bending moments (M_x, M_y), a torsional moment (M_z), shear forces (F_x, F_y), and an axial force (F_z). Many functional activities induce diaphysial stresses that are generated primarily by moments. Diaphysial moments are engendered by joint forces and moments as well as by muscular attachments to the bone. **(b)** Depiction of stresses acting on a given unit cube within the bone. Normal stresses (σ) act perpendicular to the faces of the cube and compress or elongate the cube. Shear stresses (τ) that are primarily produced by shear forces and torsional moments cause a change in angles in the cube.

In vivo strain data

One problem encountered in quantifying the *in vivo* stress (strain) environment of bone is that the forces and moments acting on the bone are unknown, and stresses engendered cannot be computed directly. Bonding strain gauges directly on the periosteal surface of bone represents one means of overcoming this deficiency. The use of this method has been mostly limited to animal experiments, however, two studies have reported *in vivo* strain data from humans (Burr *et al.*, 1996; Lanyon *et al.*, 1975). Information from strain gauges is limited to their sites of attachment. Linear beam theory (Rybicki *et al.*, 1974) or finite elements (Brown *et al.*, 1992) can be employed to calculate a more complete description of the mechanical milieu of bone.

Analysis of *in vivo* strain gauge data reveals that peak strains induced in limb bones during functional loading (e.g. running at maximum speed) are remarkably similar across a variety of species, including humans (2000–3500 $\mu\varepsilon$) (Burr *et al.*, 1996; Rubin and Lanyon, 1982). This phenomenon has been referred to as 'dynamic strain similarity' (Rubin and Lanyon, 1984). For functionally engendered strains during vigorous activities, bone's safety factor to yield is about 2–3 and the safety factor to fracture is approximately 6–7 (Rubin, 1984). These safety factors were calculated using 6800 $\mu\varepsilon$ for yield strain of and 15 700 $\mu\varepsilon$ for ultimate tensile strain (Carter *et al.*, 1981).

Effect of geometry on bone stresses

Many functional activities, including running, induce stresses in the middiphysis of long bones that are generated to a large extent by bending and torsional moments (Judex *et al.*,

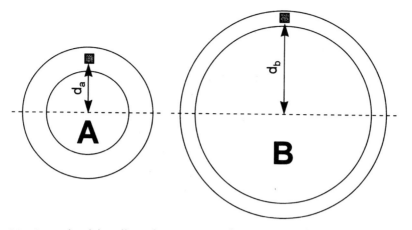

Figure 4.5   Example of the effect of cross-sectional geometry on bending induced maximal stresses. Both long bones depicted possess the same cross-sectional area, but bone A has a smaller medullary area. The same applied bending moment generates 50 per cent larger peak stresses in bone A. The moment of inertia (I) of a given area (grey square) about the neutral axis is proportional to the square of the distance (d) from the neutral axis. The bending induced neutral axis (zero stress) is represented by the dashed line. Thus, bone B is subjected to smaller stresses because more bone tissue is distributed further away from the neutral axis ($d_b > d_a$).

1997; Rubin, 1984). Stresses induced by moments are highly dependent on the cross-sectional shape of the bone section. The following example demonstrates the potent effect of geometry and reinforces the concepts of material and structural properties.

Consider two prismatic long bones that exhibit the same material properties (Figure 4.5). Both bones have a cylindrical cross-section and the same cross-sectional area (295 mm²), but the second bone has a larger periosteal diameter (40 mm versus 25 mm) and a corresponding larger endosteal diameter (35 mm versus 15.8 mm). Pure axial loading would produce the same stresses in the two bones. However, similar bending moments applied to both bones would generate dramatically different responses. The maximal generated stress in the second bone would be only 50 per cent of the maximal stress produced in the first bone. Thus, not only bone mass and bone quality are important for the prevention of bone fractures but also bone's relative distribution. This concept is expressed quantitatively in the second moment of inertia (I). Values of I increase as the square of the distance between a given area of bone and the loading induced neutral axis (line of zero stress) (Figure 4.5). Consequently, changing the ratio between periosteal and endosteal diameter provides a means for bone to increase its bending or torsional stiffness without adding additional bone mass or changing bone mineral density.

BONE FRACTURES

Why does bone fracture?

Currey and Alexander (1985) defined mechanically optimised bone, requiring that it be:

(1)   strong enough not to yield, under the greatest bending moments likely to act on it;

(2)   strong enough not to fail by fatigue, under the greatest bending moments expected to act repeatedly on it;

(3)   strong enough not to fracture, under the greatest bending moments likely to act on it;

(4)   stiff enough in bending; and

(5)   strong enough in bending under impact loading.

Obviously, healthy bone tissue satisfies these requirements during functional (but not excessive) loading conditions. The high incidence of bone fractures demonstrates, however, that safety margins are not sufficient for all loading environments.

In simplest terms, a bone fractures when it cannot withstand the applied load. Bone fracture mechanics, however, is a complex combination of the applied loading environment, material and structural properties of the bone, and type of bone involved. In particular, the interactions among complex loading conditions, viscoelastic characteristics, anisotropic effects, and bone porosity and geometry make the analysis of fracture anything but simple. Different aspects of the mechanical loading environment determine, to a large extent, the potential for fracture and the type of fracture generated. Either large magnitude single loads or smaller repetitive loads may induce a fracture. The predominant type of load can usually determine the fracture type. For instance, long bones subjected primarily to torsional loads, produce a oblique (spiral) fracture line. This kind of loading often causes fracture in skiing accidents when the ski acts as an extended moment arm for applying torque. Axial loads tend to induce transverse fracture lines. A range of fracture types and their corresponding mechanisms are depicted in Figure 4.6.

Characterisation of bone fractures

Most bone fractures can be characterised as *direct injuries* occurring close to the site of load application. In contrast, a fracture is labeled an *indirect injury* if the fracture stems from forces transmitted through other tissues; an example for an indirect injury is an avulsion fracture that occurs when large tendinous or ligamentous forces are transferred to their bony attachment site and cause a piece of bone to be pulled out. The viscoelastic properties of both bone and tendon (or ligament) play a large role when excessive forces act on tendons or ligaments. In general, when the load is applied slowly, the bone tends to be the weaker element, but if the load is applied rapidly, then the likelihood of a tendon or ligament rupture is increased.

Once a fracture has been diagnosed, it is commonly characterised by (Whiting and Zernicke, 1998):

(1)   Injury site – location, such as diaphyseal, epiphyseal, or metaphyseal.

(2)   Extent of injury – complete or incomplete, depending on whether the fracture line(s) completely or partially traverse the bone.

(3)   Configuration – shape of the fracture. If a single line is present it may be either transversely, obliquely, or spirally oriented. In the case of multiple fracture lines, the fracture may be characterised as a comminuted or butterfly fracture.

(4)   Fragment relations – displaced or undisplaced. Fragments can be displaced in many ways, including angulated displacement, rotational displacement, distraction, over-riding, impaction, and sideway shifting (Figure 4.7).

(5)   Environmental relations – open or closed fractures depending on whether the skin is penetrated or not.

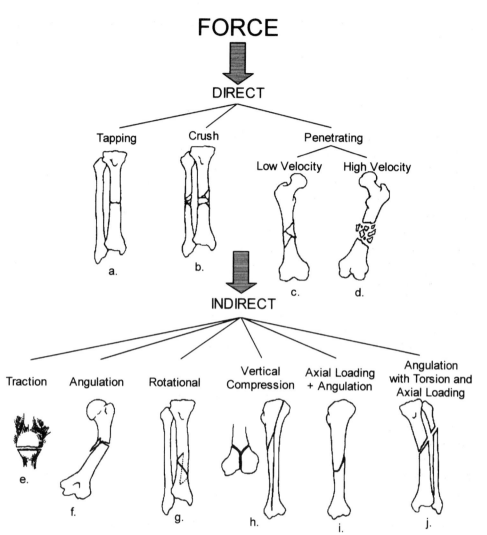

Figure 4.6 Frequent clinically encountered bone fractures characterised by their injury mechanism: (a–d) direct force, (e–j) indirect force. **(a)** Tapping mechanism producing a transverse fracture by inducing relatively small forces over a small area. **(b)** Crushing from large forces distributed over a large area causing an extensive comminuted fracture. **(c–d)** Comminuted fracture from penetration (large force acting on a small area) induced (c) at low velocity and (d) at high velocity. **(e)** Tensile force related traction mechanism producing transverse or avulsion fracture. **(f)** Bending moment induced angulation resulting in angulated or butterfly fracture. **(g)** Torque induced rotational mechanism causing spiral fracture. **(h)** Vertical compression resulting in oblique fracture. **(i)** Combination of axial compression and angulation. **(j)** Combination of angulation with torsion and axial loading resulting in complex fracture pattern (from Harkess *et al.*, 1996, with permission).

(6) Complications – immediate, early, and/or late complications may accompany a bone fracture. Visceral, vascular, neurological, and muscular injuries are examples of immediate complications. Tissue necrosis, infection, and tetanus represent early complications and osteoarthritis, growth disturbances, and re-fracture are late complications.

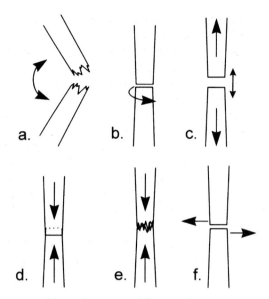

Figure 4.7   Displacement of bone fragments following fracture. (**a**) Bending induced angular displacement. (**b**) Torque induced rotational displacement. (**c**) Tension induced distraction. (**d**) Compression induced overriding. (**e**) Compression induced impaction. (**f**) Shearing induced lateral shifting.

(7)   Aetiology – predisposing factors that may influence progression to a fracture as seen in stress fractures or pathological fractures. Examples are bone diseases or inflammatory disorders.

High impact fractures

Occupational injuries, vehicle–pedestrian accidents, and sports-related high-energy impacts frequently lead to traumatic fractures of long bones. Bone is a viscoelastic material and increases its ultimate strength when loads are applied rapidly. At higher strain rates, it can store much more energy (area under the load–deformation curve) before it fractures. At the point of fracture, this large quantity of energy creates multiple fractures to absorb the energy released (law of conservation of energy).

Stress fractures

Stress fractures, common in occupational and athletic injuries, are related to material fatigue. The fatigue-related microcracks seem to be focused within specific areas of the bone matrix (Burr *et al.*, 1997) probably reflecting the imposed non-uniform mechanical environment. If microcrack damage is not excessive, bone has the ability to repair these microcracks by resorbing material around the cracks and depositing new tissue (remodelling). Whether increased remodelling activity in the area of microcracks is initiated by the presence of microcracks themselves or by the mechanical environment that induced them is unclear.

Theoretically, this remodelling repair process could give bone an indefinite fatigue life. However, if the mechanical environment that induced the microcracks persists, the repair process may also accelerate progression to a stress fracture. Greater remodelling increases the number and size of porosities in the affected areas as osteoclasts first remove bone before osteoblasts follow to fill the excavated cones. If these porosities unduly weaken the bone before new material is deposited, then stress fractures can develop. This phenomenon may explain, in part, the discrepancy between *in vitro* studies which indicate that millions of loading cycles at physiological strain magnitude and strain rates are necessary to induce a stress fracture (Schaffler *et al.*, 1990) and *in vivo* data that suggest that a much smaller number of cycles can lead to stress fractures (e.g., stress fractures in military recruits typically occur within the first six weeks of training).

Tibial stress fractures account for up to 50 per cent of all stress fractures observed clinically. The location of stress fractures depends on the activity that induced the fracture, emphasising that different activities generate different mechanical environments. Tibial stress fractures, for instance, occur most commonly between the middle and distal thirds of the diaphysis in runners, in the proximal diaphysis in basketball and volleyball players, and in the middiaphysis in dancers (Montelone, 1995).

RELEVANCE TO ERGONOMICS

Although work-related injuries are commonly associated with damage to soft tissues or joints (e.g. repetitive strain injuries), the prevalence of bone fractures is still high. In 1995, 2.04 million non-fatal workplace injuries occurred in private industry in the United States (Bureau of Labor Statistics, 1997). Fractures accounted for 6.1 per cent of total injuries causing a mean of 18 days away from work per person (Bureau of Labor Statistics, 1997). Primary means for preventing fractures should consist of eliminating situations that may generate high risk mechanical environments. The workplace related mechanical environment should be adjusted to have a minimal impact on the worker. Minimisation of forces and moments acting on bones may be accomplished by educating employees about better techniques or by using improved equipment. Secondary prevention of occupational, bone-related injuries should emphasise the enhancement of bone quantity and quality, muscular strength, and proprioception. Regular physical exercise, a balanced diet rich in calcium, and 'normal' hormonal levels are the optimal means to achieve this goal.

References

BROWN, T.D., PEDERSON, D.R., GRAY, M.L., BRAND, R.A. and RUBIN C.T., 1992, Toward an identification of mechanical parameters initiating periosteal remodeling: a combined experimental and analytical approach, *Journal of Biomechanics*, **23**, 893–905.

BUREAU OF LABOR STATISTICS, 1997, *Lost-Worktime Injuries: Characteristics and Resulting Time Away from Work, 1995*, US Department of Labor, Washington, DC.

BURR, D.B., MILGROM, C., FYHRIE, D., FORWOOD, M., NYSKA, M., FINESTONE, A., *et al.*, 1996, In vivo measurement of human tibial strains during vigorous activity, *Bone*, **18**, 405–410.

BURR, D.B., FORWOOD, M.R., FYHRIE, D.P., MARTIN, R.B., SCHAFFLER, M.B. and TURNER, C.H., 1997, Bone microdamage and skeletal fragility in osteoporotic and stress fractures, *Journal of Bone and Mineral Research*, **12**, 6–15.

CARTER, D.R. and HAYES, W.C., 1977, The compressive behavior of bone as a two-phase porous structure, *Journal of Bone and Joint Surgery*, **59**, 954–962.

CARTER, D.R., CALER, W.E., SPENGLER, D.M. and FRANKEL, V.H., 1981, Fatigue behavior of adult cortical bone: the influence of mean strain and strain range, *Acta Orthopaedica Scandinavia*, **52**, 481–490.

CURREY, J.D., 1969, The mechanical consequences of variation in the mineral content of bone, *Journal of Biomechanics*, **2**, 1–11.

CURREY, J.D., 1979, Mechanical properties of bone tissues with greatly differing functions, *Journal of Biomechanics*, **12**, 313–319.

CURREY, J.D., 1988, The effect of porosity and mineral content on the Young's modulus of elasticity of compact bone, *Journal of Biomechanics*, **21**, 131–139.

CURREY, J.D. and ALEXANDER, R.McN., 1985, The thickness of walls of tubular bones, *Journal of Zoology* (London), **206**, 453–468.

GIBSON, L.J., 1985, The mechanical behavior of cancellous bone, *Journal of Biomechanics*, **18**, 317–328.

GOLDSTEIN, S.A., WILSON, D.L., SONSTEGARD, D.A. and MATHEWS, L.S., 1983, The mechanical properties of human tibial trabecular bone as a function of metaphyseal location, *Journal of Biomechanics*, **16**, 965–969.

GROSS, P.M., HEISTAD, D.D. and MARCUS, M.L., 1979, Neurohumeral regulation of blood flow to bones and marrow, *American Journal of Physiology*, **236**, H440–H448.

HARKESS, J.W., RAMSEY, W.C. and HARKESS, J.W., 1996, Principles of fractures and dislocations, in ROCKWOOD, C.A., GREEN, D.P., BUCHOLZ, R.W. and HECKMAN, J.D. (Eds), *Rockwood and Green's Fractures in Adults*, 4th edn, Philadelphia, PA: Lippincott-Raven.

JUDEX, S., GROSS, T.S. and ZERNICKE, R.F., 1997, Strain gradients correlate with sites of exercise-induced bone forming surfaces in the adult skeleton, *Journal of Bone and Mineral Research*, **12**, 1737–1745.

KATZ, J.L., YOON, H.S., LIPSON, S., MAHARIDGE, R., MEUNIER, A. and CHRISTEL, P., 1984, The effects of remodeling on the elastic properties of bone, *Calcified Tissue International*, **36**, 31–36.

KEAVENY, T.M. and HAYES, W.C., 1993, Mechanical properties of cortical and trabecular bone, in Hall, B.K. (Ed.), *Bone*, Vol. 3, Boca Raton, FL: CRC Press, 285–344.

LANYON, L.E., HAMPSON, W.G.L., GOODSHIP, E. and SHAH, J.S., 1975, Bone deformation recorded in vivo from strain gauges attached to the human tibial shaft, *Acta Orthopaedica Scandinavia*, **46**, 256–268.

MARTIN, R.B. and BURR, D.B., 1989, *Structure, Function, and Adaptation of Compact Bone*, New York: Raven Press.

McELHANEY, J.H., 1966, Dynamic response of bone and muscle tissue, *Journal of Applied Physiology*, **21**, 1231–1236.

MONTELONE, G.P., 1995, Stress fractures in the athlete, *Orthopedic Clinics of North America*, **26**, 423–432.

NORDIN, M. and FRANKEL, V., 1989, Biomechanics of bone, in Nordin, M. and Frankel, V. (Eds), *Basic Biomechanics of the Musculoskeletal System*, 2nd edn, Malvern, PA: Lea & Febiger, 3–29.

REILLY, D.T. and BURSTEIN, A.H., 1975, The elastic and ultimate properties of compact bone tissue, *Journal of Biomechanics*, **8**, 393–405.

RIGGS, B.L., HODGON, S.F. and O'FOLLON, W.M., 1990, Effects of fluoride treatment on the fracture rate in postmenopausal women with osteoporosis, *New England Journal of Medicine*, **322**, 802–809.

RUBIN, C.T., 1984, Skeletal strain and the functional significance of bone architecture, *Calcified Tissue International*, **36**, S11–S18.

RUBIN, C.T. and LANYON, L.E., 1982, Limb mechanics as a function of speed and gait: a study of functional strains in the radius and tibia of horse and dog, *Journal of Experimental Biology*, **101**, 187–211.

RUBIN, C.T. and LANYON, L.E., 1984, Dynamic strain similarity in vertebrates: an alternative to allometric bone scaling. *Journal of Theoretical Biology*, **107**, 321–327.

RYBICKI, E.F., SIMONEN, F.A., MILLS, E.J., HASSLER, C.R., SCOLES, P., MILNE, D. and WEIS, E.B., 1974, Mathematical and experimental studies on the mechanics of plated transverse fractures, *Journal of Biomechanics*, **7**, 377–384.

SCHAFFLER, M.B., RADIN, E.L. and BURR, D.B., 1990, Long-term fatigue behavior of compact bone at low strain magnitude and rate, *Bone*, **11**, 321–326.

SNYDER, S.M. and SCHNEIDER, E., 1991, Estimation of mechanical properties of cortical bone by computed tomography, *Journal of Orthopaedic Research*, **9**, 422–431.

SOGAARD, C.H., MOSEKILDE, L., SCHWARTZ, W., LEDIG, G., MINNE, H.W. and ZIEGLER, R., 1995, Effects of fluoride on rat vertebral body biomechanical competence and bone mass, *Bone*, **16**, 163–169.

TURNER, C.H., AKHTER, M.P. and HEANEY, R.P., 1992, The effects of fluoridated water on bone strength, *Journal of Orthopaedic Research*, **10**, 581–587.

WHITING, W.C. and ZERNICKE, R.F., 1998, *Biomechanics of Musculoskeletal Injury: Human Kinetics*.

CHAPTER FIVE

Muscle mechanics in ergonomics

JACQUES BOBET

INTRODUCTION

How should an ergonomist design a task so it is safe, easy, and comfortable? How should he/she instruct the worker who must do the task? There is no simple answer, but for many tasks a good answer requires that the ergonomist understand the physics of muscle. The ergonomist who sets out to design a physical task, or instruct a worker in this task, without understanding muscle is like the captain who sails without knowing the physics of water, or the pilot who flies without knowing the physics of flight. Muscle mechanics, the study of muscle force and its effects, is key to the health, safety, and effectiveness of workers. It is central to such questions as: How to reduce the stresses on the body? How to optimise performance of a task? How to prevent fatigue? How to make a task less demanding? How to prevent pain and injury to muscle? What muscles are active in a given task, and why? Does a worker have the 'strength' needed for a task?

This chapter is a review and tutorial in muscle mechanics for ergonomists. It has two parts. The first, 'Basics of muscle mechanics', explains muscle force, stiffness, and power. The second, 'Workplace implications of muscle mechanics', discusses the implications of muscle mechanics for workplace problems. The chapter ignores the molecular or bio-physical mechanisms of muscle contraction (see Geeves, 1991, for these). It also omits many details of muscle mechanics (see the book edited by Winters and Woo, 1990 for more detail).

BASICS OF MUSCLE MECHANICS

Workplace tasks require that muscles exert force, develop stiffness, and generate power. Each of these will be discussed separately.

Muscle force

Your muscles cause useful movement by exerting force on your bones. This force, some-times called 'tension', determines whether your movement will be effective or ineffective, comfortable or painful, easy or tiring. For example, writing with your right hand is easy, restful, and effective – if you are right-handed. If you are not, writing with your right hand is difficult, tiring, and ineffective. The difference lies in the actions of the muscles, in the size and timing of the forces they exert.

A muscle's force depends on many factors. (These have been studied extensively, and several good reviews are already available. See Winter (1990) or Lieber and Bodine-Fowler (1993) for an elementary treatment. See reviews by Zajac (1989) and in Winters and Woo (1990) for more detail.) The most important of these are: muscle length, muscle velocity, and muscle activation.

You can feel the effect of muscle length on force when you lift yourself from a pool onto the deck. If you place your hands at shoulder width on the poolside, you will easily rasie your body. If you place your hands close together or far apart, however, you will struggle. The weight you hoist is the same wherever you put your hands, but the force available to do so is not. Your arms are strongest when the shoulders and elbows are at certain angles, i.e. when the muscles of the chest and arms lie at certain lengths. Placing your hands incorrectly puts the joints at unfavourable angles, the muscles at unfavourable lengths.

The effect of length on tension is most obvious in an isolated muscle (Figure 5.1A). Muscle is strongest when its sarcomeres lie at an intermediate length. If the experimenter measures the length and tension of a single muscle fibre, taking care to keep its sarcomeres even, the relation of force to length shows sharp changes in slope. Under these artificial conditions, the locations of these changes match the lengths of the actin and myosin filaments within the muscle (Gordon *et al.*, 1966) (Figure 5.1A). Under natural conditions, the relation of muscle force to length is smoother and broader (Gareis *et al.*, 1992), due to the action of factors other than filament length (Ettema and Huijing, 1994b; Gareis *et al.*, 1992; Huijing *et al.*, 1994) (Figure 5.1B).

In addition to varying with its length, a muscle's force also varies with its speed. The faster a muscle shortens, the less force it produces. If you pedal a bicycle in too low a gear, for example, your legs will whirl at great speed but you will exert little force on the pedals. Shifting to a higher gear slows your legs, allowing you to push effectively on the pedals. By slowing the movement, you return the muscle to shortening speeds at which it can exert force. Hill (1938) referred to this relationship as the muscle *force–velocity characteristic*.

Of course, muscle can exert force to resist lengthening, as well as to produce shortening. For example, if you lower a box onto a table, you allow its weight to exceed the upward force from your hands. The box descends, lengthening the 'contracting' muscles of the upper limb. These 'eccentric' contractions are now considered part of the force–velocity properties of muscle. An isolated muscle exerts more force while it is being lengthened than it does while shortening. A typical force–velocity characteristic, for cat muscle, is shown in Figure 5.2. Note that the characteristic changes with the rate of stimulation.

In cats, measuring a single muscle's force and velocity is easy. In humans, it is not. The force–velocity relation of a human muscle can be estimated from the relation of torque and angular velocity (speed of limb rotation) (see reviews by Gulch, 1994; Kannus, 1994). The torque–velocity relation in humans behaves mostly as you would expect, given the force–velocity characteristic in isolated muscle. Human muscle torque falls with increasing speeds of shortening, and rises with increasing speeds of lengthening (Hill, 1922; Perrine and Edgerton, 1978; Thorstensson *et al.*, 1976; Wickiewicz *et al.*, 1984; Wilkie, 1950). There are two surprises, however. One is that torque decreases with

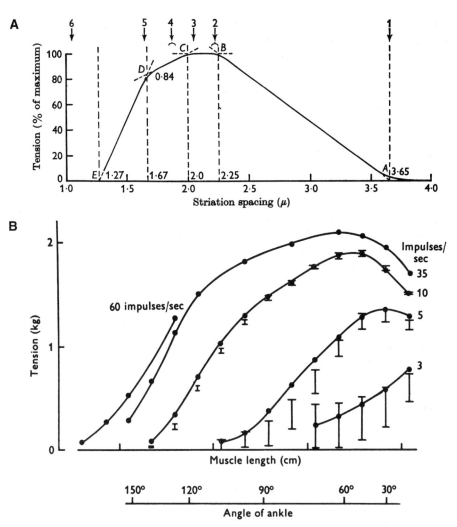

Figure 5.1 Dependence of muscle force on muscle length. **(A)** In single frog fibres, under artificial conditions, the force is highest at mid-lengths. The relation has sharp changes in slope (letters A–E), which occur at specific sarcomere lengths (numbers above x-axis), and which correspond to length-dependent changes in overlap of the thick and thin filaments (numbers 1–6, at top) (from Gordon *et al.*, 1966, by permission of the *Journal of Physiology*). **(B)** Under more natural conditions, force is still higher at mid-lengths, but the relation is smoother and broader, and depends on the level of activation. These data are for cat soleus muscle (from Rack and Westbury (1969), by permission of the *Journal of Physiology*).

velocity of stretch at high stretching velocities (Dudley *et al.*, 1990); in other words, very fast stretches generate less torque than moderately fast ones. The other is that torque rises with velocity when muscle is shortening slowly (Perrine and Edgerton, 1978; Wickiewicz *et al.*, 1984). In other words, if you contract slowly, you get more torque than if you hold a fixed angle. This 'flat spot' in the human torque-velocity curve arises because the nervous system cannot fully activate the muscle at low speeds of shortening (Dudley *et al.*, 1990; Perrine and Edgerton, 1978; Wickiewicz *et al.*, 1984). Other authors have not found this flat spot, however (e.g. Thorstensson *et al.*, 1976).

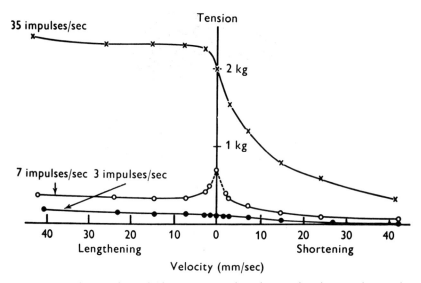

Figure 5.2   Dependence of steady force on muscle velocity, the 'force–velocity character-istic'. Positive velocities indicate shortening. Cat soleus muscle (from Joyce and Rack (1969), by permission of the *Journal of Physiology*).

While length and velocity affect muscle force, so does muscle activation. The human nervous system uses two mechanisms to vary muscle force (Milner-Brown *et al.*, 1973a, 1973b). It activates motor units within the muscle in order of size, enlisting small units at low force levels and increasingly big ones at high force levels ('recruitment'). It also sets the rate at which motor units fire, driving them slowly when they are first recruited, then faster as more force is needed ('rate coding') (see review by Clamann, 1993).

Developing stiffness

Many tasks require that the muscles keep the limb in a desired *position*, rather than exerting a desired force. To hammer a nail, for example, you need both elbow and wrist muscles. The elbow muscles provide *force*, moving the hammer onto the nail. The wrist muscles provide *stiffness*, preventing the wrist from 'breaking' on impact. All of the structures crossing a joint contribute to its stiffness, but the muscles at that joint have the largest effect.

If you push someone's foot, making it rotate about the ankle, you will feel a resist-ance. The structures spanning the joint, and the foot itself, oppose your movement. If you measure the torque which resists you, you will find that it depends on the movement you impose (Kearney and Hunter, 1982a, 1982b):

$$T = I \, d^2\theta/dt^2 + b \, d\theta/dt + k\theta \tag{5.1}$$

Equation 5.1 indicates that this torque (T) depends on the size of the imposed angular displacement (θ), the angular velocity ($d\theta/dt$), and the angular acceleration ($d^2\theta/dt^2$). The effect of each of these depends on three constants: the inertia I, the viscosity b, and the stiffness k. Their values differ from person to person and joint to joint. Two of these constants (b and k) also vary with joint angle, and increase with muscle force (Kearney and Hunter, 1982a, 1982b). Note that equation 5.1 also holds if the opposite experiment

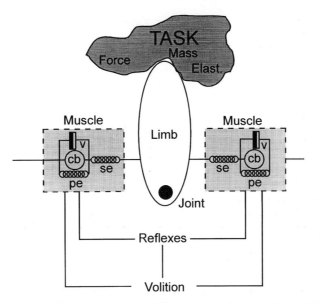

Figure 5.3 Factors that affect the worker's ability to maintain a position while doing a task. The limb rotates around the joint, under control of at least one agonist and one antagonist muscle. Each muscle contributes passive elasticity (pe), crossbridge force (cb), elasticity from structures in series with the crossbridges (se), and viscosity (v). Its activity is controlled by reflexes and volition. The limb has inertia. The task itself may exert forces on the limb, or load the limb with extra mass or elasticity (modified from Winters *et al.*, 1988).

is performed: applying a known torque to the joint and recording its movement (Agarwal and Gottlieb, 1977; Lakie *et al.*, 1984). More detail can be found in the reviews by Kearney and Hunter (1990) and Gottlieb (1996).

Muscle stiffness and viscosity arise mostly from its crossbridges (Ford *et al.*, 1977; Rack and Westbury, 1974) (Figure 5.3). These crossbridges are elastic, and any movement that lengthens the muscle must stretch them; this gives an apparent stiffness. Also, the crossbridges detach and reattach in a way that depends on the speed of stretch; this gives an apparent viscosity. Some of the stiffness arises from the presence of the stretch reflex, which activates a muscle when it is lengthened, increasing its resistance to stretch (Nichols and Houk, 1973). The stretch reflex is most important at low to intermediate values of force. Some also arises from muscle's passive elasticity. When a muscle is inactive and unloaded, it assumes a certain length (its 'rest length'). If you stretch the muscle beyond its rest length, for example by hanging a weight on it, the muscle exerts a force opposing the stretch. If the muscle crosses a joint, this force causes a torque at that joint. This torque is familiar to you if you have ever tried to increase your 'flexibility' – you will have felt a strong resistance as you tried to rotate the joint beyond its normal range. The passive muscle torque around human joints is different for different joints, but always tends to restore the muscle towards its rest length. It increases sharply at the ends of the range of motion (Mansour and Audu, 1986; Yoon and Mansour, 1982). Passive forces are not constant, and the joint tends to become less stiff if it is stretched repeatedly (Lakie *et al.*, 1984); this effect, called 'thixotropy', arises from the properties of both muscle and joint (Wiegner, 1987). Passive elasticity does not affect stiffness much, except at the extremes of the range of motion.

Generating power

Some tasks require the right muscle force. Others require the right muscle stiffness. Still others, however, require the right muscle *power*. 'Power' has various meanings in everyday use, but in physics it has a specific meaning: it is the rate of doing work. Work, in physics, also has a specific meaning: the work W done by a force F is defined as:

$$W = \int F dx \qquad\qquad (5.2)$$

where dx is the displacement (in the direction of the force) of the point at which the force is applied. Work is larger for larger forces, or for larger displacements in the direction of the force.

Climbing a hill is a simple illustration of work and power. If you walk straight up a steep hill, your heart pounds, you sweat, and your legs tire. But if you crisscross the hill, gaining a little altitude on each pass, you reach the top fresh and rested. The work done is the same in both cases: you have raised your body to the top of the hill. But the metabolic and fatigue consequences are not. Climbing straight up a hill, you do work (raising your body from bottom to top of the hill) in a short time. Your average power is high. Crisscrossing the hill, your average power is low. In both cases, this power comes from the muscle.

The major factor affecting muscle power is the velocity of contraction. A muscle generates its greatest power when it shortens at speeds around one-third of the maximum speed at which it can still generate force (Ivy *et al.*, 1981). Because muscle power depends on the product of muscle force and velocity, muscle power varies with muscle force.

In theory, an ergonomist can reduce the energy and power demands of a task by exploiting the elasticity of muscle. The idea is simple: muscle contains elastic structures which are capable of storing and releasing energy. By exploiting this elasticity, you can provide additional power or energy to a movement (see review by Cavagna, 1977). Muscle's action is analogous to that of a bow. You can impart a lot more power to an arrow by firing it from a bow than by throwing it from your hand. When you draw the bowstring, you store work in the bow's elastic structures (its springiness). When you release the bow, your work is transferred from the bow to the arrow. Because you do the work slowly but release it quickly, you get a lot of power. Because muscle is elastic, you can store and release energy in it, in much the same way.

WORKPLACE IMPLICATIONS OF MUSCLE MECHANICS

How much force is a muscle exerting?

As noted above, muscle force dictates whether a task is easy or hard, effective or ineffective, tiring or restful. How can it be measured?

Before discussing this, it is important to distinguish between muscle force and the force exerted by a limb on an external object. Muscle does not act directly on a tool; rather, the muscle force turns the limb, pressing it onto the tool. In sawing, for instance, the muscles of the shoulder and elbow pull on the bones, rotating the arm; the arm's rotation then pushes the saw onto the wood. The distinction is important: the force of the hand on the saw, while easily measured, is not the same as the force the muscles exert on the arm.

A researcher can measure muscle force in several ways. In animals, the muscle can be cut and tied to a force transducer, then stimulated with electric current. Stimulation methods that mimic normal activation by the nervous system are now available (Baratta *et al.*, 1989). Cutting the tendon and attaching it to a device is helpful for studying muscle mechanics, but cannot be used in humans.

Other methods must be used in humans. For muscle groups whose nerve is superficial, such as the ankle flexors or extensors, the researcher can stimulate the nerve electrically, passing current through the skin to produce contraction. He/she can then measure the torque about the ankle, by recording the force exerted by the foot on a force transducer. Since this torque is caused by only one muscle, he/she can estimate the muscle's force as long as its moment arm is known. (Note that this approach does not work with a voluntary contraction. In voluntary contractions, the torque cannot be attributed to a single muscle's force.) If the muscle has a long tendon, the researcher can place a force transducer around it and measure muscle force directly (reviewed in Komi, 1990). This approach requires surgery. For superficial muscles, he/she can estimate a muscle's force from its electrical activity (its electromyogram, or EMG). To do this, he/she places recording electrodes in or over the muscle. If the joint angle is not changing, and the muscle's force is steady, the level of EMG is proportional to the force. If the joint angle is changing, or muscle force is not constant, then the level of EMG can still relate to force, once the influences of muscle length, velocity, and dynamic response have been removed.

Force can also be estimated from the fluid pressure within the muscle ('intramuscular pressure'). The researcher inserts a small pressure sensor through the skin and into the muscle. Intramuscular pressure increases as muscle force increases, even if the muscle length or velocity is changing (Ballard *et al.*, 1992, 1993; Korner *et al.*, 1984). This approach has several disadvantages, however. The device must be inserted into the muscle. Pressures at different sites within the muscle are different. Also, pressure may not correlate with force if the muscle lies in tight bony or fascial compartments (Sejersted and Hargens, 1995).

Overall, there is no ideal device for measuring muscle force in the workplace. Measures based on electromyography are the best choice at present. The measurement of intramuscular pressure may prove useful in future.

How can muscle force be increased?

Many tasks require more force than a worker can exert. Transferring a heavy patient from bed to wheelchair, for instance, may require more force than the nurse can muster. Can a muscle's force be increased?

The ergonomist can increase muscle force by exploiting what is known about muscle length, velocity, and activation. Muscles are strongest at certain joint angles, and at certain joint velocities. The ergonomist should therefore design tasks so that the worker can position his joints at the 'strongest angles'. He/she should ensure that the speeds needed are low, or even negative (i.e., eccentric contractions). He/she can also manipulate activation by training and motivation. Highly trained, highly motivated subjects can activate the muscle maximally.

Of course, the ergonomist can also increase a worker's strength by using exercise. This topic is beyond the scope of this review (see Fitts and Widrick, 1996).

Note that increasing the force produced by the muscle, by whatever means, will increase the stresses on the body. This may increase the risk of injury. Reducing the force required by the task is preferable.

How can muscle force demands of a task be lessened?

If muscle forces are large, the worker will quickly become fatigued, sore, and ineffective. How can the muscle forces required by a task be lessened?

One obvious way is to reduce the force demands of the task itself. Digging weeds out of a dry lawn, for example, is a slow process which rapidly becomes fatiguing and painful. In a wet lawn, however, much lower forces are required, and the task can be done more quickly, more easily, and more effectively. Here, the muscle can get away with less force, because the forces needed for the task itself are less. Another obvious way is to let stronger muscle groups do the task. For example, putting a long handle and a footplate on a weed digger allows the large muscles of the lower limb, rather than the smaller muscles of the upper limb, to drive the digger into the ground. A third way is to exploit what is known about muscle length and velocity. Muscles are strongest at certain joint angles. Forces which are near maximal at one joint angle may be greatly submaximal at another. Similarly, muscles are strongest at certain velocities. Forces which are near-maximal at one velocity may be greatly submaximal at a slower one.

It is important to remember that the force required of the muscles depends on the torque required of the joint. Often, a task can be redesigned to require less torque from a joint. For instance, a heavy weight held at arm's length will produce a large torque about the shoulder. The shoulder muscles will have to contract mightily to counter this torque and keep the arm up. The same weight held close to the chest will produce less torque, and spawn less muscle force. The force on the weight is the same in both cases, but the muscle force is less (see Lieber and Bodine-Fowler, 1993, for more on torque).

How best to maintain a position against a disturbing force?

As noted above, many tasks require that the worker maintain a position despite a perturbing force. How can muscle mechanics be exploited to do so?

A worker's success at holding a position against a force depends on that force. Small, brief forces perturb least. In jackhammering, for example, the worker's muscles must maintain the body's position against the hammer's force. Reducing this force and its duration will make the task easier.

Holding a position can also be made easier by increasing the limb's moment of inertia. This can be done by augmenting the amount of mass that the force must rotate, or by changing the way this mass is distributed around the axis of rotation. If the worker holds the jackhammer at arm's length, with shoulders relaxed, the jackhammer's force will move only the arms. It will easily move this tiny inertia. But if the worker holds the shoulders stiffly, and leans forward, the jackhammer's force will now have to rotate the entire body about the ankle. It will produce much less movement of this larger inertia. Another way to increase the moment of inertia is to increase the mass of the body segments, by loading them with weights. These weights should be placed far from the axis of rotation for maximum effect (see Winter, 1990, for a discussion of moment of inertia).

In addition to depending on inertia, the ability of a limb to maintain its position depends on joint stiffness and viscosity. These two arise mostly from muscle, and the worker can set both by contracting the muscles at a joint. The stiffnesses and viscosities of muscles crossing a joint are additive, so he/she will make the joint stiffest and most viscous by contracting them all. The higher he/she can make these, the less displacement, since the jackhammer must overcome joint stiffness and viscosity to produce movement.

ACKNOWLEDGEMENTS

This work was supported by the Natural Sciences and Engineering Research Council of Canada. The author thanks Walter Herzog for helpful comments.

References

AGARWAL, G.C. and GOTTLIEB, G.L., 1977, Oscillation of the human ankle joint in response to applied sinusoidal torque on the foot, *Journal of Physiology*, **268**, 151–176.

BALLARD, R., ARATOW, M., CRENSHAW, A., STYF, J., KAHAN, N., WATENPAUGH, D. and HARGENS, A., 1992, Intramuscular pressure measurement as an index of torque during dynamic exercise, *Physiologist*, **35**, S115–S116.

BALLARD, R., ARATOW, M., CRENSHAW, A., STYF, J., KAHAN, N., WATENPAUGH, D. and HARGENS, A., 1993, Intramuscular pressure and electromyography as indexes of force during isokinetic exercise, *Journal of Applied Physiology*, **74**, 2634–2640.

BARATTA, R.V., ICHIE, M., HWANG, S. and SOLOMONOW, M., 1989, Method for studying muscle properties under orderly stimulated motor units with tripolar nerve cuff electrode, *Journal of Biomedical Engineering*, **11**, 141–147.

CAVAGNA, G.A., 1977, Storage and utilization of elastic energy in skeletal muscle, *Exercise and Sport Sciences Reviews*, **5**, 89–129.

CLAMANN, H.P., 1993, Motor unit recruitment and the gradation of muscle force, *Physical Therapy*, **73**, 830–843.

DUDLEY, G.A., HARRIS, R.T., DUVOISIN, M.R., HATHER, B.M. and BUCHANAN, P., 1990, Effect of voluntary vs artificial activation on the relationship of muscle torque to speed, *Journal of Applied Physiology*, **69**(6), 2215–2221.

ETTEMA, G. and HUIJING, P.A., 1994a, Skeletal muscle stiffness in static and dynamic contractions, *Journal of Biomechanics*, **27**, 1361–1368.

ETTEMA, G.J. and HUIJING, P.A., 1994b, Effects of distribution of muscle fiber length on active length-force characteristics of rat gastrocnemius medialis, *Anatomical Record*, **239**, 414–420.

FITTS, R.H. and WIDRICK, J.J., 1996, Muscle mechanics: adaptations with exercise-training, *Exercise and Sport Sciences Reviews*, **24**, 427–473.

FORD, L., HUXLEY, A. and SIMMONS, R., 1977, Tension responses to sudden length change in stimulated frog muscle fibres near slack length, *Journal of Physiology*, **269**, 441–515.

GAREIS, H., SOLOMONOW, M., BARATTA, R., BEST, R. and D'AMBROSIA, R., 1992, The isometric length-force models of nine different skeletal muscles, *Journal of Biomechanics*, **8**(25), 903–916.

GEEVES, M., 1991, The dynamics of actin and myosin association and the crossbridge model of muscle contraction, *Biochemical Journal*, **274**, 1–14.

GOTTLIEB, G.L., 1996, Muscle compliance: implications for the control of movement, *Exercise and Sport Sciences Reviews*, **24**, 1–34.

GORDON, A.M., HUXLEY, A.F. and JULIAN, F.J., 1966, The variation in isometric tension with sarcomere length in vertebrate muscle fibres, *Journal of Physiology*, **184**, 170–192.

GULCH, R., 1994, Force-velocity relations in human skeletal muscle, *International Journal of Sports Medicine*, **15**, S2–S10.

HILL, A., 1922, The maximum work and mechanical efficiency of human muscles, and their most economical speed, *Journal of Physiology*, **56**, 19–41.

HILL, A., 1938, The heat of shortening and the dynamic constants of muscle, *Proceedings of the Royal Society of London. Series B: Biological Sciences*, **126**, 136–195.

HUIJING, P.A., NIEBERG, S., VAN DEN VEEN, E. and ETTEMA, G., 1994, A comparison of rat extensor digitorum longus and gastrocnemius medialis muscle architecture and length-force characteristics, *Acta Anatomica*, **149**, 111–120.

IVY, J., WITHERS, R., BROSE, G., MAXWELL, B. and COSTILL, D., 1981, Isokinetic contractile properties of the quadriceps with relation to fiber type, *European Journal of Applied Physiology and Occupational Physiology*, **47**, 247–255.

JOYCE, G.C. and RACK, P.M., 1969, Isotonic lengthening and shortening movements of cat soleus muscle, *Journal of Physiology*, **204**, 475–491.

KANNUS, P., 1994, Isokinetic evaluation of muscular performance: implications for muscle testing and rehabilitation, *International Journal of Sports Medicine*, **15**, S11–S19.

KEARNEY, R.E. and HUNTER, I.W., 1982a, Dynamics of human ankle stiffness: variation with mean ankle torque, *Journal of Biomechanics*, **15**, 747–752.

KEARNEY, R.E. and HUNTER, I.W., 1982b, Dynamics of human ankle stiffness: variation with displacement amplitude, *Journal of Biomechanics*, **15**, 753–756.

KEARNEY, R.E. and HUNTER, I.W., 1990, System identification of human joint dynamics, *CRC Critical Reviews in Biomedical Engineering*, **18**, 55–87.

KOMI, P.V., 1990, Relevance of *in vivo* force measurements to human biomechanics, *Journal of Biomechanics*, **23** (suppl 1), 23–34.

KORNER, L., PARKER, P., ALMSTROM, C., ANDERSSON, G., HERBERTS, P., KADEFORS, R., et al., 1984, Relation of intramuscular pressure to the force output and myoelectric signal of skeletal muscle, *Journal of Orthopaedic Research*, **2**, 289–296.

LAKIE, M., WALSH, E. and WRIGHT, G., 1984, Resonance at the wrist demonstrated by the use of a torque motor: an instrumental analysis of muscle tone in man, *Journal of Physiology*, **353**, 265–285.

LIEBER, R.L. and BODINE-FOWLER, S.C., 1993, Skeletal muscle mechanics: implications for rehabilitation, *Physical Therapy*, **73**, 844–856.

MANSOUR, J.M. and AUDU, M., 1986, The passive elastic moment at the knee and its influence on human gait, *Journal of Biomechanics*, **5**, 369–373.

MILNER-BROWN, H.S., STEIN, R.B. and YEMM, R., 1973a, Changes in firing rate of human motor units during linearly changing voluntary contractions, *Journal of Physiology*, **230**(2), 371–390.

MILNER-BROWN, H.S., STEIN, R.B. and YEMM, R., 1973b, The orderly recruitment of human motor units during voluntary isometric contractions, *Journal of Physiology*, **230**(2), 359–370.

NICHOLS, T.R. and HOUK, J.C., 1973, Reflex compensation for variations in the mechanical properties of a muscle, *Science*, **181**(95), 182–184.

PERRINE, J.J. and EDGERTON, V.R., 1978, Muscle force-velocity and power-velocity relationships under isokinetic loading, *Medicine and Science in Sports and Exercise*, **10**, 159–166.

RACK, P. and WESTBURY, D., 1969, The effects of length and stimulus rate on tension in the isometric cat soleus muscle, *Journal of Physiology*, **204**, 443–460.

RACK, P.M. and WESTBURY, D.R., 1974, The short range stiffness of active mammalian muscle and its effect on mechanical properties, *Journal of Physiology*, **240**, 331–350.

SEJERSTED, O. and HARGENS, A., 1995, Intramuscular pressures for monitoring different tasks and muscle conditions, in S.C. Gandevia *et al.* (Eds), *Fatigue*, New York: Plenum Press, pp. 339–350.

THORSTENSSON, A., GRIMBY, G. and KARLSSON, J., 1976, Force-velocity relations and fiber composition in human knee extensor muscles, *Journal of Applied Physiology*, **40**, 12–16.

WICKIEWICZ, T.L., ROY, R.R., POWELL, P.L., PERRINE, J.J. and EDGERTON, V.R., 1984, Muscle architecture and force-velocity relationships in humans, *Journal of Applied Physiology*, **57**, 435–443.

WIEGNER, A.M., 1987, Mechanism of thixotropic behaviour at relaxed joints in the rat, *Journal of Applied Physiology*, **62**, 1615–1621.

WILKIE, D., 1950, The relation between force and velocity in human muscle, *Journal of Physiology*, **110**, 249–280.

WINTER, D.A., 1990, *Biomechanics and Motor Control of Human Movement*, 2nd edition, New York: Wiley.

WINTERS, J.M. and WOO, S.L.-Y. (Eds), 1990, *Multiple Muscle Systems*, New York: Raven.

WINTERS, J., STARK, L. and SEIF-NARAGHI, A.-H., 1988, An analysis of the sources of musculoskeletal system impedance, *Journal of Biomechanics*, **21**, 1011–1025.

YOON, Y. and MANSOUR, J., 1982, The passive elastic moment at the hip, *Journal of Biomechanics*, **15**(12), 905–910.

ZAJAC, F.E., 1989, Muscle and tendon: properties, models, scaling, and application to biomechanics and motor control, *CRC Critical Reviews in Biomedical Engineering*, **17**, 359–411.

PART TWO

Upper Extremity

CHAPTER SIX

Functional anatomy of
the upper limb

REUBEN FELDMAN

THE HAND

The hand is the part of the limb which permits tactile contact between the individual and the environment. All the movements of the shoulder, elbow and wrist facilitate this contact allowing for a very large area in which the hand can operate in space, reaching not only all parts of the body with little difficulty but also areas in space limited only by the effect of elbow extension and forward flexion of the body.

The movements of the hand are governed structurally by the presence of a transverse metacarpal arch, a line between the heads of all of the metacarpophalangeal joints with the uppermost portion of the arch being the metacarpal head of the third finger. It is this arch which permits extension and abduction to occur on contraction of the finger extensor muscles and permits grasp to occur with all fingers touching their adjacent neighbours on contraction of the finger flexors.

The intrinsic muscles of the hand are responsible for maintaining this arch-like configuration. Lack of function of the intrinsic muscles results in a flattening of the hand. This can result in severe disability and dysfunction of the hand.

The transverse metacarpal arch is an extension of a similar arch proximally passing through the distal wrist. There is also a longitudinal arch stretching from the proximal wrist and having as its axis the second, third and fourth fingers.

The hand performs activities in a most remarkable fashion. With sensation intact, it is able to differentiate between most environmental surfaces and temperatures instantaneously and allows for immediate motor response to these sensations. In lengths of time measured in microseconds, movement of the muscles of the hand can be initiated in response to whatever need is required, providing not only speed but quality of effective movement of all the fingers and the thumb. It is an interesting observation to realise that while most of the joints have been effectively replaced by prostheses, in the case of limb amputation, there has not yet been any satisfactory attempt at replacing the quality of movement of the hand by prosthetic devices despite all attempts at computerisation and the use of the most recent technologies.

In order to achieve the functions of power grip, precision grip and the ability for the hand to conform to all surfaces with which it will make contact, there are three anatomical arches that permit this versatility to occur. The most important is the transverse metacarpal arch which follows the dorsal surface of the metacarpal heads and has as its peak, the third metacarpal head. This is the distal transverse arch. The proximal arch is formed by the distal wrist with the capitate as its peak. In addition, there is a longitudinal arch following the palmar surface of the fingers which is formed by the contours of the fingers and the carpus. These anatomical arches are held in place primarily by the intrinsic muscles of the hand. Paralysis of these muscles results in flattening of the hand, distortion of its contours and marked hand dysfunction.

It is the existence of the transverse metacarpal arch which permits all the finger tips to meet their adjacent counterparts on flexion of the metacarpophalangeal and interphalangeal joints, permitting function to occur in any position of flexion. This, then, allows for a very effective power grip.

The existence of the transverse arch also permits each finger to contact the base of the thumb individually, thereby allowing for precision grip to occur, particularly between the tip of the thumb and that of the second and third fingers.

The function of the hand is enhanced immeasurably by the ability of the thumb to move particularly through its carpometacarpal joint, providing both opposition and rotation of the thumb as it moves towards the ulnar side of the hand. The ability to perform the movements of adduction, abduction, flexion and extension as well as opposition provides the opportunity for precision as well as for increased power of grip when the thumb is placed on the dorsum of the second and third fingers after they have been flexed to achieve a power grip. The existence of the thumb in that position provides additional stability of this grip.

The extrinsic muscles of the hand, originating as they do from the forearm, provide the function of flexion and extension of the fingers. These are augmented by wrist movements which have already been described. Increased power of flexion of the fingers can be achieved with the addition of wrist extension.

Stability of flexion of the interphalangeal joints is achieved by a network of flexor tendon sheath pulley systems which facilitate and stabilise flexion of these joints.

The intrinsic muscles are all anatomically present within the hand. Their function is to modify the basic movements as well as provide anatomical stability within the hand. It is the coordinated movement of the intrinsic and extrinsic systems which allows for satisfactory function of the hand.

Anatomically, the extensor tendons end by developing into an extensor assembly or mechanism over the interphalangeal joints. A trifurcation occurs at the end of the long extensor tendon with one middle and two lateral bands being produced. The middle band runs over the dorsum of the proximal phalanx and inserts into the base of the middle phalanx while the lateral bands form the terminal tendon after merging on the dorsum of the middle phalanx and inserting into the dorsum of the distal phalanx. Additional ligaments from the terminal tendon link into the proximal phalanx. This anatomical conformation permits precise movement by release of the distal phalanx when the finger is flexed at the proximal interphalangeal joint. This allows for pulp-to-pulp pinch and intermittent changing from pulp-to-pulp to tip-to-tip pinch with precision.

The flexor mechanism of the fingers with its tendon sheath pulley system is composed of the flexor superficialis and flexor profundus muscles. The flexor superficialis inserts on the middle phalanx while the profundus inserts on the distal phalanx. Pulleys allow for a smooth movement of the tendons with the sheaths providing protection for the tendon so as to avoid injury from bony irregularities during movement. Pulleys also reduce the stress which can occur otherwise between the tendons and their sheaths. While function of the flexor superficialis is individualised to all the fingers, a common tendon provides profundus movement without individualised possibilities.

The intrinsic muscles, as mentioned, provide moderation of the forces between flexors and extensors. Of particular interest is the lumbrical muscle which counteracts the clawing effect found in intrinsic muscle palsy. The lumbricals allow for the interphalangeal joints to function in extension during opening of the hand at the same time as the metacarpophalangeal joints are flexed. In addition, they allow for closing of the hand with interphalangeal joint flexion occurring at the same time or just behind metacarpophalangeal joint flexion.

For prehension of the hand to occur, there must be mobility of the carpometacarpal joint of the thumb and of the fourth and fifth metacarpophalangeal joints. Rigidity of the second and third carpometacarpal joints is necessary as is stability of the longitudinal arches. Synergy is established between the antagonistic movements of the long flexors and extensors by the presence of the intrinsic muscles. Over-riding all of these requirements is an adequate sensory input into all portions of the hand (Napier, 1956).

The patterns of prehension of the hand include power grip and precision grip. In power grip, the fingers are flexed at all three of their joints allowing for prehension to occur between the palmar surface of the fingers and the palm of the hand and the thumb is then positioned along the palmar surface of the object being held. If the object is cylindrical or smaller in size, the thumb can achieve a position in which the pulp of the tip of the thumb is in contact with the dorsal surface of the distal phalanx of the index and the third finger. Enhancement of this movement is achieved by ulnar deviation and extension of the wrist so as to increase the tension placed on the object by the flexor tendons.

Precision grip is achieved by establishing contact between the thumb and the index finger. The types of precision grip that can be established include tip-to-tip pinch in which there is contact between the pulp of the thumb and that of the index finger, palmar pinch in which the pulp of the thumb contacts the palmar surface of the distal phalanx of the index finger and lateral pinch in which the pulp of the thumb makes contact with the lateral aspect of the middle and distal phalanges of the index finger. Usually there is an object in between the surfaces of the fingers permitting this precision activity to occur. In this way, manipulation of small objects requiring fine finger movement can be achieved. The fingers are usually partially flexed while the thumb is abducted and in opposition.

Power grip is usually achieved by the production of two jaws with one of them being the fingers and the other the palmar surface held in place by the thumb wrapped around the fingers. Precision grip is characterised by the so called three-jaw chuck in which there is interaction between the thumb, the tip of the index and the tip of the third finger. Increased power of these grasps is achieved by an increase in wrist extension.

By the interaction of extrinsic and intrinsic muscles in the hand as described, well coordinated, quickly responsive and very selective movements can be achieved, resulting in purposeful and useful hand function.

THE WRIST

The wrist anatomically contains a number of bones and soft tissue structures that permit the transfer of loads between the forearm and the hand in both distal and proximal directions. In addition, the wrist also allows for changes in orientation of the hand relative to the forearm so as to allow the hand to be placed in positions such that its function can be assured. It is as a result of this anatomical and kinematic relationship that the hand can perform activities of daily living, grasp and placement in space in such a way as to permit it to achieve whatever functions are required of it.

In addition, the wrist is traversed by long flexors and extensors to the fingers. Function of these structures is assured by the relative stability of the wrist.

A discussion of the anatomy of the wrist can be found in any textbook on the subject. Similarly, the complex disposition of the ligaments of the wrist divided, as they are, between extrinsic and intrinsic ligaments, is best seen in a treatise of anatomy. However, the wrist is surrounded by ten wrist tendons of which only one, the flexor carpi ulnaris, inserts on the pisiform. All other tendons traverse the wrist and its carpal bones to insert on the metacarpal bones of the hand.

In so doing, these muscles contribute to the function of flexion and extension of the wrist with ulnar and medial deviation of the hand as well as providing pronation and supination of the forearm.

From the neutral position of the wrist, flexion can normally be achieved to 85–90° while extension is normal between 75 and 80°. These values would be the average of those that have been identified by various workers attempting to determine the exact normal range of these movements.

Pronation and supination of the forearm occurs when the radius rotates on the underlying ulna through the proximal and distal radioulnar joints. With the neutral position placing the hand in a vertical position, normal pronation is 90° while supination would be considered normal at 70–80°. Finally, radial deviation is normal at approximately 15–20° while ulnar deviation is normal at 35°.

While these values are considered to be normal values, adequate function of the wrist can be achieved, allowing for normal activities of daily living, even with marked compromise of wrist function. This is because of the compensatory actions of the many joints in the wrist which permit movement even in the presence of decreased function of some of these joints. As has been shown by Brumfield and Champoux (1984), it is sufficient to have 10° of flexion and 35° of extension of the wrist to allow for the performance of normal activities of daily living. A review of the amount of wrist motion required for the performance of selected daily activities is presented in Table 6.1.

Table 6.1 Amount of wrist motion required for performance of selected daily activities.

Activity	Mean extension (degrees)		
	Minimum	Maximum	Arc
Lift glass to mouth	11.2	24.0	12.8
Pour from pitcher	8.7	29.7	21.0
Cut with knife	−3.5	20.2	23.7
Lift fork to mouth	9.3	36.5	27.2
Use telephone	−0.1	42.6	42.7
Read newspaper	1.7	34.9	33.2
Rise from chair	0.6	63.4	62.8

Negative values indicate flexion.
Data from Brumfield and Champoux (1984).
N = 19: 12 men and 7 women, age 25 to 60 years (mean 33 years).

Despite its presence between the long forearm bones and the hand, the wrist maintains its stability by a balance of forces between those created by the long flexors and extensors which traverse the wrist and the ligamentous structures together with the articular surface conformation which counterbalance the long tendon forces. In this way, a fine balance is created between extrinsic and intrinsic forces, allowing for dynamic stability to be present. Steindler, in 1955, studied the forces created by the various components of the stabilising effect and noted the presence of antagonistic groupings of motor forces between extensors and flexors of the fingers.

The most important function of the wrist is that of providing proper positioning so as to facilitate movement of the fingers and the hand. In this way, wrist extension facilitates finger flexion in prehension by shortening the flexors, thereby promoting efficient and appropriate grasp. This is demonstrated on viewing the functional position of the hand which includes wrist extension, with finger and thumb flexion.

In the same manner, flexion of the wrist facilitates finger extension by providing stretch on the extensors and resulting in separation of the fingers in extension.

Electromyographic studies have demonstrated that grip strength was at its greatest when wrist extension was at 20°. Extension beyond 20° did not substantially change the amount of grip strength that was achieved (Volz et al., 1980).

Finally, the tenodesis effect is achieved in wrist extension. When the fingers are relaxed and the wrist is extended there is passive movement and approximation between the tip of the thumb and the distal phalanx of the index finger. With slight flexion of the thumb, a three-point prehension is possible with the thumb making contact with the distal phalanges of the index and third fingers. This tenodesis effect is used to provide rudimentary prehension in individuals who are quadriplegic. The force of prehension can be increased by a number of orthotic devices which add force to this type of prehension, thereby faciltating upper limb function in the high spinal cord injured patient.

THE ELBOW

The elbow serves to augment the ability of the shoulder to bring the hand and finger tips into various areas of a person's spatial environment. It acts as a second link in the shoulder–elbow–wrist complex, allowing contact between the person and the environment. More specifically, as a result of elbow motion, the height and length of the upper extremity can be adjusted. In addition, with the ability to pronate and supinate the forearm, the hand can be placed in the most effective position so that function can occur.

The anatomy of the elbow is such that it consists of three joints, the humeroulnar, humeroradial and proximal radioulnar joints.

These three joints permit two movements to occur. The first is flexion and extension. This movement occurs simultaneously between the humeroulnar and humeroradial joints with the axis of flexion and extension being a line through the trochlea of the distal humerus (Volz et al., 1980). This line forms the carrying angle which in men is 10–15° and in women 20–25°. The normal range of motion in flexion and extension of the elbow is 0–140° with 0° representing full extension and 140° representing full flexion.

The second of the two motions which the elbow can perform is pronation–supination. For this to be performed, the radius must be able to rotate around the ulna for a total of 140°. This movement is done in the proximal and distal radioulnar joints simultaneously. Stability for the proximal radioulnar joint is achieved by the presence of the annular ligament which allows for close association between the components of this joint and good joint congruity, present both distally and proximally, to have its major effect.

Despite the presence of three joints in the elbow, excellent stability can be maintained. This stability is achieved by mechanisms which include the interlocking of all bony parts by placement of the ligaments in their maximum amount of tension at full extension position.

The presence of the radial (lateral) collateral ligament, the ulnar (medial) collateral ligament and the annular ligament help to achieve this stability. In addition, the interosseous ligament between the radius and ulna helps in this function.

While joint congruity is excellent in most areas of the elbow, there is some incongruity, particularly in flexion in the area of the medial condyle of the humerus. This allows for some instability to occur and permits passive adduction and abduction of the elbow. This is not achieved actively.

The movements which occur in the elbow are dependent upon a number of different muscle groups. In flexion, the major muscle involved is the brachialis muscle, which, on active movement, permits flexion and on relaxation permits extension with the help of gravity. The brachialis functions irrespective of the position of the forearm. This muscle is helped by both the brachioradialis muscle and to a lesser extent the biceps muscle (Basmajian and Latif, 1957).

Extension is achieved by the use of the triceps muscle as well as a small triangular posterior placed muscle called the anconeus which initiates extension and when extension is full, maintains the fully extended position of the elbow.

The major supinator of the arm is the biceps, and it is this function which is a major function of the biceps muscle. In addition, the supinator provides additional movement in that direction. The biceps functions only when the elbow is in the flexion position and only if the forearm is supinated or in the neutral position.

Pronation is performed by the use of two muscles. The pronator teres is situated proximally across the anterior portion of the elbow joint from the medioproximal to the laterodistal portion of the joint and is particularly active during elbow extension. During elbow flexion it is much more relaxed and therefore has a much lesser role in pronation.

The pronator quadratus, situated on the anterior distal forearm between the radius and the ulna is active in pronation whether the elbow is in the flexed position or in the extended position. This distinction provides an interesting method by which a study of pronation and supination could be done so as to determine which muscles are most effective in providing this movement (Basmajian and Travil, 1961).

In summary, the elbow, which contains its own sophisticated inherent stability, is composed of three articulations, which provide the opportunity for two movements with the help of a variety of different muscles acting at different times during the process of flexion and extension. This permits placement of the hand more precisely in space as well as positioning of the wrist to allow for improved hand function.

References

BASMAJIAN, J.V. and LATIF, M., 1957, Integrated action and function of the chief flexors of the elbow, *J Bone Joint Surg.* **39A**, 1106–1118.

BASMAJIAN, J.V. and TRAVIL, A., 1961, Electromyography of the pronator muscles of the forearm, *Anat Rec*, **139**, 45–49.

BRUMFIELD, R.H. and CHAMPOUX, J.A., 1984, A biomechanical study of normal functional wrist motion, *Clin Orthop*, **187**, 23–25.

MOREY, B.F. and CHAD, E.Y.S., 1976, Passive motion of the elbow joint. A biomechanical analysis, *J Bone Joint Surg*, **38B**, 902–913.

NAPIER, J.R., 1956, The prehensile movements of the human hand, *J Bone Joint Surg*, **38B**, 902–913.

STEINDLER, A., 1955, *Kinesiology of the Human Body*, Springfield: Charles C. Thomas, p. 534.

VOLZ, R.G. *et al.*, 1980, Biomechanics of the wrist, *Clin Orthop*, **149**, 112–117.

CHAPTER SEVEN

Hand grasping, finger pinching and squeezing

SHEIK N. IMRHAN

INTRODUCTION

The method of grasping an object, the degree of manipulation offered by a particular grasp, and the strength and endurance of grasping are of great importance to ergonomists for the design of tasks and equipment, especially hand tools and other hand-operated devices (Konz, 1990; Kroemer *et al.*, 1994), prosthetic devices (An *et al.*, 1985), and complex mechanical devices such as robotic hands (Mason and Salisbury, 1985). It is also useful for evaluating hand disability (Fiedmann and Abbs, 1990; Mai *et al.*, 1988). Napier (1956) identified two distinct movements of the hand – prehensile and non-prehensile – and Landsmeer (1962) provides further discussions of Napier's classifications. In prehensile movements, an object is seized and held partly or wholly within the compass of the hand; and in non-prehensile movements or handling, seizing does not occur but the whole hand or finger applies pressure on the object, as in pressing the flat of the hand against a door when pushing. Napier (1956) further identified two main kinds of prehensile movements: power grip (grasp) and precision grip (grasp). In the power grasp, the object is held in the palm of the hand with the force from the thumb opposed by the combined forces from the other fingers, and muscular force application is dominant. In the precision grasp, the object is held between the flexor aspects of the fingers and the opposing thumb, and muscular force application is limited. Pinch is defined by Long *et al.* (1970) as compression between the thumb and index and thumb and first two fingers. These definitions create some confusion when distinguishing between grasps that create appreciable muscular forces (or power) and those that do not. In many industrial tasks, the finger pinching is used both for control/precision and for the application of great forces or power (relative to the strength capacity of the fingers). To avoid confusion in this paper, Napier's power grip will be called 'hand grasping' to allow the concept of muscular power to be applied to pinching. Moreover, tool design characteristics, especially for the industrial workplace, create such a variety of grasps that further subclassification is necessary for describing tasks. The established classification of pinches in section, 'Types of precision grasps' and the more recent classification by Kroemer

(1986) fulfil most of these needs. In this chapter, the biomechanical aspects of hand grasping and pinching will be discussed; personal and demographic aspects are not addressed.

GRASPING OVER-EXERTION OF THE HAND

The nature of industrial work often calls for pinching and power grasping activities that impose tremendous strain in the hands, either through the exertion of great forces or from highly repetitive or sustained contractions. Powerful or repetitive hand and finger activities have been linked to the incidence of soft tissue cumulative trauma disorders of the hand, such as carpal tunnel syndrome, trigger finger, etc. (Armstrong and Chaffin, 1979; Eastman Kodak, 1986; Putz-Anderson, 1988) and degeneration of the distal interphalangeal joint (DIP) (Hadler, 1978; Moran *et al.*, 1985). One approach towards mitigating cumulative strains is to minimise grasp forces in tasks. Therefore an understanding of the nature of grasping and grasp forces is necessary.

Hand grasp and finger pinch forces (compressive, thrust or rotational) may be required for holding and stabilising an object or system, squeezing mechanical parts together or helping to create torques on handles, but the type of hand grasp or pinch used by a person and the amount of force applied depend on several factors, among the most important of which are the intended activity and the size, weight, and shape of the object. In the industrial workplace other factors, such as frictional properties at the hand–object contact or stability of the object may also modify the type of grasp and amount of muscular force generated (Bucholz *et al.*, 1988; Kinoshita *et al.*, 1996a). The influential factors do not necessarily act independently of each other. A short cylinder (jar lid), for example, may be grasped differently from a long one (screwdriver handle) for the same activity (generating torque, for example); and the hand may change from a power grasp to a precision grasp according to the force requirements (Napier, 1956).

TYPES OF PREHENSILE GRASPS

Ayoub *et al.* (1976) classify some common task-related prehensile grasps for ergonomic use; Smith (1985) lists common terms for pinches used by clinicians; and Kroemer (1986) provides alternative classifications for grasps that have not been properly described in the literature. These, together with the classification from Napier (1956) and Landsmeer (1962) provide the following practical, though not exhaustive, classification:

(1) *Hand grasp*: The object is held between the flexor aspects of the fingers and palm of the hand with the flexion force of the thumb opposed by the flexion forces of the other fingers. This is also known as the power grasp. There are variations in the hand grasp:
- the spherical grasp – used on a spherical object in the palm of the hand (e.g. door knob or cricket ball);
- the cylindrical grasp – used on a cylindrical object around its circumference (e.g. a hammer handle);
- the disc grasp – used on a disc shaped object (e.g. a jar lid); and
- and the hook grasp – the handle is hooked by digits II–V (index, middle, ring and little fingers) at the region of the knuckles or proximal interphalangeal joints (PIP), but the thumb does not apply counter force to digits II–V (e.g. in carrying a briefcase).

Note that the spherical and disc grasps also function for control and manipulation of the object as in the initial and terminal stages of screwing and unscrewing a disc-shaped or spherical screw-top jar lid onto or off a jar.

(2) *Pinch grasp*: The prevailing definitions and classifications of pinches described by Smith (1985) are based on early work among clinicians and have been adopted by ergonomists. Three most well-known pinches are the pulp, chuck and lateral pinches. In the pulp pinch, the pad of the distal phalange of thumb opposes the pad of the distal phalange of another finger in the same hand; in the tip pinch, the tip of the thumb opposes the tip of another finger; in the lateral pinch (key pinch), the thumb opposes the radial lateral aspect of index finger in the clenched fist. The chuck pinch is similar to the pulp and tip pinches except that the thumb opposes both the index and middle fingers simultaneously. Furthermore, there are different types of pulp pinches, as follows:

■ pulp-2 pinch: the thumb opposes the index finger;
■ pulp-3 pinch: the thumb opposes the middle finger;
■ pulp-4 pinch: the thumb opposes the ring finger; and
■ pulp-5 pinch: the thumb opposes the little finger.

This terminology is not rigid. Smith (1985) gives alternative names for pinches and their frequency of use among clinicians. The hand-contact area available or chosen, the amount of force that must be applied to the object, and the intended activity determine the type of pinch a person uses; for example, pulp-2 pinch for small areas and activities of high precision such as threading a needle or picking up small coins, and the chuck or lateral pinches for larger areas or greater forces. For simple compression forces, pulp pinches are preferred and for rotation, as in turning a key, the lateral pinch.

FORCE DEVELOPMENT AND TRANSMISSION

The extrinsic muscles of the hand are responsible for forceful contractions in grasping and the intrinsic muscles, for control and manipulation activities. The major force-producing muscles are the flexor digitorum profundus (FDP) and the flexor digitorum superficialis (FPS) which run along the foream from the elbow to the fingers. Long *et al.* (1970) describe in detail the roles of the extrinsic and intrinsic muscles in grasping objects in a variety of ways; and a few researchers (An *et al.*, 1979, 1985; Chao *et al.*, 1976) have developed two- and three-dimensional biomechanical models to explain and predict individual muscle forces while grasping, for clinical applications. Armstrong and Chaffin (1979) and Armstrong (1982) have used model information from Chao *et al.* (1976) and LeVeau (1977) to develop biomechanical models for explaining cumulative trauma disorders of the hand and for influencing ergonomic designs of hand tools and tasks.

BIOMECHANICAL FACTORS INFLUENCING PINCH STRENGTH

Because of differences in subject samples and measurement instruments and methods, pinch strength values in published studies vary considerably (Imrhan and Rahman, 1995). For example, the lateral pinch using traditional clinical methods of measurement varies from about 6.3 kgf (Swanson *et al.*, 1970) to 11.6 kgf (Mathioweitz *et al.*, 1985a) in males. The majority of these studies, however, show a range of 8.2–10.1 kgf for males and 6.4–8.0 kgf for females. The strengths of the other pinches can be estimated from the ratios stated below.

Maximal voluntary contraction (MVC) pinch strength depends on a number of bio-mechanical factors including the type of pinch, the width of pinch (separation distance of the thumb from the other fingers), wrist angle, finger joint angle, and finger–object contact area. Most published strength values are based on testing methods established in the clinical fields and the application of their results for ergonomic designs have limitations (Imrhan and Rahman, 1995). In clinical testing, the width of pinch grasp on pinch gauges is limited to about 16–18 mm, the hand–object (pinch gauge) contact area to about 20 × 14 mm, and the finger joints are typically flexed. For these restrictive pinching conditions, the order of strength magnitudes fall into four groups: (1) chuck and lateral; (2) pulp-2 and pulp-3; (3) pulp-4; and (4) pulp-5. The strength ratio of each type compared with the lateral pinch is approximately 0.7 for pulp-2/lateral, 0.7 for pulp-3/lateral, 0.45 for pulp-4/lateral, and 0.3 for pulp-5/lateral. Handgrip/lateral pinch ratio is approximately 4.5 (Imrhan and Loo, 1989). Imrhan and Rahman (1995), in an investigation of lateral, chuck and pulp-2 pinches over a pinch width range of 20–140 mm, have shown that for large contact areas for the finger pads and when the thumb is allowed to hyperextend, the above stated ratios no longer hold. Instead, the chuck pinch is always stronger than the lateral and pulp-2 pinches; the lateral is stronger than the pulp-2 from 20–56 mm but weaker from 68–92 mm. At 68 mm people experience great difficulty in executing the lateral pinch due to the sharp abduction of the metacarpal–phalangeal joint of the thumb and excessive stretching of its tendons, and beyond 92 mm, most people cannot execute this pinch. In addition, at 20 mm, the lateral pinch is 1.2 times as strong as the pulp-2 pinch and the chuck pinch is 1.2 times as strong as the lateral pinch. These 20 mm ratios, compared with the above ones, emphasise the effects of the different test conditions. Dempsey and Ayoub (1996) investigated pinches over a 10–70 mm width, using traditional clinical methods, and found the 50 mm pinch width strength to be the strongest; and Apfel (1986) found an increase in lateral pinch with the hyperextended versus the flexed thumb.

Wrist position

Putz-Anderson (1988) cites several studies linking hand force and wrist position to cumulative trauma disorders of the hand. For a sufficient amount of bending of the wrist away from its natural position, pinch strength declines. The greatest degrading effect occurs for flexion (palmar flexion), followed by extension (dorsiflexion), ulnar deviation and radial deviation. Decrements found in various studies were: 14 per cent (Kraft and Detels, 1972), 32–43 per cent (Imrhan, 1991), 9–38 per cent (Fernandez et al., 1991), 6–26 per cent (Hallbeck and McMullin, 1993); 15–22 per cent (Kamal et al., 1992); and 9–24 per cent (Dempsey and Ayoub, 1996). Some of this variation was due to different degrees of bending.

Degradation of pinch strength in deviated wrist positions is due to a combination of mechanisms: leverage – the change in the angle between the finger tendon and bone at the point of attachment on the finger (Hazleton et al., 1975); length–tension properties of the musculotendinous finger flexors – tendon excursion and increase in the length of musculotendinous units beyond their optimal force-producing length (Bunnell, 1944; Gordon et al., 1966; Hazleton et al., 1975; Pryce, 1980); and compression of the finger flexor tendons against the carpal tunnel wall and intra-wrist structures (Armstrong and Chaffin, 1979; Pryce, 1980; Smith *et al.*, 1977; Tichauer, 1966), leading to inefficient contraction.

Body posture, and forearm and hand configurations

Tests on forearm orientation (Hallbeck *et al.*, 1992; Mathioweitz *et al.*, 1985b; Palanisami *et al.*, 1994; Woody and Mathioweitz, 1988) have shown small changes but their direction (positive or negative) is not consistent enough for any firm generalisation. Catovic *et al.* (1989, 1991) found that right-handed pinch strengths are slightly greater with the hand just left of centre in front of the body in the transverse plane; and Mathioweitz *et al.* (1985b) found that, compared to the 180 degree elbow angle, the 90 degree elbow angle yielded pinch strengths only 3 per cent stronger with the right hand and 2.5 per cent stronger with the left hand. Data from Catovic *et al.* (1989, 1991), Swanson *et al.* (1970) and Palanisami *et al.* (1994) are not in complete agreement on the the effects of forearm support and body posture (sitting versus standing) on pinch strength, but most agree that standing provides greater strength. Hook and Stanley (1986) demonstrated that pinching was much stronger with the non-pinching fingers flexed compared to extended.

Hand–handle contact area

Theoretically, a small area for finger–object contact should restrict pinch force if the pressure on the fingers is at some critical value. This crictical value is unknown and has not been tested systematically. The data from Imrhan and Rahman (1995) when compared to other data, such as Imrhan and Loo (1989), suggest that larger hand–object contact areas are associated with greater pinch forces. They found that when the whole pad of the thumb contacts the object pinch forces were 1.5–1.8 times those generated on the limited contact area on traditional pinch meters for lateral, chuck and pulp-2 pinches. Imrhan and Sundararajan (1992) also showed that when pinching and pulling (as in tearing open plastic wrappers), a slightly greater contact area for the pinching fingers increased pull forces by 4, 19 and 18 per cent for lateral, chuck, and pulp-2 pinches, respectively.

Distribution of forces in individual fingers and phalanges

The relative contributions of the fingers in a gripping action do not seem to be greatly affected by factors such as the level of contraction (maximal or submaximal), or the shape, size or weight of the object, at least for weights from 0.2 to 2.0 kgf (Kinoshita *et al.*, 1995, 1996a; Radwin *et al.*, 1992). Most studies show the index and middle fingers sharing about 60 per cent of the load, and the ring and little fingers about 40 per cent – for the hook grip with digits II–V (Hazleton *et al.*, 1975; Ohtsuki *et al.*, 1981a, 1981b), 5-finger prismatic pinch grasps on a flat plate (Radwin *et al.*, 1992), hand (power) grasp on a power-tool handle (Lee and Cheng, 1995), prismatic (pinch) grasp on cylinders (Amiss, 1987), and hand (power) grasp on cylinders (Radhakrishnan and Ravindra, 1989). Kinoshita *et al.* (1995, 1996a, 1996b) show a higher percentage (approximately 70 per cent) for 5-finger prismatic pinch on flat plates but only about 40 per cent for circular (disc-type) grasp on cylinders above one face. Moreover, as the cylinders get larger and heavier and the finger separation widens, the ring and little fingers assume the extra load.

The contributions of the individual phalanges are also uneven – the distal phalange contributing less (about 68 per cent) than the middle phalange in the hook grip (Hazleton et al., 1975). Radhakrishnan and Ravindra (1989) and An et al. (1980) showed that, in the power grip on cylinders, the relative contributions of the phalanges depend on the size of the grasp (diameter of the cylinder). The distal phalange contributes more than the middle and proximal phalanges for smaller diameters, and the middle phalange, the most for larger diameters, at least in the diameter range 30–75 mm. Pinch forces required to hold an object against shear forces at the finger–object contact have been investigated by Bucholz et al. (1988) and Kinoshita et al. (1996b). Results show that the total pinch force increases with the weight of the object and decreases with greater finger–object friction, as expected, but the proportional contributions of the individual fingers do not depend on these two factors.

HAND (POWER) GRASPING

As mentioned earlier, the hand (power) grip is preferred to the precision grip when great muscular forces must be transferred to the object being held. The association of handgrip force exertions with CTDs of the hand has been discussed by Silverstein et al. (1987); the uses of handgrip strength for ergonomic designs have been emphasised by Kroemer et al. (1994), Konz (1990) and Eastman Kodak (1986); and the application of handgrip strength to disability rating and pre-placement evaluations has been stated by Kirpatrick (1956) and Patterson (1965). The biomechanical aspects of handgrip strength, therefore, warrant discussion.

Traditional power grasp strength (handgrip strength) measurements (Bechtol, 1954; Cotton and Bonnell, 1969; Cotton and Johnson, 1970; Eastman Kodak, 1986; Hertzberg, 1955; Montoye and Faulkner, 1965; Petrofsky et al., 1980) refer to MVC forces measured on standard handgrip dynamometers with two straight parallel or slightly curved handles. The grip resembles a combination of the cylindrical and hook grips. However, it is recognised that handgrips used in the workplace and the shape of hand-held objects often do not resemble those used for standardised testing. Some MVC tests have, therefore, been performed on cylindrical handles (Radhakrishnan and Ravindra; 1989) and angulated handles (Fellows and Freivalds, 1991; Fitzhugh, 1973a, 1973b; Fransson and Winkel, 1991). Other biomechanical factors, apart from handle design and grip type, influence handgrip strength. The most important are the size of the grasp (grip), wrist position, forearm position and body posture.

Size of grip

Strength magnitudes vary widely across studies, largely because of subject samples and test conditions in general; adult male handgrip strength falls in the range 400–600 N and females, 50–65 per cent of those values. Grip strength varies with handgrip size over a sufficiently large range of grip spans. The trend is typically increasing–decreasing without a clearly defined maximum. Data show an optimal range of 50–65 mm for males, and about 5 mm less for females, for MVC isometric contractions on parallel or slightly curved handles (Bechtol, 1954; Cotton and Bonnell, 1969; Cotton and Johnson, 1970; Hertzberg, 1955; Montoye and Faulkner, 1965; Petrofsky et al., 1980). For the pistol grip on a tool handle, the optimal range has been found to be 50–60 mm (Lee and Cheng, 1995; Oh and Radwin, 1993); for angulated handles and dynamic contraction, 64–89 mm (Fitzhugh, 1973a, 1973b; Fransson and Winkel, 1991; Greenberg and Chaffin, 1997); and for angulated handles and isometric contraction, 50–65 mm (Fransson and Winkel, 1991). At an optimal grasp span, the muscle fibre sarcomeres are stretched to the length that maximises the number of crossbridges between actin and myosin filaments and, hence, maximises the muscle fibres' contractile capacities (Petrofsky et al., 1980); and at small and large grasp spans, the major finger flexors, the FDP and FDS, lose some of their tension–length advantage for force production. For the power grasp on cylinders, grasp force data from Radhakrishnan and Ravindra (1989) did not show an optimum in the 50–70 mm diameter range, but shear forces derived from torque data by Pheasant and O'Neill (1976) suggest an optimum in the range 30–50 mm. Similar shear force data from torques using disc and lateral pinch grasps on jar lids also suggest an optimum in the range 55–74 mm for jar lids in the elderly (Imrhan and Loo, 1988).

Wrist and forearm positions, and body posture

Several studies have shown that handgrip strength is influenced by wrist position (Anderson, 1965; Hazleton et al., 1975; Kattel et al., 1996; Kraft and Detels, 1972; Pryce, 1980; Terrell and Purswell, 1976) and most of these studies give the order of strength magnitude for the various wrist positions as neutral, ulnar and radial deviation, dorsiflexion (extension), and palmar flexion (flexion), in decreasing order. For the hook grasp, Hazleton et al. (1975) reported that the 30 degree ulnar deviation position was the strongest. However, for dorsiflexion, the degree of wrist bending must be appreciable (more than 30 degrees) for any sharp decrease of strength to occur as shown in the data of Kraft and Detels (1972) and Pryce (1980). This is because the natural (resting) position of the wrist is about 35 degrees in dorsiflexion (Taylor and Scharwz, 1955) where the biomechanical mechanisms stated below are most efficient. Strength decrements are usually around 30, 22, 18 and 15 per cent, respectively for flexion, extension, radial deviation and ulnar deviation, though Terrell and Purswell (1976) and Kattel et al. (1996) found decrements as great as 40 per cent.

The losses of strength in bent wrist positions are due to a number of possible mechanisms: length–tension properties of muscles (Gordon et al., 1966; Hazleton, et al., 1975) – in the bent wrist, especially in flexion – the powerful flexor tendons shorten and lose some of their tension producing capability; pressure of the tendons against the carpal wall, due to carpal tunnel size reduction with a bent wrist, decreases the efficiency of tendon pull; and partial loss of the buttressing actions of the thenar and hypothenar emininences offered with a natural or undeviated wrist.

The effects of forearm orientation on handgrip strength have been investigated by Fitzhugh (1973a, 1973b) and Terrell and Purswell (1976). The former found no difference between the pronated and supinated positions, but the latter found a 12 per cent decrease in the pronated position compared to the supinated and mid-oriented positions (which were of about equal strength) for the neutral position of the wrist. Similar decreases were observed for most of the other wrist positions tested by Terrell and Purswell (1976). The data of Kattel et al. (1996) support Terrell and Purswell (1976). Body posture has also been implicated in the loss of grip strength, though to a mild degree. Teraoka (1979) found that handgrip strength was 6 per cent stronger when standing compared to sitting and 4 per cent stronger when sitting compared to lying supine.

Types of gasp strengths

There is little data for comparing the traditional dynamometric hook grasp measurements with others, such as cylindrical grasp, spherical grasp, or an irregular grasp. Fransson and Winkel (1991), however, found that the normal 'forward' grasp was stronger than a reverse grasp for spans between 41 and 67 mm on angulated handles, but there was no difference in strength above 67 mm.

Gloves

Grip strength is reduced by both regular working gloves (Cochran and Riley, 1986; Hertzberg, 1955, 1972; Lyman and Groth, 1958; Sudhakar *et al.*, 1988), and pressurised gloves used in extra-vehicular activity (EVA) in the space environment (Bishu and Kim, 1995), the reduction depending on the type of gloves. The decrease with working gloves ranges from about 7 to 30 per cent, depending on test conditions while the decrease with EVA gloves is almost 50 per cent.

Hand grasping for other tasks

In industrial activities, gripping is seldom an independent task but is often a precursor and requirement for the completion of other tasks, such as torquing, lifting, pulling, pushing, etc. via handles. Poor grip strength in people can be offset by designs that minimise grip force, such as using an optimum diameter cylindrical handle for torquing, or a lever handle instead of a spherical one on water faucets for the elderly, etc. The largest degree of hand–handle contact with the power grip produces the greatest forces but placement of the handle influences grip force (Fothergill *et al.*, 1992). However, if handgrip is ineffective, placement makes little difference (Fothergill *et al.*, 1992).

Pheasant and O'Neill (1976) showed that turning torque on a cylindrical handle is the product of handle diameter, coefficient of friction at the hand–handle contact, and grip force, and that loss in grip force at large diameter handles leads to decreased torquing ability. Imrhan and Loo (1989) and Imrhan and Farahmand (1998) suggested that, for small disc-type or cylindrical handles, stronger grip forces are used on small handles to compensate for loss in leverage in gripping. Loss of friction on smooth or slippery (grease- or oil-smeared) handles may also lead to stronger grips for compensation. Gloves have been found to decrease torquing force due, most likely, to decrease grip strength, especially for stiff gloves. It also seems that the disturbance of tactile feedback from significant padding on handles can lead to stronger grip force, as a compensation, when using tools, as found by Fellows and Freivalds (1991).

CONCLUSIONS

Confusion on grasping terminology must be resolved because established classifications and definitions may not distinguish among the myriad of grasps used in the workplace. While maximal forces for pinching and hand grasping have been investigated over the years, more data are still needed to further the understanding of the effects of several factors on grasping strength, such as hand-contact areas, handle geometry, and object characteristics. The recent thrust in research on submaximal forces and grasp types for real or simulated tasks has improved our understanding on how the hand works in the workplace, and the continuation of such research is necessary for influencing the design of equipment and tasks and enhancing the understanding of cumulative strains from hand work. The difficulties in applying three dimensional hand models to ergonomic designs should indicate the depth of further research needed in modelling but it should not be a deterrent for further research in the less realistic two-dimensional modelling.

References

AMISS, A.A., 1987, Variation in finger forces in maximal isometric grasp tests on a range of cylinders, *Journal of Biomechanical Engineering*, **9**, 313–320.

AN, K.-N., CHAO, E.Y., COONEY, W.P. and LINSHEID, R.L., 1979, Normative model of human hand for biomechanical analysis, *Journal of Biomechanics*, **12**, 775.

AN, K.-N., CHAO, E.Y. and ASKEW, L.J., 1980, Hand strength measurement instruments, *Archives of Physical Medicine and Rehabilitation*, **61**, 366–368.

AN, K.N., CHAO, E.Y., COONEY, W.P. and LINSHEID, R.L., 1985, Forces in the normal and abnormal hand, *Journal of Orthopaedic Research*, **3**, 202–211.

ANDERSON, C.T., 1965, Wrist Joint Position Influences Normal Hand Function, unpublished master's thesis, University of Iowa, Iowa City, IA.

APFEL, E., 1986, The effect of thumb interphalangeal joint position on strength of key pinch, *Journal of Hand Surgery*, **11A**, 47–51.

ARMSTRONG, T.J., 1982, Development of a biomechanical hand model for the study of manual activities, in Easterby, R., Kroemer, K.H.E. and Chaffin, D.B. (Eds), *Anthropometry and Biomechanics: Theory and Application*, New York: Plenum Press, 183–192.

ARMSTRONG, T.J. and CHAFFIN, D.B., 1979, Some biomechanical aspects of the carpal tunnel, *Journal of Biomechanics*, **12**, 567–570.

AYOUB, M.M., MACKENZIE, H.J. and DEIVANAYAGAM, S., 1976, *Training Manual in Occupational Ergonomics*, Texas Tech University, Lubbock, TX.

BECHTOL, C.O., 1954, Grip test: the use of a dynamometer with adjustable handle spacings, *The Journal of Bone and Joint Surgery*, **36A**, 820–832.

BISHU, R.R. and KIM, B., 1995, Force-endurance relationship: does it matter if gloves are donned?, *Applied Ergonomics*, **26**(3), 179–185.

BUCHOLZ, B., FREDRICK, L.J. and ARMSTRONG, T.J., 1988, An investigation of human palmar skin friction and the effects of materials, pinch force and moisture, *Ergonomics*, **31**(3), 317–325.

BUNNELL, S., 1944, *Surgery of the Hand*, Philadelphia, PA: J.B. Lippincott Co.

CATOVIC, A., KOSOVEL, Z., CATOVIC, E. and MUFTIC, O., 1989, A comparative investigation of the influence of certain arm positions on hand pinch grips in the standing and sitting positions of dentists, *Applied Ergonomics*, **20**(2), 109–114.

CATOVIC, E., CATOVIC, A., KRALJEVIC, K. and MUFTIC, O., 1991, The influence of arm position on the pinch grip strength of female dentists in standing and sitting positions, *Applied Ergonomics*, **22**(3), 163–166.

CHAO, E.Y., OPGRANDE, J.D. and AXMEAR, F.E., 1976, Three dimensional force analysis of finger joints in isometric hand functions, *Journal of Biomechanics*, **9**, 387–396.

COCHRAN, D.J. and RILEY, M.W., 1986, The effects of handle shape and size on exerted forces, *Human Factors*, **28**, 253–256.

COTTON, D.J. and BONNELL, L., 1969, Investigation of the T-5 cable tensionmeter grip attachment for measuring strength of college women, *Research Quarterly*, **40**, 848–850.

COTTON, D.J. and JOHNSON, A., 1970, Use of the T-5 cable tensionmeter grip attachment for measuring strength of college men, *Research Quarterly*, **41**, 454–456.

DEMPSEY, P.G. and AYOUB, M.M., 1996, The influence of gender, grasp type, pinch width and wrist position on sustained pinch strength, *International Journal of Industrial Ergonomics*, **17**(3), 259–273.

EASTMAN KODAK COMPANY, 1986, *Ergonomic Design for People at Work, Volume 2*, New York: Van Nostrand Reinhold Company.

FELLOWS, G.L. and FREIVALDS, A., 1991, Ergonomics evaluation of a foam rubber grip for tool handles, *Applied Ergonomics*, **22**(4), 225–230.

FERNANDEZ, J.E., DAHALAN, J.B., HALPERN, C.A. and VISWANATH, V., 1991, The effect of wrist posture on pinch strength, in *Proceedings of the Human Factors Society 35th Annual Meeting*, Human Factors Society, Santa Monica, California, pp. 748–752.

FIEDMANN, M. and ABBS, J.H., 1990, Precision grip in Parkinsonian patients: Parkinson's disease: anatomy, pathology and therapy, *Advances in Neurology*, **53**, 191–195.

FITZHUGH, F.E., 1973a, *Dynamic Aspects of Grip Strength*, Technical Report, University of Michigan.

FITZHUGH, F.E., 1973b, *Grip Strength Performance in Dynamic Gripping Tasks*, Technical Report, University of Michigan.

FOTHERGILL, D.M., GRIEVE, D.W. and PHEASANT, S.T., 1991, Human strength capabilities during one handed maximum voluntary exertions in the fore and aft plane, *Ergonomics*, **35**, 203–212.

FOTHERGILL, D.M., GRIEVE, D.W. and PHEASANT, S.T., 1992, The influence of some handle designs and handle height on the strength of the horizontal pulling action, *Ergonomics*, **35**(2), 203–212.

FRANSSON, C. and WINKEL, J., 1991, Hand strength: the influence of grip span and grip type, *Ergonomics*, **34**, 881–892.

GORDON, A.M., HUXLEY, A.F. and JULIAN, F.J., 1966, Variation in isometric tension with sarcomere length in vertebrate muscle fibers, *Journal of Physiology*, **184**, 170.

GREENBERG, L. and CHAFFIN, D., 1997, *Workers and their Tools*, Ann Arbor, MI: University of Michigan Press.

HADLER, N.M., 1978, Hand structure and function in an industrial setting: influence of three patterns of stereotyped, repetitive usage, *Arthritis Rheum*, **21**, 210.

HALLBECK, M.S. and McMULLIN, D.L., 1993, Maximal power grasp and three-jaw chuck pinch force as a function of wrist position, age, and glove type, *International Journal of Industrial Ergonomics*, **11**, 195–206.

HALLBECK, M.S., KAMAL, A.H. and HARMON, P.E., 1992, The effects of forearm posture, wrist posture, gender, and hand on three peak pinch force types, in *Proceedings of the Human Factors Society 36th Annual Meeting*, Human Factors Society, Santa Monica, CA, pp. 801–805.

HAZLETON, F.T., SMIDT, G.L., FLATT, A.E. and STEPHENS, R.I., 1975, The influence of wrist position on the force produced by the finger flexors, *Journal of Biomechanics*, **8**, 301–306.

HERTZBERG, T., 1955, Some contributions of applied physical anthropology to human engineering, *Annals of the New York Academy of Science*, **63**, 616–629.

HERTZBERG, H.T.E., 1972, Engineering anthropology, in Van Cott, H.P. and Kinkade, R.G. (Eds), *Human Engineering Guide to Equipment Design*, Washington, DC: US Government Printing Office, pp. 467–584.

HOOK, W.E. and STANLEY, J.K., 1986, Assessment of thumb to index pulp to pulp pinch grip strengths, *The Journal of Hand Surgery*, **11B**(1), 91–92.

IMRHAN, S.N., 1991, The influence of wrist position on different types of pinch strength, *Applied Ergonomics*, **22**(6), 379–384.

IMRHAN, S.N. and FARAHMAND, K., 1999, Male torque strength in simulated oil rig tasks: the effects of grease-smeared gloves and handle length, diameter and orientation, *Applied Ergonomics* (in press).

IMRHAN, S.N. and JENKINS, G.D., 1999, Flexion-extension hand torque strengths: applications in maintenance tasks, *International Journal of Industrial Ergonomics* (in press).

IMRHAN, S.N. and LOO, C.H., 1988, Modeling wrist-twisting strength of the elderly, *Ergonomics*, **31**(12), 1807–1819.

IMRHAN, S.N. and LOO, C.H., 1989, Trends in finger pinch strength in children, adults, and the elderly, *Human Factors*, **31**(6), 689–701.

IMRHAN, S.N. and RAHMAN, R., 1995, The effects of pinch width on pinch strengths on adult males using realistic pinch-hand coupling, *International Journal of Industrial Ergonomics*, **16**, 123–134.

IMRHAN, S.N. and SUNDARARAJAN, K., 1992, An investigation of finger pull strengths, *Ergonomics*, **35**(3), 289–299.

IMRHAN, S.N., JENKINS, G. and TOWNES, M., 1992, The effect of forearm orientation on wrist-turning strength, in Kumar, S. (Ed.), *Advances in Industrial Ergonomics and Safety IV*, London: Taylor and Francis, pp. 687–691.

KAMAL, A.H., MOORE, B.J. and HALLBECK, M.S., 1992, The effects of wrist position/glove type on peak lateral pinch force, in Kumar, S. (Ed.), *Advances in Industrial Ergonomics and Safety IV*, London: Taylor and Francis, pp. 701–708.

KATTEL, B.P., FREDRICKS, T.K., FERNANDEZ, J.E. and LEE, D.C., 1996, The effect of upper extremity posture of maximum grip strength, *International Journal of Industrial Ergonomics*, **18**(5–6), 423–430.

KINOSHITA, H., KAWAI, S. and IKUTA, K., 1995, Contribution and coordination of individual fingers in multiple finger prehension, *Ergonomics*, **38**(6), 1212–1230.

KINOSHITA, H., KAWAI, S., IKUTA, K. and TERAOKA, T., 1996a, Individual finger forces acting on a grasped object during shaking actions, *Ergonomics*, **39**(2), 243–256.

KINOSHITA, H., MURASE, T. and BANDOU, T., 1996b, Grip posture and forces during holding cylindrical objects with circular grips, *Ergonomics*, **39**(9), 1163–1176.

KIRPATRICK, J.E., 1956, Evaluation of grip loss, *California Medicine*, **85**(5), 314–320.

KONZ, S., 1990, *Work Design: Industrial Ergonomics*, 3rd edn, Worthington, OH: Publishing Horizons.

KRAFT, G.H. and DETELS, P.E., 1972, Position function of the wrist, *Archives of Physical Medicine and Rehabilitation*, **53**, 272–275.

KROEMER, K.H.E., 1986, Coupling the hand with the handle, *Human Factors*, **28**, 337–339.

KROEMER, K.H.E., KROEMER, H.B. and KROEMER-ELBERT, K.E., 1994, *Ergonomics: How to Design for Ease and Efficiency*, Englewood Cliffs, NJ: Prentice Hall.

LANDSMEER, J.M.F., 1962, Power grip and precision handling, *Annals of Rheumatic Diseases*, **21**, 164–170.

LEE, Y.-H. and CHENG, S.-L., 1995, Trigger force and measurement of maximal finger flexion, *International Journal of Industrial Ergonomics*, **15**, 167–177.

LEVEAU, B., 1977, *Williams and Lissner: Biomechanics of Human Motion*, Philadelphia, P.A: W.B. Saunders Co.

LONG, C.H., CONRAD, P.W., HALL, E.A. and FURLER, S.L., 1970, Intrinsic-extrinsic muscle control of the hand in power grip and precision handling, *Journal of Bone and Joint Surgery*, **52a**(5), 853–867.

LYMAN, J. and GROTH, J., 1958, Prehension force as a measure of psychomotor skill for bare and gloved hands, *Journal of Applied Psychology*, **42**(1), 18–21.

MAI, N., BOLSINGER, P., AVARELLO, M., DIENER, H.C. and DICHGANS, J., 1988, Control of isometric finger force in patients with cerebellar disease, *Brain*, **111**, 973–988.

MASON, M.T. and SALISBURY, J.K., 1985, *Robot Hands and the Mechanics of Manipulation*, Cambridge, MA: MIT Press.

MATHIOWETZ, V., WEBER, K., VOLLAND, G. and KASHMAN, N., 1984, Reliability and validity of grip and pinch strength evaluations, *Journal of Hand Surgery*, **9A**(2), 222–226.

MATHIOWETZ, V., KASHMAN, N., VOLLAND, G., WEBER, K., DOWE, M. and ROGERS, S., 1985a, Grip and pinch strength: normative data for adults, *Archives of Physical Medicine and Rehabilitation*, **66**, 69–74.

MATHIOWETZ, V., RENNELLS, C. and DONAHOE, L., 1985b, Effects of elbow position on grip and key pinch strength, *The Journal of Hand Surgery*, **10A**(5), 694–696.

MORAN, J.M., HEMANN, J.H. and GREENWALD, A.S., 1985, Finger joint contact areas and pressures, *Journal of Orthopaedic Research*, **3**, 49.

MONTOYE, J.J. and FAULKNER, J.A., 1965, Determination of the optimum setting of an adjustable dynamometer, *Research Quarterly*, **35**(1), 29–36.

NAPIER, J.R., 1956, Prehensile movement of the human hand, *Journal of Bone and Joint Surgery*, **38-B**, 902–913.

OH, S. and RADWIN, R.G., 1993, Pistol grip power tool handle and trigger size effects on grip exertions and operator preference, *Human Factors*, **35**(3), 551–569.

OHTSUKI, T., 1981a, Inhibition of individual fingers during grip strength exertion, *Ergonomics*, **24**(1), 21–36.

OHTSUKI, T., 1981b, Description in grip strength induced by simultaneous bilateral exertion with reference to finger strength, *Ergonomics*, **24**(1), 37–48.

PALANISAMI, P., NARASIMHAN, T.M. and FERNANDEZ, J.E., 1994, The effect of sitting on peak pinch strength, in Aghazadeh, F. (Ed.), *Advances in Industrial Ergonomics and Safety VI*, London: Taylor and Francis, pp. 587–594.

PATTERSON, H.M., 1965, Grip measurements as part of the pre-placement evaluation, *Industrial Medicine and Surgery*, **34**, 555–557.

PETROFSKY, J.S., WILLIAMS, C., KAMEN, G. and LIND, A.R., 1980, The effect of handgrip span on isometric exercise performance, *Ergonomics*, **23**, 1129–1135.

PHEASANT, S.T. and O'NEILL, D., 1976, Performance in gripping and turning: a study in hand/handle effectiveness, *Applied Ergonomics*, **6**, 205–208.

PRYCE, J.C., 1980, The wrist position between neutral and ulnar deviation that facilitates the maximum power grip strength, *Journal of Biomechanics*, **13**, 505–511.

PUTZ-ANDERSON, V., 1988, *Cumulative Trauma Disorders: A Manual for Musculoskeletal Diseases of the Upper Limb*, UK: Taylor and Francis, London.

RADHAKRISHNAN, S. and RAVINDRA, M.N., 1989, Biomechanical assessment of hand strength, in Sahay, K.B. and Saxena, R.K. (Eds), *Biomechanics*, New York: John Wiley and Sons, pp. 182–189.

RADWIN, R.G., OH, S., JENSON, T.R. and WEBSTER, J.G., 1992, External finger forces in submaximal five-finger static pinch prehension, *Ergonomics*, **35**, 278–288.

SILVERSTEIN, B.A., FINE, L.J. and ARMSTRONG, T.J., 1987, Occupational factors and carpal tunnel syndrome, *American Journal of Industrial Medicine*, **43**, 779–784.

SMITH, R.O., 1985, Pinch and grasp strength: standardization of terminology and protocol, *The American Journal of Occupational Therapy*, **39**(8), 531–535.

SMITH, R.O. and BENGE, M.W., 1985, Pinch and grasp strength: standardization of terminology and protocol, *The American Journal of Occupational Therapy*, **39**(8), 531–535.

SMITH, E., SONSTEGARD, D. and ANDERSON, W., 1977, Contribution of the finger flexor tendons to the carpal tunnel syndrome, *Archives of Physical Medicine and Rehabilitation*, **58**, 379–385.

STOKES, H.M., 1983, The seriously uninjured hand – weakness of grip, *Journal of Occupational Medicine*, **25**(9), 683–684.

SUDHAKAR, L.R., SCHOEMARKLIN, R.W., LAVENDER, S.A. and MARRAS, W.S., 1988, The effects of gloves on grip strength and muscle activity, in *Proceedings of the Human Factors Society 32nd Annual Meeting*, Santa Monica, California, pp. 647–650.

SWANSON, A.B., MATEV, I.B. and DE GROOT, G., 1970, The strength of the hand, *Bulletin of Prosthetics Research*, **9**, 387–396.

TERAOKA, T., 1979, Studies on the peculiarity of grip strength in relation to body positions and aging, *Kobe Journal of Medical Science*, **25**, 1–17.

TAYLOR, C.L. and SCHWARTZ, R.J., 1955, The anatomy and mechanics of the human hand, *Artificial Limbs*, **2**(2), 22–35.

TERRELL, R. and PURSWELL, J.L., 1976. The influence of forearm and wrist orientation on static grip strength as a design criterion for hand tools, in *Proceedings of the 20th Annual Meeting of the Human Factors Society*, Santa Monica, California, pp. 28–32.

TICHAUER, E.R., 1966, Some aspects of stress on forearm and hand in industry, *Journal of Occupational Medicine*, **8**, 63–71.

WOODY, R. and MATHIOWEITZ, V., 1988, Effects of arm position on pinch strength measurements, *Journal of Hand Therapy*, **1**(2), 124–126.

CHAPTER EIGHT

Hand tools

ANIL MITAL AND ARUNKUMAR PENNATHUR

INTRODUCTION

Hand tools have been in existence for a long time. Early human primates, some million years ago, dug, pounded, cut, and scraped objects using stone tools (Leaky, 1960; Washburn, 1960). Hand tools evolved with evolution of the human race; handles were added to the hand tools to facilitate handling. The development, first of the screw system, and later the screwdriver, ten thousand years ago, were other important milestones in the development of specialised hand tools (Fraser, 1980). The variety in hand tools during those times was necessitated by the growth of specialised occupations such as agriculture, manufacturing, construction, etc.

Since the time hand tools were first developed and refined, there have been just a few major changes in the basic types and designs of common hand tools (e.g., the axe and the hammer have still to undergo major changes in their basic design). There has however been a virtual proliferation in the variety of commercially available hand tools among the common types of tools. The variety in the commercial forms of these tools indicates, among other things, that these tools have yet to reach an optimal form. More importantly, the health and productivity problems posed by the use of such a variety of tools indicates the lack of sufficient testing and evaluation of these tools from an ergonomics perspective.

The goals of this chapter are to highlight the importance and scope of the hand tool design problem, review the important factors affecting hand tool design, and recommend hand tool design and usage guidelines. This chapter is organised into five major sections. The remainder of this section highlights the scope and importance of the hand tool design problem. The scope of the problem is presented through a brief description of the operator–hand tool system. The importance of the problem is highlighted by presenting data from the recent Bureau of Labor Statistics (BLS) findings about hand tool injuries and illnesses in the United States. The second section contains a brief description of the anatomy of the human hand and the forearm. The tool- and task-related factors involved in the operator–hand tool system are discussed in the third section. The operator-related factors in the operator–hand tool system are discussed in the fourth section. The fifth section concludes the chapter with remarks regarding important activities in the design and use of hand tools.

Scope of the problem – the operator–hand tool system

The operator–hand tool system is conceptualised to consist of three major components: the human operator, the tool, and the task the operator performs with the tool (Kriefeldt and Hill, 1975). These three components interact with each other, and involve several factors which influence the efficiency of the system. The human operator-related factors include such factors as age, gender, strength, body size, technique, experience, and posture. The tool- and task-related factors include such factors as the type of tool, grip/handle shape and size, gloves, wrist orientation, reach distance, force/torque requirements of the task, and duration of application of force/use. For the operator-hand tool system to perform efficiently, it is essential that the effect of these different factors on system performance be known and accounted for in design.

The overall goal in designing hand tools is to optimise the relationship between the human worker and the hand tool. This goal implies designing jobs and/or hand tools to alleviate common physiological and musculoskeletal problems such as those discussed in the following section, associated with the use of hand tools. The selection and use of hand tools is a function of the workpiece design, and the force/torque requirements of the job. It is desirable that the force/torque generated by the equipment, with or without an external power source, be greater (but not excessive to damage the workpiece) than the force/torque required for the job. Therefore, the force/torque exertion capabilities of humans with various hand tools should be known, and jobs requiring the use of hand tools by human workers must be designed to be within these capabilities.

Importance of the problem

The extent of use of hand tools, both for common daily activities as well as for industrial activities makes the hand tool design problem important. In addition, reports of musculoskeletal injuries and illnesses due to poorly designed hand tools, and the need for employers to reduce their worker compensation costs, have made good hand tool design a necessity.

Tables 8.1 and 8.2 present the current BLS classification of different types of non-powered and powered hand tools in use in the USA. Tables 8.3–8.33 (Bureau of Labor

Table 8.1 Non-powered hand tools included in the Bureau of Labor Statistics' survey of occupational injuries and illnesses in the USA.

Major class of non-powered hand tool	Specific tools
Boring hand tools	Augers, braces, drills
Cutting hand tools	Axes, hatchets, bolt cutters, chisels, knives, saws, scissors, snips, shears
Digging hand tools	Hoes, picks, shovels, trowels
Gripping hand tools	Pliers, tongs, vises, clamps
Measuring hand tools	Calipers, micrometers, dividers, gauges, levels, rulers, tape measures, squares
Striking and nailing hand tools	Hammers, mallets, punches, counter punches, counter sinks, sledges
Surfacing hand tools	Files, planes, sanders, sharpening stones and wheels
Turning hand tools	Screwdrivers, wrenches
Other non-powered hand tools	Brooms, mops, crowbars, pitchforks, spading forks, rakes, stapling tools

Table 8.2 Powered hand tools included in the Bureau of Labor Statistics' survey of occupational injuries and illnesses in the USA.

Major class of powered hand tool	Specific tools
Boring hand tools	Augers, drills, routers and moulders
Cutting hand tools	Chainsaws, chisels, knives, other saws
Striking and nailing hand tools	Hammers, jackhammers, punches, riveters
Surfacing hand tools	Buffers, polishers, waxers, hand grinders, sanders, sandblasters
Turning hand tools	Bolt setters, impact wrenches, screwdrivers
Welding and heating hand tools	Blow torches, soldering irons, welding torches
Other powered hand tools	Nail guns, scrubbers, paint sprayers, electric or pneumatic stapling tools

Table 8.3 Non-fatal occupational injuries due to hand tools in major US industry divisions.

Industry	1993		1994	
	Total number	Due to hand tools	Total number	Due to hand tools
Private industry	2 252 591	105 478	2 236 639	99 322
Agriculture, forestry and fishing	44 826	3 274	41 020	3 209
Mining	21 090	1 463	20 734	1 499
Construction	204 769	17 399	218 835	17 874
Manufacturing	583 841	32 166	584 254	32 583
Transportation and public utilities	232 998	4 560	241 703	3 849
Wholesale and retail trade	569 524	29 692	560 360	25 207
Finance, insurance and real estate	60 158	2 233	55 342	1 813
Services	535 386	14 692	514 390	13 287

Statistics, 1995, 1996) summarise the most recent and comprehensive data (1993 and 1994) on injuries and illnesses in the USA due to hand tools. The main highlights of this data are presented in the remainder of this section. It is assumed that the injury trends shown continued in year 1995 and beyond.

Number and incidence of injury due to hand tools

In 1993, in all US private industry, nearly 5 per cent of all occupational injuries and illnesses were due to hand tools. Of this, approximately 3.2 per cent of injuries were due to non-powered hand tools, and 1.2 per cent due to powered hand tools. These numbers were 4.4 per cent, 2.9 per cent and 1.2 per cent respectively in 1994 (Tables 8.3, 8.5 and 8.7). The overall incidence rates for injuries due to hand tools in all private industry fell to 12.3 in 1994 from 13.4 in 1993. Non-powered hand tools had a higher incidence rate than powered hand tools, indicating that not only were non-powered hand tools in greater

Table 8.4 Incidence rates for non-fatal occupational injuries due to hand tools in major US industry divisions.

Industry	1993		1994	
	Total incidence	Due to hand tools	Total incidence	Due to hand tools
Private industry	285.6	13.4	277.0	12.3
Agriculture, forestry and fishing	421.3	30.8	385.1	30.1
Mining	334.1	23.2	329.0	23.8
Construction	490.5	41.7	486.2	39.7
Manufacturing	326.1	18.0	319.7	17.8
Transportation	425.9	8.3	423.9	6.8
Wholesale and retail trade	275.8	14.4	266.9	12.0
Finance, insurance and real estate	99.1	3.7	88.7	2.9
Services	233.6	6.4	220.4	5.7

Incidence rates represent the number of injuries and illnesses per 10 000 full-time workers and are computed as follows:

Incidence rate = (N/EH × 20 000 000), where
   N is the number of injuries and illnesses
   EH is the total hours worked by all employees during the calendar year
   20 000 000 is the base for 10 000 equivalent full-time workers (working 40 hours per week, 50 weeks per year).

use than powered hand tools, but they also contributed more to injuries than powered hand tools. The incidence rates for non-powered hand tools fell from 9.0 in 1993 to 8.1 in 1994. The corresponding numbers for powered hand tools were 3.4 and 3.2 (Tables 8.4, 8.6 and 8.8).

Industries affected by hand tool injuries

In 1993, nearly 31 per cent of all hand tool injuries occurred in the manufacturing industry, and nearly 6 per cent of all injuries in the manufacturing industry were due to hand tools. Wholesale and retail trade accounted for nearly 28 per cent of all hand tool injuries in 1993, which was 5 per cent of all injuries in that industry. Seventeen per cent of all hand tool injuries were in the construction industry, with nearly 8.5 per cent of all injuries in the construction industry due to hand tools. Even when only 2.7 per cent of all injuries in the service sector were due to hand tools, among the different US industries, the service sector reported nearly 14 per cent of all hand tool injuries. The same trend continued in all US industries in 1994 as well (Table 8.3). The prevalence of hand tool injuries in the construction industry is further reinforced by the hand tool injury incidence rates for that industry – the highest among all other industry divisions in 1993 and 1994. For 1993 and 1994, agriculture, forestry and fishing had the second highest hand tool injury incidence rates, followed by mining, manufacturing, and trade, in that order. Since incidence rates take into account the actual number of employees in a particular industry, they are a better reflection of the relative severity of hand tool injuries among the different US industries (Table 8.4).

Table 8.5 Non-fatal occupational injuries in the USA due to different types of non-powered hand tools classified by major US industry divisions.

Tool type	Total number		Agriculture, forestry and fishing		Mining		Construction		Manufacturing		Transportation and public utilities		Wholesale trade		Retail trade		Finance, insurance and real estate		Services	
	1993	1994	1993	1994	1993	1994	1993	1994	1993	1994	1993	1994	1993	1994	1993	1994	1993	1994	1993	1994
A	2 252 591	2 236 639	44 826	41 020	21 090	20 734	204 769	218 835	583 841	584 254	232 998	241 703	160 934	165 742	408 590	394 619	60 158	55 342	535 386	514 390
B	141 794	133 347	3 834	3 734	1 782	1 781	21 428	22 959	37 832	38 570	9 261	7 549	6 828	6 722	30 194	24 127	3 303	2 615	27 332	25 290
C	70 721	65 300	2 166	1 788	1 209	1 162	8 876	9 434	18 408	17 887	3 162	2 802	3 382	3 755	21 646	17 360	1 465	1 351	10 407	9 761
D	688	511	21	15	–	–	279	181	216	162	13	–	50	–	15	–	–	27	90	56
E	38 462	34 016	1 129	1 034	84	107	1 973	2 041	8 066	7 608	770	597	1 719	2 124	18 172	14 120	686	611	5 862	5 774
F	6 073	6 440	417	365	20	5	2 185	2 744	1 343	1 229	590	475	215	130	344	413	158	377	801	702
G	1 787	1 673	38	–	161	55	145	85	960	1 272	61	51	82	–	178	130	–	12	155	54
H	819	650	31	9	–	31	104	93	367	294	38	19	50	–	91	–	–	–	126	138
I	6 926	7 968	292	70	194	246	1 995	2 762	2 190	2 543	469	359	464	428	489	757	46	88	788	716
J	1 010	841	19	–	–	–	94	183	309	258	11	–	–	–	250	143	107	10	194	186
K	6 367	5 929	56	68	279	327	995	600	2 580	2 272	532	643	342	583	684	901	146	64	751	472
L	8 060	6 868	158	210	426	363	959	666	2 236	2 121	625	569	407	337	1 392	834	291	155	1 566	1 613

A refers to total in all private industry
B refers to all tools, instruments, and equipment
C refers to all non-powered hand tools
D refers to non-powered boring hand tools
E refers to non-powered cutting hand tools
F refers to non-powered digging hand tools
G refers to non-powered gripping hand tools
H refers to non-powered measuring hand tools
I refers to non-powered striking and nailing hand tools
J refers to non-powered surfacing hand tools
K refers to non-powered turning hand tools
L refers to all other non-powered hand tools such as crowbars, pitchforks, etc.

Table 8.6 Incidence of non-fatal occupational injuries in the USA due to different types of non-powered hand tools classified by major industry divisions.

Tool type	All industry		Agriculture, forestry and fishing		Mining		Construction		Manufacturing		Transportation and public utilities		Wholesale trade		Retail trade		Finance, insurance and real estate		Services	
	1993	1994	1993	1994	1993	1994	1993	1994	1993	1994	1993	1994	1993	1994	1993	1994	1993	1994	1993	1994
A	285.6	277.0	421.3	385.1	334.1	329.0	490.5	486.2	326.1	319.7	425.9	423.9	280.0	281.1	274.2	261.4	99.1	88.7	233.6	220.4
B	18.0	16.5	36.0	35.0	28.2	28.3	51.3	51.0	21.1	21.1	16.9	13.2	11.9	11.4	20.3	16.0	5.4	4.2	11.9	10.8
C	9.0	8.1	20.4	16.8	19.2	18.4	21.3	21.0	10.3	9.8	5.8	4.9	5.9	6.4	14.5	11.5	2.4	2.2	4.5	4.2
D	0.1	0.1	0.2	0.1	–	–	0.7	0.4	0.1	0.1	–	–	0.1	–	–	–	–	–	–	–
E	4.9	4.2	10.6	9.7	1.3	1.7	4.7	4.5	4.5	4.2	1.4	1.0	3.0	3.6	12.2	9.4	1.1	1.0	2.6	2.5
F	0.8	0.8	3.9	3.4	0.3	0.1	5.2	6.1	0.8	0.7	1.1	0.8	0.4	0.2	0.2	0.3	0.3	0.6	0.4	0.3
G	0.2	0.2	0.4	–	2.6	0.9	0.4	0.2	0.5	0.7	0.1	0.1	0.1	–	0.1	0.1	–	–	0.1	–
H	0.1	0.1	0.3	0.1	–	0.5	0.2	0.2	0.2	0.2	0.1	–	0.1	–	0.1	–	–	–	0.1	0.1
I	0.9	1.0	2.7	0.7	3.1	3.9	4.8	6.1	1.2	1.4	0.9	0.6	0.8	0.7	0.3	0.5	0.1	0.1	0.3	0.3
J	0.1	0.1	0.2	–	–	–	0.2	0.4	0.2	0.1	–	–	–	–	0.2	0.1	0.2	–	0.1	0.1
K	0.8	0.7	0.5	0.6	4.4	5.2	2.4	1.3	1.4	1.2	1.0	1.1	0.6	1.0	0.5	0.6	0.2	0.1	0.3	0.2
L	1.0	0.8	1.5	2.0	6.7	5.8	2.3	1.5	1.2	1.2	1.1	1.0	0.7	0.6	0.9	0.6	0.5	0.2	0.7	0.7

A refers to total incidence rates due to all sources
B refers to all tools, instruments, and equipment
C refers to all non-powered hand tools
D refers to non-powered boring hand tools
E refers to non-powered cutting hand tools
F refers to non-powered digging hand tools
G refers to non-powered gripping hand tools
H refers to non-powered measuring hand tools
I refers to non-powered striking and nailing hand tools
J refers to non-powered surfacing hand tools
K refers to non-powered turning hand tools
L refers to all other non-powered hand tools such as crowbars, pitchforks, etc.

Incidence rates represent the number of injuries and illnesses per 10 000 full-time workers and are computed as follows:

Incidence rate = (N/EH × 20 000 000), where

N is the number of injuries and illnesses

EH is the total hours worked by all employees during the calendar year

20 000 000 is the base for 10 000 equivalent full-time workers (working 40 hours per week, 50 weeks per year).

Table 8.7 Non-fatal occupational injuries in the USA due to different types of powered hand tools classified by major US industry divisions.

Tool type	Total number 1993	Total number 1994	Agriculture, forestry and fishing 1993	Agriculture, forestry and fishing 1994	Mining 1993	Mining 1994	Construction 1993	Construction 1994	Manufacturing 1993	Manufacturing 1994	Transportation and public utilities 1993	Transportation and public utilities 1994	Wholesale trade 1993	Wholesale trade 1994	Retail trade 1993	Retail trade 1994	Finance, insurance and real estate 1993	Finance, insurance and real estate 1994	Services 1993	Services 1994
A	2 252 591	2 236 639	44 826	41 020	21 090	20 734	204 769	218 835	583 841	584 254	232 998	241 703	160 934	165 742	408 590	394 619	60 158	55 342	535 386	514 390
B	141 794	133 347	3 834	3 734	1 782	1 781	21 428	22 959	37 832	38 570	9 261	7 549	6 828	6 722	30 194	24 127	3 303	2 615	27 332	25 290
C	26 422	25 857	975	1 205	189	301	6 693	6 681	10 609	11 507	1 037	649	1 463	1 083	1 521	1 438	674	292	3 262	2 701
D	3 115	3 724	31	20	27	57	955	1 100	1 191	1 339	119	62	128	247	118	524	71	18	475	356
E	6 826	6 074	726	831	15	10	2 110	2 090	2 274	1 802	226	112	252	140	457	341	322	212	444	537
F	2 812	2 491	78	34	29	–	1 468	1 396	636	748	147	59	64	46	57	–	–	12	308	182
G	4 250	3 684	43	14	18	6	554	419	1 543	1 994	110	95	253	121	416	197	190	14	1 123	824
H	1 066	876	–	–	16	5	102	70	493	480	108	46	108	55	118	141	–	–	120	73
I	5 835	6 826	52	290	29	138	891	1 072	3 470	4 047	234	234	538	388	162	80	12	23	447	553
J	2 083	1 729	43	10	19	69	556	439	792	847	52	–	121	71	155	117	53	10	291	144

A refers to total in all private industry
B refers to all tools, instruments, and equipment
C refers to all powered hand tools
D refers to powered boring hand tools
E refers to powered cutting hand tools
F refers to powered striking and nailing hand tools
G refers to powered surfacing hand tools
H refers to powered turning hand tools
I refers to powered welding and heating hand tools
J refers to all other powered hand tools such as nail guns, sprayers, etc.

Table 8.8 Incidence of non-fatal occupational injuries in the USA due to different types of powered hand tools classified by major US industry divisions.

Tool type	All industry		Agriculture, forestry and fishing		Mining		Construction		Manufacturing		Transportation and public utilities		Wholesale trade		Retail trade		Finance, insurance and real estate		Services	
	1993	1994	1993	1994	1993	1994	1993	1994	1993	1994	1993	1994	1993	1994	1993	1994	1993	1994	1993	1994
A	285.6	277.0	421.3	385.1	334.1	329.0	490.5	486.2	326.1	319.7	425.9	423.9	280.0	281.1	274.2	261.4	99.1	88.7	233.6	220.4
B	18.0	16.5	36.0	35.0	28.2	28.3	51.3	51.0	21.1	21.1	16.9	13.2	11.9	11.4	20.3	16.0	5.4	4.2	11.9	10.8
C	3.4	3.2	9.2	11.3	3.0	4.8	16.0	14.8	5.9	6.3	1.9	1.1	2.6	1.8	1.0	1.0	1.1	0.5	1.4	1.2
D	0.4	0.5	0.3	0.2	0.4	0.9	2.3	2.4	0.7	0.7	0.2	0.1	0.2	0.4	0.1	0.4	0.1	–	0.2	0.2
E	0.9	0.8	6.8	7.8	0.2	0.2	5.0	4.6	1.3	1.0	0.4	0.2	0.4	0.2	0.3	0.2	0.5	0.3	0.2	0.2
F	0.4	0.3	0.7	0.3	0.5	–	3.5	3.1	0.4	0.4	0.3	0.1	0.1	0.1	–	–	–	–	0.1	0.1
G	0.5	0.5	0.4	0.1	0.3	0.1	1.3	0.9	0.9	1.1	0.2	0.2	0.4	0.2	0.3	0.1	0.3	–	0.5	0.4
H	0.1	0.1	–	–	0.2	0.1	0.2	0.2	0.3	0.3	0.2	0.1	0.2	0.1	0.1	0.1	–	–	–	–
I	0.7	0.8	0.5	2.7	0.5	2.2	2.1	2.4	1.9	2.2	0.4	0.4	0.9	0.7	0.1	–	–	–	0.2	0.2
J	0.3	0.2	0.4	0.1	0.3	1.1	1.3	1.0	0.4	0.5	0.1	–	0.2	0.1	0.1	0.1	0.1	–	0.1	0.1

A refers to total incidence rates due to all sources
B refers to all tools, instruments, and equipment
C refers to all powered hand tools
D refers to powered boring hand tools
E refers to powered cutting hand tools
F refers to powered striking and nailing hand tools
G refers to powered surfacing hand tools
H refers to powered turning hand tools
I refers to powered welding and heating hand tools
J refers to all other powered hand tools such as nail guns, scrubbers, sprayers, etc.

Incidence rates represent the number of injuries and illnesses per 10 000 full-time workers and are computed as follows:

Incidence rate = $(N/EH \times 20\,000\,000)$, where

N is the number of injuries and illnesses
EH is the total hours worked by all employees during the calendar year
20 000 000 is the base for 10 000 equivalent full-time workers (working 40 hours per week, 50 weeks per year).

Overall, non-powered hand tools caused more injuries (nearly 31 per cent) in the retail trade industry than in any other industry. Twenty-six per cent of all injuries due to non-powered hand tools occurred in the manufacturing sector. This number increased to 27 per cent in 1994, while the number for the retail trade industry fell to 26 per cent in 1994. The service industry (15 per cent in 1993 and 1994), and the construction industry (13 per cent in 1993 and 14.4 per cent in 1994) were the other industries where non-powered hand tools caused many injuries (Table 8.5). In terms of incidence rates, however, construction and agriculture had the highest incidences of injuries due to non-powered hand tools, followed by mining and retail trade. Since the types of hand tools used in a particular industry are specific to that industry (for instance, one would expect non-powered digging hand tools, such as hoes, shovels, etc., and non-powered striking and nailing hand tools, such as hammers, mallets, etc., to be more prevalent in the construction industry), the 'tools of the (respective) trades' caused more injuries than any other tool type in a particular industry. Hence, non-powered cutting hand tools caused the most injuries in the agriculture, forestry and fishing industries; non-powered hand tools such as pitchforks and crowbars, and turning hand tools such as screwdrivers and wrenches caused the most injuries in the mining industry; non-powered digging hand tools such as hoes, picks, and shovels, and non-powered striking, nailing, and cutting hand tools such as hammers, mallets, axes, hatchets, saws, and chisels, caused the most injuries in the construction industry; non-powered cutting hand tools such as such as bolt cutters, knives, saws, and shears, and non-powered turning hand tools such as screwdrivers and wrenches, caused the most injuries in the manufacturing sector; non-powered cutting hand tools caused the most injuries in the retail trade and the service industries (Table 8.6).

Manufacturing had the highest number of injuries due to powered hand tools (nearly 42 per cent in years 1993 and 1994), followed by construction (25 per cent) and services (12 per cent) (Table 8.7). In terms of injury incidence rates, however, the construction industry had the highest incidences (an average of 15.0 for 1993 and 1994 combined), followed by agriculture, forestry and fishing (an average of 10.0 for 1993 and 1994 combined). Manufacturing had an average incidence rate of 6.0 for 1993 and 1994. Among the different powered hand tools, powered cutting hand tools such as chainsaws, chisels, knives, etc., caused the most incidences of injuries in agriculture, forestry and fishing; powered welding and heating tools such as blow torches, soldering irons, welding torches, etc., caused the most injuries in the mining industry; powered cutting tools such as chainsaws, chisels, etc., and powered striking and nailing tools such as jackhammers, punches, riveters, etc., caused the most injuries in the construction industry; powered welding and heating tools such as blow torches and soldering irons, and powered cutting tools such as chainsaws, chisels, etc., caused the most injuries in manufacturing (Table 8.8).

Occupations affected by hand tool injuries

According to the BLS, in 1993 and 1994, nearly 8.5 per cent of all injuries in the farming, forestry and fishing occupations, and in the precision production, craft and repair occupations were due to hand tools. In the two years, nearly 4.5 per cent of all injuries to operators, fabricators and labourers were the result of hand tool use. Operators, fabricators and labourers accounted for nearly 41 per cent of all hand tool injuries. Workers in the precision production, craft and repair occupation had nearly 28 per cent of all hand tool injuries, and workers in the service occupations accounted for about 17 per cent of all injuries due to hand tools (Table 8.9).

Table 8.9 Number of non-fatal occupational injuries due to hand tools in major US occupations.

Occupation	1993		1994	
	Total number	Due to hand tools	Total number	Due to hand tools
All private industry	2 252 591	105 478	2 236 639	99 322
Managerial and professional specialty	123 596	1 423	118 188	1 503
Technical, sales and administrative support	344 402	6 206	335 976	7 241
Services	414 134	20 860	391 297	15 446
Farming, forestry and fishing	59 050	5 050	52 606	4 520
Precision production, craft, and repair	366 112	29 669	372 276	27 993
Operators, fabricators and labourers	925 515	41 573	950 357	42 041

Injuries due to non-powered hand tools were most prevalent among operators, fabricators and labourers (nearly 36 per cent of all injuries). Workers in the precision production, craft, and repair occupations were the next most affected by non-powered hand tools, followed by workers in the service occupations. Among the different types of non-powered hand tools, non-powered cutting hand tools were the cause for most injuries in all occupations, especially among workers in the service occupations, and among operators, fabricators and labourers. In addition to cutting hand tools, striking and nailing hand tools, and turning hand tools were among the most injury causing non-powered hand tools in precision production, craft, and repair (Table 8.10).

Injuries due to the use of powered hand tools were again most prevalent among operators, fabricators and labourers (nearly 50 per cent of all injuries due to powered hand tools were caused to this occupational group). Workers in the precision production, craft and repair occupations accounted for the majority of the rest of the injuries due to powered hand tools (about 33 per cent). Among the different types of powered hand tools, welding and heating tools caused the most injuries among operators, fabricators and labourers (nearly 33 per cent of all powered hand tool injuries among operators, fabricators, and labourers were due to welding and heating tools). Powered cutting tools, powered boring tools, powered surfacing tools, and powered welding and heating tools, were among the tools that caused most injuries in the precision production, craft and repair occupations. Powered cutting hand tools were the cause for most injuries in the farming, forestry and fishing occupations (Table 8.11).

Nature of injuries due to hand tools

In 1993 and 1994, nearly 5 per cent of all occupational traumatic injuries and disorders in the USA were caused due to the use of hand tools. Two per cent of all traumatic injuries to muscles, tendons, ligaments, joints, etc., were caused by hand tools. About 2 per cent of the sprains, strains, and tears that occur in the USA annually were due to hand tools. Hand tools caused nearly 24 per cent of all work related open wounds, nearly 27 per cent

Table 8.10 Non-fatal occupational injuries in the USA due to different types of non-powered hand tools for select US occupations.

Tool type	Total number		Managerial and professional specialty		Technical, sales and admin. support		Service		Farming, forestry and fishing		Precision production, craft and repair		Operators, fabricators and labourers	
	1993	1994	1993	1994	1993	1994	1993	1994	1993	1994	1993	1994	1993	1994
A	2 252 591	2 236 639	123 596	118 188	344 402	335 976	414 134	391 297	59 050	52 606	366 112	372 276	925 515	950 357
B	141 794	133 347	6 230	4 841	13 370	13 617	26 813	21 732	5 891	5 215	38 129	35 813	50 448	51 332
C	70 721	65 300	1 096	1 282	5 047	5 828	18 413	13 693	3 063	2 550	17 432	16 607	25 160	25 064
D	688	511	–	15	47	32	33	32	21	14	252	222	332	197
E	38 462	34 016	779	856	3 555	3 820	15 472	10 692	1 447	1 410	5 679	6 053	11 295	11 103
F	6 073	6 440	32	123	268	319	492	633	706	632	1 451	1 578	3 106	3 147
G	1 787	1 673	–	–	60	68	82	75	10	13	761	688	865	805
H	819	650	38	44	70	87	83	46	25	12	238	93	334	367
I	6 926	7 968	28	40	208	521	90	232	291	139	3 186	3 146	3 061	3 763
J	1 010	841	31	25	114	81	227	134	107	–	236	247	294	354
K	6 367	5 929	42	57	247	520	300	404	80	48	3 452	2 797	2 199	2 088
L	8 060	6 868	127	99	461	351	1 579	1 432	372	269	1 975	1 607	3 432	3 078

A refers to total in all private industry
B refers to all tools, instruments, and equipment
C refers to all non-powered hand tools
D refers to non-powered boring hand tools
E refers to non-powered cutting hand tools
F refers to non-powered digging hand tools
G refers to non-powered gripping hand tools
H refers to non-powered measuring hand tools
I refers to non-powered striking and nailing hand tools
J refers to non-powered surfacing hand tools
K refers to non-powered turning hand tools
L refers to all other non-powered hand tools such as crowbars, pitchforks, etc.

Table 8.11 Non-fatal occupational injuries in the USA due to different types of powered hand tools for select US occupations.

Tool type	Total number		Managerial and professional specialty		Technical, sales and admin. support		Services		Farming, forestry and fishing		Precision production, craft and repair		Operators, fabricators and labourers	
	1993	1994	1993	1994	1993	1994	1993	1994	1993	1994	1993	1994	1993	1994
A	2 252 591	2 236 639	123 596	118 188	344 402	335 976	414 134	391 297	59 050	52 606	366 112	372 276	925 515	950 357
B	141 794	133 347	6 230	4 841	13 370	13 617	26 813	21 732	5 891	5 215	38 129	35 813	50 448	51 332
C	26 422	25 857	234	130	627	773	1 824	1 254	1 809	1 787	8 832	8 372	12 928	13 308
D	3 115	3 724	29	18	76	265	250	97	33	–	1 488	1 916	1 217	1 372
E	6 826	6 074	54	44	151	135	298	235	1 560	1 433	2 081	1 607	2 658	2 590
F	2 812	1 064	67	–	69	29	33	26	86	418	820	202	1 727	377
G	4 250	3 684	40	15	110	61	840	600	15	–	1 338	1 180	1 902	1 791
H	1 066	876	–	–	–	44	–	–	–	–	569	439	476	379
I	5 835	6 826	19	26	128	159	117	145	26	252	1 606	1 850	3 863	4 366
J	2 083	1 729	14	–	75	47	268	147	84	36	685	621	942	831

A refers to total in all private industry
B refers to all tools, instruments, and equipment
C refers to all powered hand tools
D refers to powered boring hand tools
E refers to powered cutting hand tools
F refers to powered striking and nailing hand tools
G refers to powered surfacing hand tools
H refers to powered turning hand tools
I refers to powered welding and heating hand tools
J refers to all other powered hand tools such as nail guns, scrubbers, etc.

Table 8.12 Number of non-fatal occupational injuries due to hand tools classified by the nature of injury.

Nature of injury or illness	1993		1994	
	Total number	Due to hand tools	Total number	Due to hand tools
All private industry	2 252 591	105 478	2 236 639	99 322
Traumatic injuries and disorders	2 042 628	98 204	2 032 510	91 453
Traumatic injuries to muscles, tendons, ligaments, joints, etc.	970 466	20 081	971 248	19 135
Sprains, strains, tears	959 163	19 875	963 496	18 986
Open wounds	223 770	55 710	214 020	49 816
Cuts, lacerations	169 894	49 810	164 608	44 288
Bruises, contusions	211 179	6 159	211 952	6 016
Carpal tunnel syndrome	41 019	15	38 336	94
Bursitis	2 790	64	3 092	44
Synovitis	341	0	342	0
Tendonitis	25 026	727	25 187	709
Tenosynovitis	1 832	64	1 458	0
Ganglion/cysts	2 667	54	2 538	52

of the cuts and lacerations, almost 3 per cent of the bruises and contusions, very few (only 0.2 per cent) of the carpal tunnel syndrome cases, 1 to 2 per cent of the bursitis cases, nearly 3 per cent of the tendonitis cases, and less than 2 per cent of the ganglion/cysts in all US industries (Table 8.12). Of the different types of injuries hand tools caused, open wounds, and cuts and lacerations had the highest incidence rates (Table 8.13).

Among the different types of injuries, non-powered hand tools caused most incidence of cuts, punctures, and lacerations. Sprains and strains had the next highest incidence rates among non-powered hand tools. Bruises and fractures were the other significant injuries due to non-powered hand tools. Among the different types of non-powered hand tools, non-powered digging hand tools caused most sprains/strains, followed by other types of non-powered hand tools such as crowbars and pitchforks. The vast majority of the cuts and punctures were caused by non-powered cutting hand tools. Non-powered striking and nailing hand tools caused the most bruises (Tables 8.14 and 8.15).

Powered hand tools also caused cuts, punctures, and lacerations more than any other type of injury. Sprains and strains, and bruises were the other significant types of injuries caused by powered hand tools. The majority of cuts, punctures and lacerations were caused when using powered cutting tools. Powered surfacing tools also caused a significant incidence of cuts, punctures, and lacerations (Tables 8.16 and 8.17).

Body parts affected due to hand tool injuries

In 1993 and 1994, approximately 6 per cent of all injuries to the head were due to hand tools. Nearly 2 per cent of all injuries to the neck were due to hand tools. Hand tools also caused nearly 2.2 per cent of all injuries to the trunk including the shoulder, back, abdomen, and pelvic region, and nearly 12 per cent of the upper extremity injuries.

Table 8.13 Incidence rates for non-fatal occupational injuries due to hand tools classified by the nature of injury.

Nature of injury or illness	1993		1994	
	Total incidence	Due to hand tools	Total incidence	Due to hand tools
All private industry	285.6	13.4	277.0	12.3
Traumatic injuries and disorders	258.9	12.4	251.7	11.3
Traumatic injuries to muscles, tendons, ligaments, joints, etc.	123.0	2.6	120.3	2.4
Sprains, strains, tears	121.6	2.5	119.3	2.4
Open wounds	28.4	7.1	26.5	6.2
Cuts, lacerations	21.5	6.3	20.4	5.5
Bruises, contusions	26.8	0.8	26.2	0.8
Carpal tunnel syndrome	5.2	–	4.8	–
Bursitis	0.4	–	0.4	–
Synovitis	–	–	–	–
Tendonitis	3.2	0.1	3.1	0.1
Tenosynovitis	0.2	–	0.2	–
Ganglion/cysts	0.3	–	0.3	–

Incidence rates represent the number of injuries and illnesses per 10 000 full-time workers and are computed as follows:

Incidence rate = (N/EH × 20 000 000), where
  N is the number of injuries and illnesses
  EH is the total hours worked by all employees during the calendar year
  20 000 000 is the base for 10 000 equivalent full-time workers (working 40 hours per week, 50 weeks per year).

Among the upper extremities, hand tools were responsible for about 5 per cent of the injuries to the arm, about 4 per cent of the injuries to the wrist, about 14 per cent of the injuries to the hands except the fingers, and nearly 21 per cent of the injuries to the fingers. Hand tools also caused 2 per cent of all injuries to the lower extremities. Of all the injuries due to hand tools, nearly 8 per cent of the injuries occurred to the head, 0.8 per cent to the neck, 18 per cent to the trunk including the shoulder, back, abdomen, and pelvic region, 62 per cent to the upper extremities, and 9 per cent to the lower extremities. Among the body parts in the upper extremities, 7 per cent of the hand tool injuries occurred in the arm region, 7 per cent in the wrist region, 20 per cent in the hands except fingers, and 63 per cent to the fingers (Tables 8.18 and 8.19).

Nearly 44 per cent of all injuries due to the use of non-powered hand tools occurred to the fingers. The hand (about 13 per cent) and the back (about 12.5 per cent) were other body parts that were most affected due to non-powered hand tools. Among the different types of non-powered hand tools, non-powered cutting hand tools caused the vast majority of injuries to the finger (nearly 79 per cent), followed by non-powered striking and nailing tools (about 10.5 per cent). The majority of the injuries (nearly 75 per cent) to the hand were also caused by non-powered cutting hand tools. Non-powered digging hand tools (about 39 per cent), non-powered hand tools such as crowbars, pitchforks, etc.

Table 8.14 Number of non-fatal occupational injuries in the USA due to different types of non-powered hand tools classified by the nature of injury.

Tool type	Total number		Sprains/strains		Fractures		Cuts, punctures		Bruises		Carpal tunnel syndrome		Tendonitis		Back pain	
	1993	1994	1993	1994	1993	1994	1993	1994	1993	1994	1993	1994	1993	1994	1993	1994
A	2 252 591	2 236 639	959 163	963 496	136 478	138 545	202 464	190 890	211 179	211 952	41 019	38 336	25 026	25 187	58 385	62 228
B	141 794	133 347	33 849	33 584	7 447	7 294	57 906	51 716	11 113	9 996	35	155	950	846	1 997	2 019
C	70 721	65 300	13 318	13 094	2 870	2 656	40 653	35 955	4 176	3 953	12	81	520	444	659	806
D	688	511	165	155	174	56	155	105	115	90	–	–	–	–	9	–
E	38 462	34 016	669	643	99	88	35 790	31 566	271	267	–	–	38	68	59	41
F	6 073	6 440	4 030	4 220	88	130	385	259	203	226	–	65	124	71	258	402
G	1 787	1 673	413	376	196	134	393	260	226	286	–	–	36	34	12	12
H	819	650	309	188	59	94	102	141	156	88	–	–	–	–	17	–
I	6 926	7 968	1 339	1 740	1 152	1 039	699	955	1 671	1 583	–	–	90	103	53	67
J	1 010	841	144	193	28	53	621	462	76	33	–	–	–	–	15	–
K	6 367	5 929	2 605	2 276	494	510	1 194	1 357	545	508	–	–	79	82	51	58
L	8 060	6 868	3 357	3 125	572	518	1 185	796	895	847	–	–	139	64	189	202

A refers to all injuries in private industry
B refers to all tools, instruments, and equipment
C refers to all non-powered hand tools
D refers to non-powered boring hand tools
E refers to non-powered cutting hand tools
F refers to non-powered digging hand tools
G refers to non-powered gripping hand tools
H refers to non-powered measuring hand tools
I refers to non-powered striking and nailing hand tools
J refers to non-powered surfacing hand tools
K refers to non-powered turning hand tools
L refers to other categories of non-powered hand tools such as crowbars, pitchforks, staplers, etc.

Table 8.15 Incidence of non-fatal occupational injuries in the USA due to different types of non-powered hand tools classified by the nature of injury.

Tool type	Total incidence		Sprains/strains		Fractures		Cuts, punctures		Bruises		Carpal tunnel syndrome		Tendonitis		Back pain	
	1993	1994	1993	1994	1993	1994	1993	1994	1993	1994	1993	1994	1993	1994	1993	1994
A	285.6	277.0	121.6	119.3	17.3	17.2	25.7	23.6	26.8	26.2	5.2	4.8	3.2	3.1	7.4	7.7
B	18.0	16.5	4.3	4.2	0.9	0.9	7.3	6.4	1.4	1.2	–	–	0.1	0.1	0.2	0.2
C	9.0	8.1	1.7	1.6	0.4	0.3	5.2	4.4	0.5	0.5	–	–	0.1	–	0.1	–
D	0.1	0.1	–	–	–	–	–	–	–	–	–	–	–	–	–	–
E	4.9	4.2	0.1	0.1	–	–	4.5	3.9	–	–	–	–	–	–	–	–
F	0.8	0.8	0.5	0.5	–	–	–	–	–	–	–	–	–	–	–	–
G	0.2	0.2	–	–	–	–	–	–	–	–	–	–	–	–	–	–
H	0.1	0.1	–	–	–	–	–	–	–	–	–	–	–	–	–	–
I	0.9	1.0	0.2	0.2	0.2	0.1	0.1	0.1	0.2	0.2	–	–	–	–	–	–
J	0.1	0.1	–	–	–	–	0.1	0.1	–	–	–	–	–	–	–	–
K	0.8	0.7	0.3	0.3	0.1	0.1	0.2	0.2	0.1	0.1	–	–	–	–	–	–
L	1.0	0.8	0.4	0.4	0.1	0.1	0.2	0.1	0.1	0.1	–	–	–	–	–	–

A refers to all injuries in private industry
B refers to all tools, instruments, and equipment
C refers to all non-powered hand tools
D refers to non-powered boring hand tools
E refers to non-powered cutting hand tools
F refers to non-powered digging hand tools
G refers to non-powered gripping hand tools

H refers to non-powered measuring hand tools
I refers to non-powered striking and nailing hand tools
J refers to non-powered surfacing hand tools
K refers to non-powered turning hand tools
L refers to other categories of non-powered hand tools such as crowbars, pitchforks, staplers, etc.

Incidence rates represent the number of injuries and illnesses per 10 000 full-time workers and are computed as follows:

Incidence rate = $(N/EH \times 20\,000\,000)$, where

N is the number of injuries and illnesses
EH is the total hours worked by all employees during the calendar year
20 000 000 is the base for 10 000 equivalent full-time workers (working 40 hours per week, 50 weeks per year).

Table 8.16 Non-fatal occupational injuries in the USA due to different types of powered hand tools classified by the nature of injury.

Tool type	Total number		Sprains/strains		Fractures		Cuts, punctures		Bruises		Carpal tunnel syndrome		Tendonitis		Back pain	
	1993	1994	1993	1994	1993	1994	1993	1994	1993	1994	1993	1994	1993	1994	1993	1994
A	2 252 591	2 236 639	959 163	963 496	136 478	138 545	202 464	190 890	211 179	211 952	41 019	38 336	25 026	25 187	58 385	62 228
B	141 794	133 347	33 849	33 584	7 447	7 294	57 906	51 716	11 113	9 996	35	155	950	846	1 997	2 019
C	26 422	25 857	4 813	4 276	1 312	1 406	9 515	8 708	1 270	1 194	–	14	119	190	20	202
D	3 115	3 724	621	961	304	536	1 429	1 351	126	140	–	–	20	37	23	32
E	6 826	6 074	661	388	196	67	5 019	4 658	149	73	–	–	15	–	39	17
F	2 812	2 491	1 106	953	412	315	195	294	433	244	–	–	23	60	120	71
G	4 250	3 684	1 081	798	150	174	1 657	1 339	234	404	–	–	12	48	34	40
H	1 066	876	219	312	89	92	329	189	111	98	–	–	32	10	–	13
I	5 835	6 826	333	267	36	103	79	102	42	42	–	–	9	–	13	16
J	2 083	1 729	575	437	118	102	755	657	116	108	–	–	–	20	54	–

A refers to all injuries in private industry
B refers to all tools, instruments, and equipment
C refers to all powered hand tools
D refers to powered boring hand tools
E refers to powered cutting hand tools
F refers to powered striking and nailing hand tools
G refers to powered surfacing hand tools
H refers to powered turning hand tools
I refers to powered welding and heating hand tools
J refers to other powered hand tools such as nail guns, sprayers, etc.

Table 8.17 Incidence of non-fatal occupational injuries in the USA due to different types of powered hand tools classified by the nature of injury.

Tool type	Total incidence		Sprains/strains		Fractures		Cuts, punctures		Bruises		Carpal tunnel syndrome		Tendonitis		Back pain	
	1993	1994	1993	1994	1993	1994	1993	1994	1993	1994	1993	1994	1993	1994	1993	1994
A	285.6	277.0	121.6	119.3	17.3	17.2	25.7	23.6	26.8	26.2	5.2	4.8	3.2	3.1	7.4	7.7
B	18.0	16.5	4.3	4.2	0.9	0.9	7.3	6.4	1.4	1.2	–	–	0.1	0.1	0.2	0.2
C	3.4	3.2	0.6	0.5	0.2	0.2	1.2	1.1	0.2	0.2	–	–	–	–	–	–
D	0.4	0.5	0.1	0.1	–	0.1	0.2	0.2	–	–	–	–	–	–	–	–
E	0.9	0.8	0.1	–	–	–	0.6	0.6	–	–	–	–	–	–	–	–
F	0.4	0.3	0.1	0.1	–	–	–	–	–	–	–	–	–	–	–	–
G	0.5	0.5	0.1	0.1	–	–	0.2	0.2	–	–	–	–	–	–	–	–
H	0.1	0.1	–	–	–	–	–	–	–	–	–	–	–	–	–	–
I	0.7	0.8	–	–	–	–	–	–	–	–	–	–	–	–	–	–
J	0.3	0.2	0.1	–	–	–	0.1	0.1	–	–	–	–	–	–	–	–

A refers to all injuries in private industry
B refers to all tools, instruments, and equipment
C refers to all powered hand tools
D refers to powered boring hand tools
E refers to powered cutting hand tools
F refers to powered striking and nailing hand tools
G refers to powered surfacing hand tools
H refers to powered turning hand tools
I refers to powered welding and heating hand tools
J refers to other powered hand tools such as nail guns, scrappers, etc.

Incidence rates represent the number of injuries and illnesses per 10 000 full-time workers and are computed as follows:

Incidence rate = (N/EH × 20 000 000), where

N is the number of injuries and illnesses
EH is the total hours worked by all employees during the calendar year
20 000 000 is the base for 10 000 equivalent full-time workers (working 40 hours per week, 50 weeks per year).

Table 8.18 Number of non-fatal occupational injuries due to hand tools classified by the part of body affected.

Part of body	1993		1994	
	Total number	Due to hand tools	Total number	Due to hand tools
All private industry	2 252 591	105 478	2 236 639	99 322
Head	155 504	8 722	151 186	8 880
Neck	40 704	893	40 178	695
Trunk, including shoulder, back, abdomen and pelvic region	869 447	18 820	866 731	18 415
Upper extremities	518 703	65 537	506 792	60 428
Arm	92 209	4 625	94 949	4 637
Wrist	114 540	4 486	110 232	3 946
Hands except fingers	92 405	13 197	88 123	12 116
Fingers	192 634	41 376	187 390	38 212
Hands and fingers	6 907	697	6 777	800
Hands and wrists	5 325	329	5 553	238
Hands and arms	3 821	417	4 042	56
Lower extremities	440 016	9 313	443 751	9 149

Table 8.19 Incidence rates for non-fatal occupational injuries due to hand tools classified by part of body affected.

Part of body	1993		1994	
	Total incidence	Due to hand tools	Total incidence	Due to hand tools
All private industry	285.6	13.4	277.0	12.3
Head	19.7	1.1	18.7	1.1
Neck	5.2	0.1	5.0	0.1
Trunk, including shoulder, back, abdomen and pelvic region	110.2	2.4	107.3	2.3
Upper extremities	65.8	8.3	62.8	7.5
Arm	11.7	0.6	11.8	0.6
Wrist	14.5	0.6	13.6	0.5
Hands except fingers	11.7	1.7	10.9	1.5
Fingers	24.4	5.2	23.2	4.7
Hands and fingers	0.9	0.1	0.8	0.1
Hands and wrists	0.7	–	0.7	–
Hands and arms	0.5	–	0.5	–
Lower extremities	55.8	1.2	55.0	1.1

Incidence rates represent the number of injuries and illnesses per 10 000 full-time workers and are computed as follows:

Incidence rate $= (N/EH \times 20\ 000\ 000)$, where
  N is the number of injuries and illnesses
  EH is the total hours worked by all employees during the calendar year
  20 000 000 is the base for 10 000 equivalent full-time workers (working 40 hours per week, 50 weeks per year).

Table 8.20 Non-fatal occupational injuries in the USA due to different types of non-powered hand tools classified by the part of body affected.

Type of tool	Total number		Back		Shoulder		Finger		Hand		Wrist	
	1993	1994	1993	1994	1993	1994	1993	1994	1993	1994	1993	1994
A	2 252 591	2 236 639	615 010	606 545	105 881	109 543	192 634	187 390	92 405	88 123	114 540	110 232
B	141 794	133 347	22 687	21 564	5 025	4 795	44 978	41 510	14 786	13 405	5 517	5 092
C	70 721	65 300	8 639	8 814	1 875	2 061	31 090	28 581	9 541	8 442	2 766	2 417
D	688	511	64	77	19	38	152	87	78	50	82	36
E	38 462	34 016	268	352	168	71	24 511	21 923	7 177	6 006	1 188	996
F	6 073	6 440	3 425	3 743	278	387	171	200	135	131	300	274
G	1 787	1 673	175	245	41	36	625	537	185	175	106	77
H	819	650	180	115	17	15	101	144	38	49	31	28
I	6 926	7 968	784	797	254	367	2 527	3 039	751	915	270	354
J	1 010	841	111	82	19	19	435	325	108	99	117	78
K	6 367	5 929	1 166	1 115	550	585	1 399	1 356	518	591	327	277
L	8 060	6 868	2 320	2 156	481	518	1 134	928	454	407	309	286

A refers to all injuries in private industry
B refers to all tools, instruments, and equipment
C refers to all non-powered hand tools
D refers to non-powered boring hand tools
E refers to non-powered cutting hand tools
F refers to non-powered digging hand tools
G refers to non-powered gripping hand tools
H refers to non-powered measuring hand tools
I refers to non-powered striking and nailing hand tools
J refers to non-powered surfacing hand tools
K refers to non-powered turning hand tools
L refers to other categories of non-powered hand tools such as crowbars, pitchforks, staplers, etc.

Table 8.21 Incidence of non-fatal occupational injuries in the USA due to different types of non-powered hand tools classified by the part of body affected.

Tool type	Total incidence		Back		Shoulder		Finger		Hand		Wrist	
	1993	1994	1993	1994	1993	1994	1993	1994	1993	1994	1993	1994
A	285.6	277.0	78.0	75.1	13.4	13.6	24.4	23.2	11.7	10.9	14.5	13.6
B	18.0	16.5	2.9	2.7	0.6	0.6	5.7	5.1	1.9	1.7	0.7	0.6
C	9.0	8.1	1.1	1.1	0.2	0.3	3.9	3.5	1.2	1.0	0.4	0.3
D	0.1	0.1	–	–	–	–	–	–	–	–	–	–
E	4.9	4.2	–	–	–	–	3.1	2.7	0.9	0.7	0.2	0.1
F	0.8	0.8	0.6	0.5	0.4	–	–	–	–	–	–	–
G	0.2	0.2	–	–	–	–	0.1	0.1	–	–	–	–
H	0.1	0.1	–	–	–	–	–	–	–	–	–	–
I	0.9	1.0	0.1	0.1	–	–	0.3	0.4	0.1	0.1	–	–
J	0.1	0.1	–	–	–	–	0.1	–	–	–	–	–
K	0.8	0.7	0.2	0.1	0.1	0.1	0.2	0.1	0.1	–	–	–
L	1.0	0.8	0.3	0.3	0.1	0.1	0.1	0.1	0.1	–	–	–

A refers to injury incidence in all industries
B refers to injury incidence due to all tools, instruments and equipment
C refers to injury incidence due to all non-powered hand tools
D refers to injury incidence due to non-powered boring hand tools
E refers to injury incidence due to non-powered cutting hand tools
F refers to injury incidence due to non-powered digging hand tools
G refers to injury incidence due to non-powered gripping hand tools
H refers to injury incidence due to non-powered measuring hand tools
I refers to injury incidence due to non-powered striking and nailing hand tools
J refers to injury incidence due to non-powered surfacing hand tools
K refers to injury incidence due to non-powered turning hand tools
L refers to injury incidence due to other non-powered hand tools such as crowbars, pitchforks

Incidence rates represent the number of injuries and illnesses per 10 000 full-time workers and are computed as follows:

Incidence rate = $(N/EH \times 20\ 000\ 000)$, where
  N is the number of injuries and illnesses
  EH is the total hours worked by all employees during the calendar year
  20 000 000 is the base for 10 000 equivalent full-time workers (working 40 hours per week, 50 weeks per year).

(about 26 per cent), and non-powered turning hand tools (about 13 per cent) caused the most incidence of injuries to the back (Tables 8.20 and 8.21).

The body parts most significantly affected by the use of powered hand tools include the fingers (nearly 27 per cent of injuries due to powered hand tools occurred to the fingers). The hand (about 9.3 per cent) and the back (about 10 per cent) were the other body parts affected by powered hand tools. Among the different types of powered hand tools, powered striking and nailing hand tools caused the most injuries to the back; powered cutting hand tools, and powered boring hand tools caused the most injuries to the fingers; powered cutting hand tools caused the most injuries to the hand (Tables 8.22 and 8.23).

Table 8.22 Non-fatal occupational injuries in the USA due to different types of powered hand tools classified by part of body affected.

Type of tool	Total number		Back		Shoulder		Finger		Hand		Wrist	
	1993	1994	1993	1994	1993	1994	1993	1994	1993	1994	1993	1994
A	2 252 591	2 236 639	615 010	606 545	105 881	109 543	192 634	187 390	92 405	88 123	114 540	110 232
B	141 794	133 347	22 687	21 564	5 025	4 795	44 978	41 510	14 786	13 405	5 517	5 092
C	26 422	25 857	2 760	2 325	578	612	7 179	6 183	2 466	2 630	1 369	1 178
D	3 115	3 724	163	378	98	85	1 296	1 467	491	462	259	316
E	6 826	6 074	484	296	53	100	2 982	2 308	611	886	304	287
F	2 812	2 491	916	714	112	112	407	410	95	161	132	144
G	4 250	3 684	616	408	90	148	1 334	903	423	415	374	174
H	1 066	876	61	92	53	60	336	293	191	112	76	100
I	5 835	6 826	173	214	44	26	277	350	231	274	63	44
J	2 083	1 729	298	177	108	54	460	369	362	245	137	82

A refers to all injuries in private industry
B refers to all tools, instruments, and equipment
C refers to all powered hand tools
D refers to powered boring hand tools
E refers to powered cutting hand tools
F refers to powered striking and nailing hand tools
G refers to powered surfacing hand tools
H refers to powered turning hand tools
I refers to powered welding and heating hand tools
J refers to other powered hand tools such as nail guns, scrappers, etc.

Table 8.23 Incidence of non-fatal occupational injuries in the USA due to different types of powered hand tools classified by the part of body affected.

Tool type	Total incidence		Back		Shoulder		Finger		Hand		Wrist	
	1993	1994	1993	1994	1993	1994	1993	1994	1993	1994	1993	1994
A	285.6	277.0	78.0	75.1	13.4	13.6	24.4	23.2	11.7	10.9	14.5	13.6
B	18.0	16.5	2.9	2.7	0.6	0.6	5.9	5.1	1.7	1.7	0.7	0.6
C	3.4	3.2	0.4	0.3	0.1	0.1	0.9	0.8	0.3	0.3	0.2	0.2
D	0.4	0.5	–	–	–	–	0.2	0.2	0.1	0.1	–	–
E	0.4	0.8	0.1	–	–	–	–	0.3	–	0.1	–	–
F	0.4	0.3	0.1	0.1	–	–	–	–	–	–	–	–
G	0.5	0.5	0.1	–	–	–	0.2	0.1	–	–	–	–
H	0.1	0.1	–	–	–	–	–	–	–	–	–	–
I	0.7	0.8	–	–	–	–	–	–	–	–	–	–
J	0.3	0.2	–	–	–	–	0.1	–	–	–	–	–

A refers to total injury incidence for all private industry
B refers to injury incidence due to all tools, instruments and equipment
C refers to injury incidence due to all powered hand tools
D refers to injury incidence due to powered boring hand tools
E refers to injury incidence due to powered cutting hand tools
F refers to injury incidence due to powered striking and nailing hand tools
G refers to injury incidence due to powered surfacing hand tools
H refers to injury incidence due to powered turning hand tools
I refers to injury incidence due to powered welding and heating hand tools
J refers to injury incidence due to all other powered hand tools such as nail guns, scrubbers, sprayers, etc.

Incidence rates represent the number of injuries and illnesses per 10 000 full-time workers and are computed as follows:

Incidence rate = (N/EH × 20 000 000), where
    N is the number of injuries
    EH is the total hours worked by all employees during the calendar year
    20 000 000 is the base for 10 000 equivalent full-time workers (working 40 hours per week, 50 weeks per year).

Events/exposure leading to hand tool injuries

In 1993 and 1994, the most significant event or exposure leading to injury due to the use of non-powered hand tools was being struck by objects. Nearly 61 per cent of the non-powered hand tool injuries happened in this manner. Overexertion was the next leading cause of non-powered hand tool injuries (nearly 23 per cent). Being struck against objects (9 per cent), and being caught in objects (2 per cent) were the other significant events leading to non-powered hand tool injuries. Non-powered cutting hand tools caused nearly 70 per cent of all cases of being struck by objects. Non-powered digging hand tools, other non-powered hand tools such as crowbars, pitchforks, etc., and non-powered turning hand tools caused the most cases of overexertion injuries. Non-powered cutting hand tools, again, caused the most exposures of being struck against objects, and being caught in objects (Tables 8.24 and 8.25).

Table 8.24 Non-fatal occupational injuries in the USA due to different types of non-powered hand tools classified by the event/exposure leading to injury.

Tool type	Total number		Struck by object		Struck against object		Caught in object		Overexertion	
	1993	1994	1993	1994	1993	1994	1993	1994	1993	1994
A	2 252 591	2 236 639	294 177	292 609	161 753	162 269	98 846	96 840	635 802	613 251
B	141 794	133 347	64 277	60 608	14 670	12 576	6 886	6 919	37 746	35 497
C	70 721	65 300	42 880	40 629	6 709	5 308	1 690	1 305	15 958	15 391
D	688	511	188	149	93	38	134	36	162	156
E	38 462	34 016	30 042	27 691	5 129	3 918	399	185	812	778
F	6 073	6 440	658	592	177	193	21	–	4 920	5 432
G	1 787	1 673	630	416	172	264	397	398	510	485
H	819	650	283	264	129	101	32	42	308	172
I	6 926	7 968	4 934	5 898	229	112	56	51	1 568	1 764
J	1 010	841	589	387	132	163	16	31	214	204
K	6 367	5 929	2 606	2 931	130	97	278	213	3 172	2 542
L	8 060	6 868	2 794	2 153	505	418	349	329	4 018	3 660

A refers to all injuries in private industry
B refers to all tools, instruments, and equipment
C refers to all non-powered hand tools
D refers to non-powered boring hand tools
E refers to non-powered cutting hand tools
F refers to non-powered digging hand tools
G refers to non-powered gripping hand tools
H refers to non-powered measuring hand tools
I refers to non-powered striking and nailing hand tools
J refers to non-powered surfacing hand tools
K refers to non-powered turning hand tools
L refers to other categories of non-powered hand tools such as crowbars, pitchforks, staplers, etc.

Table 8.25 Incidence of non-fatal occupational injuries in the USA due to different types of non-powered hand tools classified by the event/exposure leading to injury.

Tool type	Total incidence		Struck by object		Struck against object		Caught in object		Overexertion		Repetitive motion	
	1993	1994	1993	1994	1993	1994	1993	1994	1993	1994	1993	1994
A	285.6	277.0	37.3	36.2	20.5	20.1	12.5	12.0	80.6	76.0	12.0	11.5
B	18.0	16.5	8.2	7.5	1.9	1.6	0.9	0.9	4.8	4.4	–	–
C	9.0	8.1	5.4	5.0	0.8	0.7	0.2	0.2	2.0	1.9	–	–
D	0.1	0.1	–	–	–	–	–	–	–	–	–	–
E	4.9	4.2	3.8	3.4	0.6	0.5	–	–	0.1	0.1	–	–
F	0.8	0.8	0.1	0.1	–	–	–	–	0.6	0.7	–	–
G	0.2	0.2	0.1	–	–	–	–	–	0.1	0.1	–	–
H	0.1	0.1	–	–	–	–	–	–	–	–	–	–
I	0.9	1.0	0.6	0.7	–	–	–	–	0.2	0.2	–	–
J	0.1	0.1	0.1	–	–	–	–	–	–	–	–	–
K	0.8	0.7	0.3	0.4	–	–	–	–	0.4	0.3	–	–
L	1.0	0.8	0.4	0.3	0.1	–	–	–	0.5	0.4	–	–

A refers to injury incidence in all private industry
B refers to injury incidence due to all tools, instruments, and equipment
C refers to injury incidence due to all non-powered hand tools
D refers to injury incidence due to non-powered boring hand tools
E refers to injury incidence due to non-powered cutting hand tools
F refers to injury incidence due to non-powered digging hand tools
G refers to injury incidence due to non-powered gripping hand tools
H refers to injury incidence due to non-powered measuring hand tools
I refers to injury incidence due to non-powered striking and nailing hand tools
J refers to injury incidence due to non-powered surfacing hand tools
K refers to injury incidence due to non-powered turning hand tools
L refers to injury incidence due to all other non-powered hand tools such as crowbars, pitchforks, stapling tools etc.

Incidence rates represent the number of injuries and illnesses per 10 000 full-time workers and are computed as follows:

Incidence rate = $(N/EH \times 20\,000\,000)$, where
   N is the number of injuries and illnesses
   EH is the total hours worked by all employees during the calendar year
   20 000 000 is the base for 10 000 full-time workers (working 40 hours per week, 50 weeks per year).

Being struck by objects was the most significant event or exposure leading to injuries due to use of powered hand tools. Nearly 31 per cent of all hand tool injuries due to powered hand tools were caused by being struck by objects. Overexertion was the next major event/exposure leading to injury (about 20 per cent). Powered cutting hand tools caused most cases struck by objects (nearly 38 per cent), followed by powered surfacing hand tools (about 18 per cent). For cases reporting being struck against objects, and being caught in objects, again, powered cutting hand tools and powered surfacing hand tools resulted in most injuries. Powered striking and nailing hand tools (21 per cent), and

Table 8.26 Non-fatal occupational injuries in the USA due to different powered hand tools classified by the event/exposure leading to injury.

Tool type	Total number		Struck by object		Struck against object		Caught in object		Overexertion	
	1993	1994	1993	1994	1993	1994	1993	1994	1993	1994
A	2 252 591	2 236 639	294 177	292 609	161 753	162 269	98 846	96 840	635 802	613 251
B	141 794	133 347	64 277	60 608	14 670	12 576	6 886	6 919	37 746	35 497
C	26 422	25 857	8 861	7 951	2 546	2 505	2 736	3 179	5 431	4 447
D	3 115	3 724	1 487	1 130	227	277	495	1 068	697	971
E	6 826	6 074	3 222	3 093	1 318	1 400	1 119	790	698	464
F	2 812	2 491	846	766	65	104	249	306	1 189	890
G	4 250	3 684	1 601	1 503	712	500	504	533	1 176	826
H	1 066	876	540	377	42	15	88	91	339	313
I	5 835	6 826	126	129	27	62	73	177	392	334
J	2 083	1 729	923	759	149	139	158	159	727	476

A refers to all injuries in private industry
B refers to all tools, instruments, and equipment
C refers to all powered hand tools
D refers to powered boring hand tools
E refers to powered cutting hand tools
F refers to powered striking and nailing hand tools
G refers to powered surfacing hand tools
H refers to powered turning hand tools
I refers to powered welding and heating hand tools
J refers to other powered hand tools such as nail guns, scrappers, etc.

Table 8.27 Incidence of non-fatal occupational injuries in the USA due to different types of powered hand tools classified by the event/exposure leading to injury.

Tool type	Total incidence		Struck by object		Struck against object		Caught in object		Overexertion		Repetitive motion	
	1993	1994	1993	1994	1993	1994	1993	1994	1993	1994	1993	1994
A	285.6	277.0	37.3	36.2	20.5	20.1	12.5	12.0	80.6	76.0	12.0	11.5
B	18.0	16.5	8.2	7.5	1.9	1.6	0.9	0.9	4.8	4.4	–	–
C	3.4	3.2	1.1	1.0	0.3	0.3	0.4	0.4	0.7	0.6	–	–
D	0.4	0.5	0.2	0.1	–	–	0.1	0.1	0.1	0.1	–	–
E	0.9	0.8	0.4	0.4	0.2	0.2	0.1	0.1	0.1	0.1	–	–
F	0.4	0.3	0.1	0.1	–	–	–	–	0.2	0.1	–	–
G	0.5	0.5	0.2	0.2	0.1	0.1	0.1	0.1	0.2	0.1	–	–
H	0.1	0.1	0.1	–	–	–	–	–	–	–	–	–
I	0.7	0.8	–	–	–	–	–	–	–	–	–	–
J	0.3	0.2	0.1	0.1	–	–	–	–	0.1	0.1	–	–

A refers to injury incidence in all private industry
B refers to injury incidence due to all tools, instruments, and equipment
C refers to injury incidence due to all powered hand tools
D refers to injury incidence due to powered boring hand tools
E refers to injury incidence due to powered cutting hand tools
F refers to injury incidence due to powered striking and nailing hand tools
G refers to injury incidence due to powered surfacing hand tools
H refers to injury incidence due to powered turning hand tools
I refers to injury incidence due to powered welding and heating hand tools
J refers to injury incidence due to all other powered hand tools such as nail guns, scrubbers, sprayers, etc.

Incidence rates represent the number of injuries and illnesses per 10 000 full-time workers and are computed as follows:

Incidence rate = (N/EH × 20 000 000), where
   N is the number of injuries and illnesses
   EH is the total hours worked by all employees during the calendar year
   20 000 000 is the base for 10 000 equivalent full-time workers (working 40 hours per week, 50 weeks per year).

powered surfacing hand tools (20 per cent) were the leading categories of powered hand tools causing overexertion injuries (Tables 8.26 and 8.27).

Age and hand tool injuries

In 1993 and 1994, nearly 35 per cent of all injuries due to non-powered hand tools happened to workers in the age group 25 to 34 years. Also, about 22 per cent of workers in the age group 35 to 44 years were affected by non-powered hand tool injuries. About 19 per cent of the workers in the 20 to 24 years age group were affected by non-powered hand tool injuries. For the most severely affected age group (25 to 34 years), a majority of the injuries (nearly 53 per cent) were due to non-powered cutting tools. Non-powered striking and nailing hand tools (about 11 per cent), and non-powered digging hand tools (about 9 per cent) also significantly contributed to injuries in this age group. Non-powered cutting hand tools caused nearly 40 per cent of all injuries due to non-powered hand tools in the 35 to 44 years worker age group. Most of the other injuries in this age group were caused by other types of non-powered hand tools such as crowbars, pitchforks, etc. (about 15 per cent), and non-powered turning hand tools (about 12 per cent) (Table 8.28).

Powered hand tools, again, affected mostly the 25 to 34 years (nearly 37 per cent of all injuries), and the 35 to 44 years (nearly 24 per cent of all injuries) age groups. The age group 20 to 24 years (about 18 per cent of all injuries) was also significantly affected due to the use of powered hand tools. The use of powered cutting hand tools caused the most injuries in the 25 to 34 years age group (about 29 per cent of the injuries). Powered welding and heating hand tools closely followed, causing nearly 28 per cent of all injuries to this age group. Among the workers in the 35 to 44 years age group, powered welding and heating tools, powered cutting hand tools, and powered surfacing hand tools, all caused equally significant numbers of injuries (between 16 and 21 per cent of all injuries) (Table 8.29).

Gender and hand tool injuries

Overall, in 1993 and 1994, non-powered hand tool injuries affected nearly 80 per cent men and about 20 per cent women in the workforce. Among men, injuries due to non-powered cutting hand tools accounted for nearly 50 per cent of the total number of injuries due to non-powered hand tools. Non-powered striking and nailing tools (about 12 per cent), non-powered turning hand tools (about 11 per cent), and non-powered hand tools such as crowbars, pitchforks, etc. (about 10 per cent), accounted for the rest of the injuries due to non-powered hand tools. Among women also, most of the injuries due to non-powered hand tools (about 69 per cent) were due to non-powered cutting tools. Other types of non-powered hand tools such as crowbars and pitchforks accounted for a majority (about 14 per cent) of the rest of the injuries to women (Table 8.30). Powered hand tools affected nearly 90 per cent of the men, and nearly 10 per cent of the women. Among men, powered cutting hand tools (nearly 26 per cent of all injuries due to powered hand tools), powered welding and heating hand tools (about 26 per cent), powered surfacing hand tools (about 10 per cent), powered boring hand tools (about 11 per cent), and powered striking and nailing hand tools (nearly 9 per cent) caused the most injuries. Among women, the use of powered surfacing hand tools (nearly 23 per cent of the injuries due to powered hand tools), and the use of powered cutting hand tools (about 17 per cent) caused the most occupational injuries (Table 8.31).

Days away from work due to hand tool injuries

On an average, in 1993 and 1994, due to the use of non-powered hand tools, workers stayed away from work for only one day in nearly 24 per cent of the cases. In nearly 21 per cent of the cases, the days away from work due to non-powered hand tool injury was reported as between three and five days. In nearly 14 per cent of the cases, workers stayed away from work for six to ten days due to non-powered hand tool injuries. For injuries due to non-powered boring hand tools, workers in nearly 23 per cent of the cases stayed away from work for a day, and in nearly 16 per cent of the cases they stayed away from work for 31 days or more. About 20 per cent of the non-powered boring hand tool injury cases stayed away from work for three to five days. Workers injured due to non-powered cutting hand tools stayed away from work for a day in nearly 27 per cent of the cases, and

Table 8.28 Non-fatal occupational injuries in the USA due to different types of non-powered hand tools classified by the age of the affected hand tool user.

Tool type	A		Under 14 years		14 to 15 years		16 to 19 years		20 to 24 years		25 to 34 years		35 to 44 years		45 to 54 years		55 to 64 years		65 years and older	
	1993	1994	1993	1994	1993	1994	1993	1994	1993	1994	1993	1994	1993	1994	1993	1994	1993	1994	1993	1994
A	2 252 591	2 236 639	23	55	889	1 181	95 790	97 262	319 708	307 775	724 354	708 047	566 429	576 932	323 503	327 911	148 249	147 474	21 604	21 050
B	141 794	133 347	–	–	61	156	8 503	8 315	25 404	23 826	50 160	44 767	30 933	31 576	16 218	15 152	6 998	6 744	722	670
C	70 721	65 300	–	–	50	130	5 895	5 138	14 280	12 457	24 838	21 790	14 206	14 849	6 923	6 559	2 978	2 851	343	245
D	688	511	–	–	–	–	21	36	103	39	263	190	155	156	111	47	12	–	–	17
E	38 462	34 016	–	–	47	65	4 680	4 273	10 320	8 265	13 241	11 072	5 593	5 933	2 663	2 384	1 119	1 060	184	115
F	6 073	6 440	–	–	–	–	236	195	764	991	2 336	2 206	1 692	1 839	619	787	337	267	10	–
G	1 787	1 673	–	–	–	–	34	14	216	137	594	548	505	597	267	242	120	78	–	32
H	819	650	–	–	–	–	35	38	111	94	314	228	155	135	120	103	70	51	–	–
I	6 926	7 968	–	–	–	62	303	182	981	1 371	2 673	2 944	1 717	1 966	700	868	376	462	43	14
J	1 010	841	–	–	–	–	72	–	217	102	351	367	249	218	46	73	26	56	–	–
K	6 367	5 929	–	–	–	–	82	77	724	568	2 218	2 142	1 773	1 733	1 005	918	465	433	28	20
L	8 060	6 868	–	–	–	–	422	293	779	851	2 653	1 993	2 232	2 134	1 306	1 080	421	381	71	38

A refers to all injuries in the private industry
B refers to all tools, instruments and equipment
C refers to all non-powered hand tools
D refers to non-powered boring hand tools
E refers to non-powered cutting hand tools
F refers to non-powered digging hand tools
G refers to non-powered gripping hand tools
H refers to non-powered measuring hand tools
I refers to non-powered striking and nailing hand tools
J refers to non-powered surfacing hand tools
K refers to non-powered turning hand tools
L refers to all other non-powered hand tools such as crowbars, pitchforks, stapling tools, etc.

Table 8.29 Non-fatal occupational injuries in the USA due to different types of powered hand tools classified by the age of the affected hand tool user.

Tool type	A		Under 14 years		14 to 15 years		16 to 19 years		20 to 24 years		25 to 34 years		35 to 44 years		45 to 54 years		55 to 64 years		65 years and older	
	1993	1994	1993	1994	1993	1994	1993	1994	1993	1994	1993	1994	1993	1994	1993	1994	1993	1994	1993	1994
	2 252 591	2 236 639	23	55	889	1 181	95 790	97 262	319 708	307 775	724 354	708 047	566 429	576 932	323 503	327 911	148 249	147 474	21 604	21 050
B	141 794	133 347	–	–	61	156	8 503	8 315	25 404	23 826	50 160	44 767	30 933	31 576	16 218	15 152	6 998	6 744	722	670
C	26 422	25 857	–	–	–	–	1 000	1 358	4 768	5 037	9 788	9 016	6 198	6 393	2 825	2 614	1 332	1 075	99	115
D	3 115	3 724	–	–	–	–	96	238	621	446	1 044	1 400	759	1 032	289	395	218	161	–	35
E	6 826	6 074	–	–	–	–	310	329	1 216	1 566	2 844	1 869	1 324	1 325	639	638	388	270	37	18
F	2 812	2 491	–	–	–	–	118	53	488	337	1 063	885	803	754	226	284	82	140	–	–
G	4 250	3 684	–	–	–	–	119	288	669	741	1 364	1 063	1 050	959	653	373	294	207	25	–
H	1 066	876	–	–	–	–	8	18	160	134	410	264	252	235	135	142	73	70	–	–
I	5 835	6 826	–	–	–	–	225	336	1 183	1 435	2 267	2 672	1 358	1 583	541	570	168	152	11	–
J	2 083	1 729	–	–	–	–	104	85	378	332	700	684	512	406	247	166	91	55	12	–

A refers to all injuries in the private industry
B refers to all tools, instruments and equipment
C refers to all powered hand tools
D refers to powered boring hand tools
E refers to powered cutting hand tools
F refers to powered striking and nailing hand tools
G refers to powered surfacing hand tools
H refers to powered turning hand tools
I refers to powered welding and heating hand tools
J refers to all other powered hand tools such as nail guns, scrubbers, sprayers, etc.

Table 8.30 Non-fatal occupational injuries in the USA due to different types of non-powered hand tools classified by the gender of the affected hand tool user.

Tool type	Total number		Men		Women	
	1993	1994	1993	1994	1993	1994
A	2 252 591	2 236 639	1 490 418	1 483 202	735 570	730 802
B	141 794	133 347	113 959	105 506	26 925	27 203
C	70 721	65 300	57 760	52 806	12 415	12 158
D	688	511	671	457	16	54
E	38 462	34 016	29 623	25 202	8 591	8 723
F	6 073	6 440	5 521	5 952	540	425
G	1 787	1 673	1 536	1 305	224	363
H	819	650	618	472	200	172
I	6 926	7 968	6 514	7 592	309	355
J	1 010	841	684	665	325	176
K	6 367	5 929	6 023	5 646	326	252
L	8 060	6 868	6 171	5 197	1 806	1 590

A refers to all private industry
B refers to all tools, instruments, and equipment
C refers to all non-powered hand tools
D refers to non-powered boring hand tools
E refers to non-powered cutting hand tools
F refers to non-powered digging hand tools
G refers to non-powered gripping hand tools
H refers to non-powered measuring hand tools
I refers to non-powered striking and nailing hand tools
J refers to non-powered surfacing hand tools
K refers to non-powered turning hand tools
L refers to all other non-powered hand tools such as crowbars, pitchforks, stapling tools, etc.

for 31 days or more only in 5 per cent of the cases. Workers injured due to non-powered digging hand tools stayed away from work for a day in 13 per cent of the cases, and for 31 days or more in nearly 19 per cent of the cases. Workers injured due to non-powered gripping hand tools stayed away from work for a day in 21 per cent of the cases, and for 31 days or more in 18 per cent of the cases. Workers injured due to non-powered measuring hand tools stayed away from work for a day in about 24 per cent of the cases, and for 31 days or more in about 12 per cent of the cases. Workers injured due to non-powered striking and nailing hand tools stayed away from work for a day in about 24 per cent of the cases, and for 31 days or more in about 11 per cent of the cases. Workers injured due to non-powered surfacing hand tools stayed away from work for a day in about 28 per cent of the cases, and for 31 days or more in about 7 per cent of the cases. Workers injured due to non-powered turning hand tools stayed away from work for a day in nearly 19 per cent of the cases, and for 31 days or more in nearly 16 per cent of the cases. Workers injured due to all other non-powered hand tools such as crowbars, pitchforks, etc., stayed away from work for a day in nearly 17 per cent of the cases, and for 31 days or more in nearly 16 per cent of the cases (Table 8.32).

Overall, workers injured due to powered hand tools missed work for a day in nearly 25 per cent of the cases, and missed work for 31 days or more in nearly 13 per cent of the

Table 8.31 Non-fatal occupational injuries in the USA due to different types of powered
hand tools classified by the gender of the affected hand tool user.

Tool type	Total number		Men		Women	
	1993	1994	1993	1994	1993	1994
A	2 252 591	2 236 639	1 490 418	1 483 202	735 570	730 802
B	141 794	133 347	113 959	105 506	26 925	27 203
C	26 422	25 857	24 299	23 467	2 027	2 307
D	3 115	3 724	2 897	3 464	207	229
E	6 826	6 074	6 445	5 675	366	395
F	2 812	2 491	2 649	2 254	158	220
G	4 250	3 684	3 761	3 163	468	516
H	1 066	876	905	694	161	182
I	5 835	6 826	5 556	6 458	248	345
J	2 083	1 729	1 778	1 438	304	290

A refers to all private industry
B refers to all tools, instruments, and equipment
C refers to all powered hand tools
D refers to powered boring hand tools
E refers to powered cutting hand tools
F refers to powered striking and nailing hand tools
G refers to powered surfacing hand tools
H refers to powered turning hand tools
I refers to powered welding and heating hand tools
J refers to all other powered hand tools such as nail guns, scrubbers, etc.

cases. These numbers were nearly 14 per cent and 12 per cent, respectively, for powered
boring hand tools; 15 per cent and 18 per cent, respectively, for powered cutting hand
tools; 19 per cent and 22 per cent, respectively, for powered striking and nailing hand
tools; 24 per cent and 10 per cent, respectively, for powered gripping hand tools; 21 per
cent and 15 per cent, respectively, for powered turning hand tools; 52 per cent and 3 per
cent, respectively, for powered welding and heating hand tools; and 19 per cent and 18
per cent, respectively, for other powered hand tools such as nail guns, scrubbers, etc.
(Table 8.33).

ANATOMY OF THE HAND AND FOREARM

The force/torque generation and exertion capabilities of the human hand depend upon the
structure of the human hand and forearm. Figure 8.1 shows the bones making up the hand
and the arm. The forearm consists of two bones – the radius and the ulna. The radius is
the lateral bone of the forearm. It has a small, flat, and round head in its proximal region.
Its distal extremity is expanded, and forms a major portion of the wrist joint. The ulna, on
the other hand, is large proximally, and narrows into a small, round head, at its distal end.
These two bones are joined by the synovial joints, both proximally and distally. The
proximal joint shares an articular capsule with the elbow joint; the distal joint shares one
with the wrist. The bones are parallel to each other in the supine position. The radius

Table 8.32 Non-fatal occupational injuries in the USA due to different types of non-powered hand tools classified by the extent of days away from work due to the injury.

Tool type	Total number		% of cases involving												
			1 day		2 days		3 to 5 days		6 to 10 days		11 to 20 days		21 to 30 days		31 days or more	
	1993	1994	1993	1994	1993	1994	1993	1994	1993	1994	1993	1994	1993	1994	1993	1994
A	2 252 591	2 236 639	16.3	16.3	13.0	12.9	20.7	21.0	13.4	13.3	11.4	11.2	6.3	6.4	19.0	18.9
B	141 794	133 347	22.5	23.1	15.3	14.7	20.1	21.6	14.4	13.4	9.6	9.8	5.0	5.2	13.0	12.2
C	70 721	65 300	23.6	24.7	16.1	14.3	21.2	22.1	15.5	14.1	9.3	9.8	4.5	4.9	9.8	10.1
D	688	511	20.4	24.5	14.8	12.1	18.9	22.7	5.6	15.2	11.1	8.2	13.8	1.4	15.5	15.8
E	38 462	34 016	26.8	29.2	18.5	15.2	21.1	24.1	17.4	14.1	8.1	8.4	3.4	3.2	4.7	5.8
F	6 073	6 440	13.5	12.8	10.6	9.6	22.2	20.7	15.9	15.9	12.9	14.9	5.3	7.5	19.6	18.6
G	1 787	1 673	21.0	25.2	15.0	16.5	19.3	23.3	9.8	10.6	10.5	10.2	5.5	5.3	18.9	8.8
H	819	650	26.2	21.2	15.5	9.5	16.9	27.6	11.5	9.7	12.8	6.5	3.5	13.5	13.6	11.9
I	6 926	7 968	23.1	24.6	16.3	15.1	22.4	17.0	11.7	13.8	10.3	10.9	5.7	7.0	10.5	11.6
J	1 010	841	21.6	28.3	18.1	14.8	24.6	25.5	22.1	12.7	2.9	3.4	4.3	8.2	6.4	7.1
K	6 367	5 929	18.8	20.7	12.7	10.4	19.7	20.1	12.1	15.5	10.7	11.6	7.8	5.8	18.4	15.9
L	8 060	6 868	22.0	16.8	12.2	17.4	21.4	19.5	13.7	13.0	9.5	10.1	4.9	6.8	16.4	16.5

A refers to total in all private industry
B refers to all tools, instruments and equipment
C refers to all non-powered hand tools
D refers to non-powered boring hand tools
E refers to non-powered cutting hand tools
F refers to non-powered digging hand tools
G refers to non-powered gripping hand tools
H refers to non-powered measuring hand tools
I refers to non-powered striking and nailing hand tools
J refers to non-powered surfacing hand tools
K refers to non-powered turning hand tools
L refers to all other non-powered hand tools such as crowbars, pitchforks, stapling tools, etc.

Table 8.33 Non-fatal occupational injuries in the USA due to different types of powered hand tools classified by the extent of days away from work due to the injury.

Tool type	Total number		% of cases involving												
			1 day		2 days		3 to 5 days		6 to 10 days		11 to 20 days		21 to 30 days		31 days or more	
	1993	1994	1993	1994	1993	1994	1993	1994	1993	1994	1993	1994	1993	1994	1993	1994
A	2 252 591	2 236 639	16.3	16.3	13.0	12.9	20.7	21.0	13.4	13.3	11.4	11.2	6.3	6.4	19.0	18.9
B	141 794	133 347	22.5	23.1	15.3	14.7	20.1	21.6	14.4	13.4	9.6	9.8	5.0	5.2	13.0	12.2
C	26 422	25 857	24.9	26.8	13.9	14.1	18.7	19.6	11.6	12.4	10.9	9.7	5.4	5.1	14.6	12.3
D	3 115	3 724	22.0	14.2	12.3	18.4	20.8	25.0	14.9	15.4	11.5	7.3	4.7	7.3	13.8	12.4
E	6 826	6 074	16.2	15.0	10.1	10.5	17.6	17.1	14.1	16.8	13.8	16.5	8.6	6.3	19.6	17.9
F	2 812	2 491	19.5	18.7	11.2	9.4	16.8	20.3	12.9	12.4	13.0	9.6	5.6	7.3	21.0	22.2
G	4 250	3 684	14.4	24.3	13.5	11.9	23.1	23.9	12.5	13.1	13.5	12.4	4.7	5.1	18.4	9.2
H	1 066	876	16.1	21.2	12.7	7.3	18.6	27.0	13.1	15.1	9.3	11.9	12.9	3.1	17.3	14.4
I	5 835	6 826	51.5	52.3	22.1	19.2	14.4	15.5	4.2	5.1	3.5	3.2	1.3	1.7	3.1	3.0
J	2 083	1 729	19.5	19.6	11.7	12.4	23.2	20.6	13.7	14.8	10.9	10.5	5.8	3.7	15.1	18.4

A refers to total in all private industry
B refers to all tools, instruments and equipment
C refers to all powered hand tools
D refers to powered boring hand tools
E refers to powered cutting hand tools
F refers to powered striking and nailing hand tools
G refers to powered gripping hand tools
H refers to powered turning hand tools
I refers to powered welding and heating hand tools
J refers to all other powered hand tools such as nail guns, scrubbers, sprayers, etc.

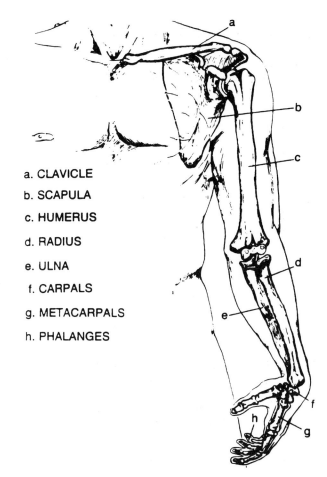

a. CLAVICLE

b. SCAPULA

c. HUMERUS

d. RADIUS

e. ULNA

f. CARPALS

g. METACARPALS

h. PHALANGES

Figure 8.1 Bones of the hand and the arm (from Putz-Anderson, 1988).

connects to the thumb side of the wrist, while the ulna connects to the little finger side of the wrist. When the hand is pronated, the radius is wrapped around the ulna. The hand also includes eight carpal bones, five metacarpals, and 14 phalanges. The bones of the carpus are arranged in two rows. Each of the digits is composed of three phalanges except the thumb, which has two. These phalanges are named according to their position as proximal, middle or medial, and distal.

There are four major nerves in the forearm and the hand. They are the median nerve, the musculocutaneous nerve, the ulnar nerve, and the radial nerve. These nerves innervate the skin and control the muscular contraction in the hand and the forearm.

The muscles that produce flexion in the wrist are called the flexor carpi radialis and flexor carpi ulnaris. Extension in the wrist is produced by the extensor carpi radialis longus, the extensor carpi radialis brevis, and the extensor carpi ulnaris. Abduction or radial deviation of the wrist is made possible by the extensor carpi radialis longus, the flexor carpi radialis, and the abductor pollicis longus. The flexor carpi ulnaris and the extensor carpi ulnaris help in the adduction or ulnar deviation of the wrist. The muscles that make hand motion possible are: lumbricals, dorsal and ventral interossei, flexor digitorum profundus, and flexor digitorum superficialis (metacarpophalangeal (MP) flexion except for the thumb); extensor digitorum (MP extension except for the thumb); dorsal

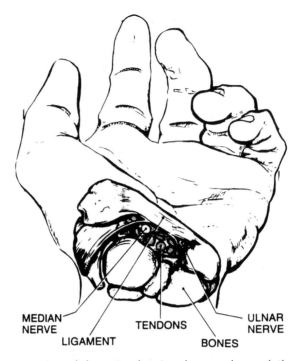

MEDIAN NERVE   TENDONS   ULNAR NERVE

LIGAMENT   BONES

Figure 8.2 A cross-section of the wrist showing the carpal tunnel (from Putz-Anderson, 1988).

interossei (digital abduction); ventral interossei (digital adduction); lumbricals, dorsal and ventral interossei (proximal interphalangeal (IP) extension); lumbrical, dorsal, and ventral interossei (distal IP extension); flexor digitorum superficialis and flexor digitorum profundus (proximal IP flexion); flexor digitorum profundus (distal IP flexion); flexor pollicis longus and brevis (thumb flexion); extensor pollicis longus and brevis (thumb extension); abductor pollicis longus and brevis (thumb abduction); adductor pollicis (thumb adduction); and opponens pollicis, abductor pollicis brevis and flexor pollicis brevis (opposition of the thumb). These muscles are connected to the bones by tendons. The tendons that are connected to the fingers pass through a channel-like structure in the wrist called the carpal tunnel. The various nerves and blood vessels also pass through this channel (Figure 8.2). The wrist joint can move only in two planes. Movement in one plane allows for ulnar and radial deviations. Movement in the second plane, perpendicular to the first plane, allows for flexion and dorsiflexion.

TOOL AND TASK RELATED FACTORS IN HAND TOOL DESIGN

Grip

Types of grips

The human hand is dexterous enough to permit different grips. The two most common grips are the power grip, and the precision grip (Napier, 1956). The power grip is used when large forces are to be exerted. In a power grip, the tool axis is perpendicular to the axis of the forearm, and the hand is fisted with four fingers on one side and the thumb on the other side. There are three classes of power grips depending on the line of direction of the force: force parallel to the forearm (e.g. saw); force at an angle to the forearm (e.g. hammer); and torque about the forearm (e.g. corkscrew).

The precision grip is primarily used for work that requires precise manipulation and control, rather than the use of large forces. In a precision grip, the tool is pinched between the thumb and fingers. There are two classes of precision grips: the internal precision grip, where the shaft of the tool is internal to the hand (e.g. a knife); and the external precision grip, where the shaft of the tool is external to the hand (e.g. pencil).

Precision grips, on an average, provide only about 20 per cent the strength of a power grip (Swanson et al., 1970). This is because precision grips use smaller muscle groups for force generation than power grips. The implication is that tools such as hammers, designed for exertion of force, should carry a power grip; tools, such as surgical knives, designed for minute manipulation, should carry a precision grip.

Angles of forearm, grip, and tool

The angles of the forearm, the grip, and the tool, are possible causative factors for upper extremity injuries and illnesses. Deviations of the wrist have been shown to result in productivity losses (Tichauer, 1976), and losses in grip strength of the individual by as much as 14–27 per cent (Terrell and Purswell, 1976). The recommended wrist orientation is a handshake (straight) orientation. If any bending is required, the tool, rather than the wrist should be bent (Tichauer and Gage, 1977). Bending the tool handles, and increasing the length of the upper portion of the handle, has been shown to result in fewer complaints of wrist stress and fatigue (Konz, 1986; Schoenmarklin and Marras, 1989a, 1989b; Tichauer, 1966a; Yoder et al., 1973). To avoid wrist deviation in the direction of the ulna when exerting large forces on a straight tool handle, the recommendation is to keep the long axis of the forearm parallel to the direction of exertion of the force (Armstrong, 1983). Further, the tool handle axis should be at 80 degrees from the long axis of the tool (as in a pistol grip) whenever large forces are to be exerted on a workpiece (Fraser, 1980). The angle of bend does not seem to influence task performance greatly (Konz, 1986; Schoenmarklin and Marras, 1989a), even though tasks such as vertical hammering seem to be more difficult, less accurate, and more stressful and fatiguing (Schoenmarklin and Marras, 1989b). In designing hand tools to be used by one hand, the finger forces have been found to be influenced by the grip posture of the hand. For good control and minimum fatigue while using the hand tool, researchers suggest using a primary control area of 10 to 13 cm from the wrist origin, and 8 to 12 cm from the wrist origin as the secondary control area (Kim et al., 1996). Further, the hand postures of the index and the middle fingers at the metacarpophalangeal joint and at the proximal interphalangeal joints become important (Kim et al., 1996).

Grip thickness

A range of grip thicknesses has been recommended for different types of grips and hand tools. Experiments with screwdriver handles (a precision grip) prompted Hunt (1934) to recommend an 8 mm diameter handle rather than a 16 mm diameter handle due to the slowing of work done with the thicker handle. Kao (1976) recommended a 13 mm diameter handle for a pen (again, a precision grip); however, Sperling (1986) recommended a 30 mm diameter handle compared to a 10 mm diameter handle for a pen due to observed lesser fatigue, lower recorded strain, and larger maximal force exertion with the 30 mm diameter handle. For power grips, hand size influences the diameter of the handle (Greenberg and Chaffin, 1977; Kilbom and Ekholm, 1991). According to Jonsson et al. (1977), power grips around a cylinder should surround more than half the circumference of the cylinder, without the fingers and the thumb meeting. Grip strength increases with increase in grip diameter up to a certain point, but decreases beyond a certain point with increase in grip diameter. Based on this observation, Hertzberg (1973) recommended an optimum grip diameter of 65 mm. Ayoub and LoPresti (1971) recommended 51 mm, and Greenberg and Chaffin (1977) recommended 50 mm. Fransson and Winkel (1991) recommended a grip diameter between 50 mm and 60 mm for females, and between 55 mm and 65 mm for males based on the maximum grip force recorded. In a recent study with Japanese subjects, Yakao et al. (1996) recommended an optimum grasping diameter of 30 to 40 mm for males, and 10 per cent less for females, for holding cylindrical tubes, based on the sensory testing of the dimensions of the length of the hand. Most published studies recommend a grip diameter between 50 and 60 mm. Also, while designing tools with power grips, it is to be remembered that people with small hands cannot use tools with grip diameters more than 60 mm. In designing cross-action tools such as plate shears and scissors, where the shafts/grips of the tool move, the recommended maximum span is 100 mm, and the recommended minimum span is 50 mm (Greenberg and Chaffin, 1977). Researchers also recommend the use of a spring to open the handles in cross-action tools as it will relieve the extensor muscles during the opening of the tool (Kilbom et al., 1993; Radonjic and Long, 1971). Despite design efforts such as weight and location compensation, grip dimensions and shapes continue to cause muscular strain (Boehlemann et al., 1994).

Grip length

Grip length of a tool is another grip-related factor that has been studied in the literature. Based on hand width ranges (which varies from 79 mm for a 1st percentile female (Garrett, 1969a, 1971) to 99 mm for a 99th percentile male (Garrett, 1969b, 1971)), Konz (1990) recommended a minimum grip length of 100 mm and a grip length of 125 mm for the grip to be comfortable. Other recommendations for grip length include 120 mm (Eastman Kodak Company, 1983), and grip lengths of 110 mm for men and 100 mm for women (Lindstrom, 1973). If the grip is enclosed, or if gloves are to be worn when using the hand tool, the minimum grip length recommended is 125 mm (Konz, 1990). The general recommendation is to have a grip length that would not limit the tool head opening, and at the same time avoid excessive compressive forces or stress concentrations on the tender parts of the palm. For external precision grip, the tool shaft must be at least 100 mm in length and must be long enough to be supported at the base of the first finger or the thumb. For internal precision grip, the tool should extend past the tender palm (Konz, 1990), and must not end close to the central part of the palm.

Grip force

Literature recommends a maximum grip force of 90 N based on the 95th percentile value (Greenberg and Chaffin, 1977). For situations requiring repeated force exertion, the recommendation is to use 40–50 per cent of the maximum handgrip strength of males and females while cutting with plate-shears for one minute without fatigue. In a study of the grip force and fatigue with three types of plate-shears (one ordinary and two shears

Table 8.34 Relationships between torque (%) and duration of repeated exertions (min) (from Mital and Channaveeraiah, 1988).

Tool	Regression equation
Pipe wrench	Torque $= 1.05 - 0.301$ (Time) $+ 0.08$ (Time)^2
Socket, crescent, and spanner wrenches	Torque $= 1.056 - 0.304$ (Time) $+ 0.104$ (Time)^2
Screwdrivers	Torque $= 1.024 - 0.138$ (Time) $+ 0.04$ (Time)^2

modified with springs and reduced grip spans), and three different types of plates (easy to cut, moderately difficult to cut, difficult to cut), Kilbom *et al.* (1993) found that females reduced their relative grip force from 65 per cent to 50 per cent when using the spring grip and the reduced grip span, and that males used 40 per cent, and females 60 per cent of their maximal grip force with the plate that was moderately difficult to cut. Further, they found that the total work was not influenced by the type of plate-shear. The productivity of male and female subjects (in terms of the cm cut per min) was strongly related to the hand size and the relative grip force used. Table 8.34 provides relationships in the form of regression equations, between torque and the duration of repeated exertions for different types of hand tools.

Grip surface characteristics

The characteristics of the grip surface is another factor that has been extensively studied in the literature. The general recommendation is to use a grip surface that is slightly compressible, non-conductive, and smooth (Konz, 1990). Compressible materials dampen vibration and allow for better distribution of pressure. Making the grip surface too soft, will, however, increase the risk of sharp objects, such as metal chips, getting embedded in the grip making it unsafe to use. Wood or plastic are desirable as grip handle materials as these do not absorb oil or other liquids, and do not conduct heat or electricity (Wu, 1975). The perception of hand fatigue has been shown to decrease when foam rubber grip is used (Fellows and Freivalds, 1991). The recommendation is to avoid metal handles, or encase metal handles in a rubber or plastic sheath (Konz, 1990). When using hand tools, the pressure–pain threshold has been reported to be around 500 kpa for females and 700 kpa for males (Mital, 1991). These pressures are even greater when exerting maximal power grips. Thus, to ensure distribution of the grip pressure, and to avoid excessive localised pressure resulting in pain in the hand, and consequent disruption of work, researchers recommend maximising the grip surface area. Another grip surface characteristic that has been studied includes the frictional characteristics of the grip surface. It has been shown that the frictional characteristics of the tool surface vary with the pressure exerted by the hand, with the smoothness and porosity of the surface and with contaminants (Bobjer, 1990; Buchholz *et al.*, 1988). Sweat increases the coefficient of friction, while oil and fat reduce it. Increase in pinch force also decreases the coefficient of friction. Adhesive tape and suede are recommended when moisture is present in the environment where the hand tools are handled (Buchholz *et al.*, 1988).

Grip shape

Grip shape has also been extensively studied in the literature. The most important consideration related to grip shapes is that the shape should maximise the area of contact between the palm and the grip in order to avoid pressure ridges and stress concentration points, especially in power grips. Grip pressure concentration under static and dynamic loading conditions has been shown to be related to vibration white finger syndrome (Gurram et al., 1993). Commercial hand tools, in general, have a cylindrical grip. Research with cylindrical grips shows that cylindrical handles with rounded ends maximise force (Rubarth, 1928). There are conflicting results regarding the relationship between torque and handle diameter. For turning action with cylindrical grips, Pheasant and O'Neill (1975) and Grieve and Pheasant (1982) reported that the torque was proportional to the diameter of the handle. Shih and Wang (1996) reported that the maximum volitional torque exertion capability of males and females for supination increased in direct proportion to the size of the handle, and that females had more effective torque exertion capability than males for handle sizes less than 44.5 mm. However, while Mital and Sanghavi (1986) reported an increase in the torque with an increase in grip diameter, it was not a proportional increase. Also, when there is no turning action on the grip and yet torque is exerted on the workpiece, torque varied with the lever arm (Mital and Channaveeraiah, 1988). Pheasant and O'Neill (1975) reported that the shape of the handle was not relevant as long as the hand did not slip around the handle. Since rectangular or triangular edges resist slippage, use of these shapes is recommended when a non-circular grip is used. Mital and Channaveeraiah (1988) compared cylindrical, triangular, and rectangular handles and reported that the torque exertion capability of individuals with triangular handle screwdrivers was greater than with cylindrical handle screwdrivers. For wrenches, the torque exertion capability was maximised when cylindrical handles were used. For supination, triangular shape was found more favourable than the square, hexagonal and circular handle shapes (Shih and Wang, 1996). Cochran and Riley (1986a), recommended a handle perimeter of 110 mm for knives; further, the thrust forces exerted with straight knives are about 10 per cent greater with triangular handles than with cylindrical or rectangular handles. For screwdrivers, a T-shaped handle is preferable than a straight handle as it prevents wrist deviation, and increases torque exertion capability by as much as 50 per cent (Pheasant and O'Neill, 1975). Further, the T-handle should be 25 mm in diameter, and should be slanted at an angle of 60 degrees to allow the wrist to be straight (Saran, 1973). For knives, a pistol grip at an angle of 78 degrees to the horizontal (Fraser, 1980) is preferable to a straight grip (Armstrong et al., 1982; Karlqvist, 1984). For poultry cutting knives, Fogleman et al. (1993) found that the traditional straight knife performed the worst. Further, a minus 30 degree blade in a dagger grip was found to be the best for a table cut (in terms of minimising the wrist extension, ulnar deviation and their ranges), and a plus 30 degree blade, held normally, was best for a hanging cut. The diameter of the knife handle was found to be insignificant.

Grooves, indentations and guards in grips

Commercially available hand tools have a variety of grooves, indentations, and guards. The literature does not recommend form fitting tools that have grooves for fingers, etc. (Tichauer and Gage, 1977). Grooves, in general, are too big or too small, and do not fit the user. This results in pressure ridges, nerve compression, and circulation impairment. Vertical grooves on the handle, provided by the designer to prevent the hand from slipping, cut into the palm of the hand and add to the pressure ridges. Such grooves and flutes should be avoided. If grooves are to be provided in the tool, it is desirable to use grooves that are small enough to avoid pressure concentration but large enough to provide good friction between the hand and the grip. For small hand tools used in precision work, regular size handles can be provided instead of grooves, for better control. The undesirability of grooves, however, does not mean that grooves should never be used. Slight and uniform surface indentations have been used and allow for greater torque exertion capabilities than smooth handles. A 50 mm diameter handle with knurled surface maximised torque exertion (Pheasant and O'Neill, 1975). Guards are used in front of the grip to prevent injuries from happening when the hand slips, or when the hand and tool collide against a sharp or rigid surface. Cochran and Riley (1986b) recommend guards of 1.52 cm height or above to ensure maximum safety to worker.

Effective weight of tool

The effective weight of a tool is the tool weight supported by the worker. Manually-operated precision tools have low effective weights and do not pose major health risks. However, many power grip tools (axes, hammers, saws), and power tools (especially with externally supplied pneumatic or electrical power), which use large muscle groups of the forearm, have high effective weights, and pose a health risk. In order to reduce fatigue, the recommended effective weight of tools is 2.3 kg (Eastman Kodak Company, 1983; Greenberg and Chaffin, 1977). Further, this weight should be reduced if the centre of gravity of the tool is far away from the wrist. This recommendation is corroborated in addition by Johnson and Childress (1988), who observed that powered screwdrivers weighing 1.12 kg or less do not produce significantly different EMG activity magnitudes. Workers subjectively rated tools weighing between 0.9 kg and 1.75 kg a 'feeling just right' (Armstrong *et al.*, 1989). Grant and Habes (1993) found that addition of flanges to handles to provide an additional source of coupling between the hand and the handle did not significantly reduce the grip force required to perform tool lifting tasks. In fact, they found that the grip force increased with increase in the effectiveness of the tool. For fine precision work, researchers recommend using much lighter tools than those used for work involving large muscle groups.

Type of tool

Wrenches enable greater torque exertion (about 10 to 20 times more) than screwdrivers as they use different muscles and lever arms (Mital, 1991). The torque exertion capability for screwdrivers, in general, increases with increase in handle diameter. The torque exertion capability for wrenches, in general, varies linearly with the lever arm. Exceptions include instances such as when more torque is exerted with a socket wrench than with a vise grip or a spanner wrench or a crescent wrench of about the same lever arm. The type of grip, and the nature of coupling between the tool and workpiece, sometimes create such situations.

Trigger

Many powered tools are started by a trigger, activated either by the thumb, or one or several of the other fingers. When triggers have to be activated repeatedly or for pro-longed periods of time, musculoskeletal problems arise as such repeated activities require precision as well as force exertion (for holding and guiding the tool). In order to avoid such musculoskeletal problems, researchers recommend designing the tool for activation by either hand (one hand operates while the other rests) (Tichauer, 1966b), or through the use of additional help from the middle finger in addition to the triggering action from the index finger (Lee and Cheng, 1995). According to Lee and Cheng (1995), the task demands for tripping a trigger should be less than 2 kg for single-finger triggering, and less than 4 kg for double-finger triggering. Also, to reduce the effect of continuous exertion of muscle force, the recommendation is to provide a latch (or other comparable locking mechanism) that can hold the trigger in place while the tool is in use. New developments in tactile sensing technologies are now enabling designers to develop zero-force triggers for use in common hand tools such as soldering guns, where, normally, forces in excess of 20 Newtons would be needed to operate the tool (Poeth and Freivalds, 1996).

Special purpose tools

In general, special purpose tools, even though more expensive than general purpose tools, are faster. The savings in labour cost, due to shorter time per use over the life of the tool, more than offset the high initial cost of the tool (Konz, 1990).

Power source of tools

The recommendation is to use power tools with external energy whenever possible (Konz, 1990). This is due to the cost-effectiveness of mechanical energy (compared to human energy), and the fact that the efficiency of machine power generation is much higher than the efficiency of human power generation. Besides, humans fatigue and machines do not. While powered hand tools add to the efficiency, they have been shown to cause adverse reaction forces and consequent operator discomfort, especially when such power tools have a shut-off mechanism that causes only a slow decline in torque when the tool is shut off (Freivalds and Eklund, 1993; Kihlberg et al., 1993).

Vibration characteristics

Using hand tools that vibrate, for short and prolonged periods, can cause vasospastic disease (Raynaud's disease) and contribute to carpal tunnel syndrome (Wasserman and Badger, 1973; NIOSH, 1983). While some researchers have questioned the existence of a direct relationship between vibration and carpal tunnel syndrome (Hammarskjoeld et al., 1991; Meagher, 1991; Taylor, 1988a, 1988b), Silverstein et al. (1987a), on the basis of extensive epidemiological evidence, suggest that the risk of cumulative trauma disorders (CTD) is increased by five times in jobs inducing high force/high repetitiveness/vibration compared to an increase by only two times in jobs inducing only high force/high repetitiveness. The recommendation of researchers is to avoid vibrations in the critical range of 40 to 130 Hz (Wasserman and Badger, 1973). According to the Technical Research Centre of Finland (1988), vibration levels for pneumatic screwdrivers and nut runners, when more than 126 dB, should not exceed eight hours of exposure time. Lundstrom and Johansson (1986) reported that exposure to vibration between 2 and 200 Hz leads to acute impairment of tactile sensibility. Since resonances of the hand–arm system do not occur above 1000 Hz (Iwata et al., 1971), it is important to avoid segmental vibration frequencies below 1000 Hz. NIOSH (1983) has provided general recommendations that are useful in practice: jobs should be redesigned to minimise the use of vibrating hand tools; powered hand tools should be redesigned to minimise vibration; and engineering controls, work practices, and administrative controls should be used to minimise vibration where jobs cannot be redesigned. A reduction in the vibration driving force, and the use of damping materials will reduce vibration (Andersson, 1990). Developments such as using the amount of energy absorbed by the hand and the arm as a basis for assessing risk to excessive vibration exposure (Burstrom and Lundstrom, 1994), and using an energy-flow hand–arm divider to reduce the magnitude of vibration transmitted to the hand (Cherian et al., 1996) augur well for the future.

Duration and repetitiveness of use

The duration and repetitiveness of use of a hand tool have been shown to increase the potential for risk of an occupational injury, either alone or in combination with some of the other factors discussed in the section on 'Effective weight of tool' (Cannon et al., 1981; Hammer, 1934; Kuorinka and Koskinen, 1979; Kurppa et al., 1979; Luopajarvi et al., 1979). Silverstein et al. (1987a, 1987b) observed that in highly repetitive work with high manual force exertions, the risk and prevalence of carpal tunnel syndrome was 15 times higher than in jobs with low repetitiveness and low force exertions. Depending on whether the demands on time are low, moderate, or high (see Sperling et al. (1991) for the set of criteria that determine what is low, moderate or high), high force or precision requirements in combination with high demands on time, or high force or precision requirements in combination with moderate demands on time, should be considered unacceptable. Duration and repetitiveness of work have been extensively studied by researchers. Greenberg and Chaffin (1977) reported that 2.5 kg held in one hand led to significant muscle fatigue within 20 minutes even with a comfortable working posture. When exertions have to be repeated, the duration of exertion, and the ensuing rest period, influence the time it takes to reach subjective fatigue. Thus, one-minute exertions with one minute rest periods lead to fatigue within four hours if 5.6 kg are held in one hand. If the weight of the object is 1.9 kg, one-minute exertions with 10 second rest breaks lead to fatigue in four hours (Greenberg and Chaffin, 1977). It has been determined that if repeated exertions are made at a self-determined pace, the maximum torque that can be exerted with screwdrivers and wrenches declines by as much as 38 per cent after 240 seconds (Mital and Channaveeraiah, 1988). This decline limits the endurance time as well. Recovery heart rate and recovery of endurance have been used to determine optimum work–rest regimes for intermittent isometric activity (Dul et al., 1990; Milner, 1985; Rohmert, 1973). Using force response to electrical simulation of the forearm muscles, and local blood flow as the criterion, it was determined that at 25 per cent MVC continuous exercise until exhaustion, recovery did not take place even after 24 hours (Bystrom and Kilbom, 1991). Several attempts have also been made to determine the maximal number of exertions per hour, or per day, that can be tolerated without fatigue or muscle-tension disorders (Luopajarvi et al., 1979; Obolenskaja and Goljanitzki, 1927). While it is difficult to set precise limits on the acceptable number of exertions per work day, it can be concluded that repetitive hand–wrist exertions distributed at a high rate over the work day introduces an increased risk of musculoskeletal disorders.

Gloves

Gloves protect the hand and forearm of the worker by resisting sharp edges, splinters, extreme temperatures, sparks, electricity, and chips. Gloves are also used to reduce transmission of vibration energy by absorbing or attenuating it. Gloves have many disadvantages as well. Gloves interfere with a person's ability to grasp objects; they also affect hand movements. Gloves change the effective dimensions of the hand. They increase the hand thickness anywhere from 8 mm to 40 mm (Damon *et al.*, 1966). Manual dexterity is reduced by the presence of the glove material over the hand (McGinnis *et al.*, 1973; Nolan and Cattroll, 1977; Plummer *et al.*, 1985). However, gloves that provide good dexterity and manipulative capabilities have been designed (Andruk *et al.*, 1976; Gianola and Reins, 1976). Gloves also reduce tactile feedback and the edges and seams of gloves cause irritation at contact points.

Human performance in the presence of gloves has, in general, been found to be mixed. Weidman (1970) studied the influence of different kinds of gloves on manual performance and observed that performance times decreased by 12.5 per cent when the gloves were made of Neoprene. With terry cloth, leather, and PVC gloves, performance decreased by 36 per cent, 45 per cent, and 64 per cent respectively. Jenkins (1958), however, reported superior performance when operating small knobs while wearing gloves. Plummer *et al.* (1985) found that the assembly of a 0.635 cm diameter bolt, nut, and washer assembly took significantly longer and resulted in more error than when assembling larger sized bolts (0.79 and 1.27 cm diameter bolts). Desai and Konz (1983) found no difference in error rates in tactile inspection of different sizes of hydraulic hoses. There are studies that report an actual increase in performance as a result of wearing gloves. Bradley (1969a, 1969b) reported an increase in speeds for control operations. Riley *et al.* (1985) also reported an increase in friction and a reduction in task strength requirements with gloves.

The force/torque exertion capability when wearing gloves is another dimension of interest to designers. When wearing gloves, a fraction of the force generated by the muscular contraction may be directed in maintaining the grip and may result in reduced force production. Such reduction in grip (grasp) force has been reported by several studies. Hertzberg (1973) reported a 20 per cent decline in the grip strength when gloves were used. Lyman (1957) and Sperling (1980) reported a 30 per cent or more decrease in strength. Cochran *et al.* (1986) reported a reduction in grasp force due to wearing gloves ranging from 7.3 per cent to 16.8 per cent when compared to work without gloves. Sudhakar *et al.* (1988) reported that the peak grip strength with rubber and leather gloves was 10 to 15 per cent lower compared to grip strength without gloves even when there was no significant difference in muscle activity between glove and no-glove conditions. Mital *et al.* (1994), however, found that the peak torque exertion capability of individuals when using hand tools such as wrenches and screwdrivers generally increased with gloves even though muscle activity did not significantly differ between the glove and the no-glove condition.

While Goel and Rim (1987) and Bingham *et al.* (1992), observed a reduction in the transmission of vibration energy in the presence of gloves, Gurram *et al.* (1994) found that wearing gloves when using hand tools was ineffective in reducing the attenuation of vibration caused by hand-held power tools.

The reduction in grip or grasp force, however, has not always been observed. Lyman and Groth (1958) reported that workers exerted more force with gloves than without gloves when inserting pins in a pegboard. Riley *et al.* (1985) also reported an increase in the maximum pull force, push force, wrist flexion torque, and wrist extension torque. Shih and Wang (1996) reported a 10 to 30 per cent increase in the maximum volitional torque exertion capability when subjects wore gloves while using hand tools. Also, the glove thickness had a positive correlation with the supination maximum volitional torque exertion.

Industrial activities such as maintenance and repair require the use of wrenches and screwdrivers, where the force exertion is mainly rotary at the periphery of the grip, in addition to the compressive (grasping) forces. Mital *et al.* (1994) used seven different hand tools and nine varieties of commercial gloves and measured peak volitional torques on a simulated workpiece. The peak torque and electromyogram of flexor digitorum profundus and supinator brevis indicated that muscle activity did not differ significantly between the glove and no-glove conditions. Further, the peak torque exertion capability of individuals increased with gloves. The magnitude of the torque was different for different gloves. Overall, it can be said that gloves are a mixed blessing. They provide safety and comfort but occasionally reduce manual performance.

OPERATOR RELATED FACTORS IN HAND TOOL DESIGN

Worker characteristics such as left/right handedness, gender, age, strength, technique, body size, and posture, have an influence on the risk of injury and decreased productivity in work with hand tools. Research in each of these factors is summarised below.

Left/right handedness

Approximately 10 per cent of the population is left-handed (Konz, 1974). Yet most tools are designed for right-handed users. Since the preferred hand is stronger by about 7–20 per cent (Miller, 1981; Shock, 1962), more dexterous (Kellor *et al.*, 1971), and faster (Konz and Warraich, 1985), a left-handed user is at a disadvantage when using a right-handed tool. Also, certain right-handed tools require a different action when used by the left hand (Capener, 1956). In many instances, tools designed for right-handed people cannot be used by left-handed people (Laveson and Meyer, 1976). The solution to this problem is to design tools for use by either hand.

Gender/age

Worker gender and age affect the strength and torque exertion capabilities of individuals, and hence the use of hand tools. The grip strength of females has been determined to be approximately 50–67 per cent of male grip strength (Chaffin and Anderson, 1984; Konz, 1990; Lindstrom, 1973). Males, on the average, can exert about 500 N force while females, on the average, are able to exert 250 N force. This difference in force exertion capability is primarily due to the females having smaller grip size and muscles. The implication is that hand tools designed on the basis of male strength and anthropometry will not work for females. Mital (1991) reported that the torque exertion capability of males with screwdrivers and wrenches is 10–56 per cent greater than females. Grip strength is also significantly affected by age (Shock, 1962). By age 65, the decline in strength is about 20–40 per cent. Etherton *et al.* (1996) report that for overhead pulling tasks in adjusting rollover protective structures for farm tractors, the older work group (55 years and older) had a mean strength of 97 per cent of that of the younger work group (55 years and younger). Further, when the task was to be done at shoulder-height, the older group's strength was only 78 per cent of that of the younger group's strength.

Strength

A significant relationship has also been observed between the isometric strengths and anthropometry, and the torque exertion capability of individuals while using hand tools. Mital and Sanghavi (1986) observed that a significant correlation existed between the isometric shoulder strength and torque exertion capability. Their overall conclusions were that heavier and stronger individuals exerted more torque than their weaker counterparts. Shoulder strength was found to be a limiting factor in torque exertion capability. Etherton et al. (1996) found that the force applied at a given wrench handle length, and the strength needed to tighten threaded fasteners became smaller as the diameter of the threaded-fastener decreased. This conclusion was based on the significant difference observed in the strength exertion capabilities of older and younger adults for pulling type tasks at or above shoulder-heights. Oertengren et al. (1991), in their study of manual screw-driving tasks found that the shoulder working height and the type of screw had an effect on the workload and torque exertion. Mital and Sanghavi (1986) and Johnson and Childress (1988) also observed that body heights, and whether or not the worker was sitting or standing, were unimportant. Fransson and Winkel (1991) found that the ability of the hand to produce force depended on the grip type used. Further, they concluded that 35 per cent of the male–female difference in hand strengths was due to the difference in the male–female hand size.

Posture

The effect of body posture on use of hand tools was studied in detail by Mital (1986) and Mital and Channaveeraiah (1988). Postures ranging from standing to lying-on-the-side were studied. It was concluded that minor posture variations were unimportant. Extreme variations, such as between standing and lying on the stomach or leaning sideways from a ladder, however, were found to cause large differences in torque exertion capabilities. Table 8.35 shows the distributions of torque exertion profiles of males and females in different postures with various wrenches and screwdrivers.

Technique/experience

Technique and experience of the worker are two other factors that have been shown to have an influence on the torque exertion capability of the workers when working with hand tools. Marras and Rockwell (1986) reported that workers experienced in spike maul use generated almost twice as much force (136 to 846 N) as the novice workers (64 to 446 N). This large difference was due to the technique used by the workers (snapping action as opposed to sustained application of force).

Table 8.35 Average minimum and maximum torques (Nm) that males and females can exert with common hand tools for different postures (from Mital and Channaveeraiah, 1988).

Tool	Gender	Torque	Posture(s)
Short screwdriver	Male	2.61	Leaning sideways from a ladder, tool axis horizontal (outward) or vertical (upward); overhead, tool axis horizontal (outward) or vertical (upward); squatting in a confined space, tool axis horizontal (outward)
		5.13	Squatting, tool axis vertical (upward)
	Female	2.02	Same as for males
		3.91	Kneeling on one or two knees, tool axis vertical (upward)
Medium screwdriver	Male	1.98	Lying on the side, tool axis horizontal (outward)
		2.64	Kneeling on one knee, tool axis vertical (upward)
	Female	1.40	Same as for males
		1.95	Squatting, tool axis vertical (downward)
Long screwdriver	Male	2.82	Same as for medium screwdriver
		3.52	Same as for short screwdriver
	Female	1.82	Lying on the side, tool axis horizontal (outward)
		2.85	Sitting, tool horizontal (outward) and at the eye level
Longest screwdriver	Male	3.40	Same as for medium screwdriver
		4.62	Standing, bent at the waist, tool axis vertical (upward)
	Female	2.46	Same as for long screwdriver
		3.58	Standing, knees bent, back supported, tool axis vertical (upward)
Crescent wrench	Male	6.41	Leaning sideways from a ladder, tool axis vertical (upward)
		34.88	Standing, tool axis horizontal (outward)
	Female	5.13	Same as for males
		24.71	Same as for males
Spanner wrench	Male	5.86	Same as for crescent wrench
		37.91	Standing, bent at the waist, tool axis horizontal (inward and outward)
	Female	4.76	Same as for crescent wrench
		25.00	Same as for males
Socket wrench	Male	7.02	Same as for crescent wrench
		43.66	Kneeling on one knee, tool axis horizontal (outward); kneeling on both knees, tool axis horizontal (outward) or vertical (upward)
	Female	5.77	Same as for crescent wrench
		31.13	Standing, tool axis horizontal (outward)
Pipe wrench	Male	6.58	Same as for crescent wrench
		46.79	Standing, tool axis horizontal (outward)
	Female	5.49	Same as for crescent wrench
		31.04	Same as for males

Reach distance

Reach distance has been determined to have an effect on the torque exertion capability as well. Mital and Sanghavi (1986) found that the torque exertion capability with wrenches and screwdrivers decreased linearly with reach distance (distance between the front of the ankles and the workpiece) between 33 cm to 58 cm in the standing posture, and between 46 cm to 71 cm in the sitting posture.

Wrist orientation

Mital and Channaveeraiah (1988) found that the orientation of the wrist played a significant role in determining the maximum torque exertion capability. They concluded that the maximum torque with wrenches was exerted when the long axis of the tool was kept horizontal. With screwdrivers, they concluded that the torque exertion was maximum when the wrist was rotated 90 degrees counterclockwise from the prone position.

CONCLUDING REMARKS

Recommendations based on research findings in hand tool design, selection, and usage have been presented in this chapter. However, it is important to realise that proper design of the hand tool alone may not be sufficient to correct any ergonomic problem. There are a number of other important activities that have to be carried out in conjunction with hand tool design, if ergonomic recommendations for hand tool design are to make any impact. These activities include problem identification (based on collected injury and risk potential data); data collection using statistical techniques, and by using ergonomic work, tool, and equipment analyses; and a complete and thorough analysis of the collected data. A number of techniques are available for identification of musculoskeletal injury hazards for the upper extremities (Mital, 1996), and these techniques should be used in addition to the comprehensive injury data collection devices instituted by the Bureau of Labor Statistics, for better overall injury prevention and control in the workplace.

Ergonomic significance of the material presented in this chapter

Humans use different types of hand tools not only in a variety of occupational settings, but also in a number of other domestic day-to-day activities. Use of hand tools has been linked to musculoskeletal disorders of the upper extremities. Decades of research with hand tools has resulted in guidelines for the design, selection, and use of hand tools, which, when adequately implemented, can provide effective engineering and ergonomic solutions to alleviate injuries to the hand tool user. This chapter highlights the injury problems due to the use of hand tools among the US workforce, and presents an up to date summary of research in the various aspects of hand tool design.

References

ANDERSSON, E.R., 1990, Design and testing of a vibration attenuating handle, *International Journal of Industrial Ergonomics*, **6**, 119–125.

ANDRUK, F.S., SHAMPINE, J.C. and REINS, D.A., 1976, *Aluminized Fireman's (Fire Proximity) Handwear: A Comparative Study of Dexterity Characteristics*, Report No. US DOD-AGFSR-76–17, Natick, MA: Navy Clothing and Textile Research Facility.

ARMSTRONG, T.J., 1983, *An Ergonomics Guide to Carpal Tunnel Syndrome*, Ohio: American Industrial Hygiene Association.

ARMSTRONG, T.J., FOULKE, J., JOSEPH, B. and GOLDSTEIN, S., 1982, Investigation of cumulative trauma disorder in a poultry processing plant, *American Industrial Hygiene Association Journal*, **43**, 103–116.

ARMSTRONG, T.J., PUNNETT, L. and KETNER, P., 1989, Subjective worker assessments of hand tools used in automobile assembly, *American Industrial Hygiene Association Journal*, **50**, 639–645.

AYOUB, M.M. and LOPRESTI, P., 1971, The determination of an optimum cylindrical handle by use of electromyography, *Ergonomics*, **14**, 103–116.

BINGHAM, M.D., SUGGS, C.W. and ABRAMS, C.F., 1992, Vibration attenuation of cushioned gloves, *Applied Engineering in Agriculture*, **8**, 4–8.

BOBJER, O., 1990, *Greppytors friktion samt upplevelsen av obehag vid beroring (Friction of grip surface and perceived discomfort upon touch)*, Preliminary report to the Swedish Work Environment Fund.

BOEHLEMANN, J., KLUTH, K., KOTZBAUER, K. and STRASSER, H., 1994, Ergonomic assessment of handle design by means of electromyography and subjective rating, *Applied Ergonomics*, **25**, 346–354.

BRADLEY, J.V., 1969a, Effect of gloves on control operation time, *Human Factors*, **11**, 13–20.

BRADLEY, J.V., 1969b, Glove characteristics influencing control manipulability, *Human Factors*, **11**, 21–35.

BUCHHOLZ, B., FREDERICK, L.J. and ARMSTRONG, T.J., 1988, An investigation of human palmer skin friction and the effects of materials, pinch force and moisture, *Ergonomics*, **31**, 317–325.

BUREAU OF LABOR STATISTICS, 1995, *Worker and Case Characteristics: Supplementary Tables to Bureau of Labor Statistics' News: Characteristics of Injuries and Illnesses Resulting in Absences From Work, 1994*, Washington, DC: US Department of Labor.

BUREAU OF LABOR STATISTICS, 1996, *Worker and Case Characteristics: Supplementary Tables to Bureau of Labor Statistics' News: Characteristics of Injuries and Illnesses Resulting in Absences From Work, 1995*, Washington, DC: US Department of Labor.

BURSTROM, L. and LUNDSTROM, R., 1994, Absorption of vibration energy in the human hand and arm, *Ergonomics*, **37**, 879–890.

BYSTROM, S. and KILBOM, A., 1991, Electrical stimulation of human forearm extensor muscles as an indicator of handgrip fatigue and recovery, *European Journal of Applied Physiology and Occupational Physiology*, **62**, 363–368.

CANNON, L., BERNACKI, E. and WALTER, S., 1981, Personal and occupational factors associated with carpal tunnel syndrome, *Journal of Occupational Medicine*, **23**, 255–258.

CAPENER, N., 1956, The hand in surgery, *The Journal of Bone and Joint Surgery*, **38B**, 128–151.

CHAFFIN, D.B. and ANDERSON, G.B.J., 1984, *Occupational Biomechanics*, New York, NY: John Wiley and Sons.

CHERIAN, T., RAKHEJA, S. and BHAT, R.B., 1996, Analytical investigation of an energy flow divider to attenuate hand-transmitted vibration, *International Journal of Industrial Ergonomics*, **17**, 455–467.

COCHRAN, D.J. and RILEY, M.W., 1986a, The effects of handle shape and size on exerted forces, *Human Factors*, **28**, 253–265.

COCHRAN, D.J. and RILEY, M.W., 1986b, An evaluation of knife handle guarding, *Human Factors*, **28**, 295–301.

COCHRAN, D.J., ALBIN, T.J., RILEY, M.W. and BISHU, R.R., 1986, Analysis of grasp force degradation with commercially available gloves, in *Proceedings of the Human Factors Society 30th Annual Meeting*, Santa Monica, California: Human Factors and Ergonomics Society, pp. 852–855.

DAMON, A., STOUDT, H.W. and McFARLAND, R.A., 1966, *The Human Body in Equipment Design*, Cambridge, MA: Harvard University Press.

DESAI, S. and KONZ, S., 1983, Tactile inspection performance with and without gloves, in *Proceedings of the Human Factors Society 27th Annual Meeting*, Santa Monica, California: Human Factors Society, pp. 782–785.

DUL, J., DOUWES, M. and SMITT, P., 1990, A work-rest model for static postures, *Biomechanics Seminars*, 117–124.

EASTMAN KODAK COMPANY, 1983, *Ergonomic Design for People at Work*, Belmont, CA: Lifetime Learning Publications.

ETHERTON, J.R., STOBBE, T.J. and WASSELL, J.T., 1996, Hand tool-task strength comparison between younger and older tractor operators using adjustable rollover protective structures, *International Journal of Industrial Ergonomics*, **17**, 247–258.

FELLOWS, G.L. and FREIVALDS, A., 1991, Ergonomics evaluation of a foam rubber grip for tool handles, *Applied Ergonomics*, **22**, 225–230.

FOGLEMAN, M.T., FREIVALDS, A. and GOLDBERG, J.H., 1993, Ergonomic evaluation of knives for two poultry cutting tasks, *International Journal of Industrial Ergonomics*, **11**, 257–265.

FRANSSON, C. and WINKEL, J., 1991, Hand strength: the influence of grip span and grip type, *Ergonomics*, **34**, 881–892.

FRASER, T.M., 1980, *Ergonomic Principles in the Design of Hand Tools*, Occupational safety and health series, No. 44, Geneva: International Labour Office.

FREIVALDS, A. and EKLUND, J., 1993, Reaction torques and operator stress while using powered nutrunners, *Applied Ergonomics*, **24**, 158–164.

GARRETT, J., 1969a, *References on Hand Anthropometry for Women*, Army Medical Research Laboratory, Wright Patterson Air Force Base, OH: AMRL Technical Report 69–42.

GARRETT, J., 1969b, *References on Hand Anthropometry for Men*, Army Medical Research Laboratory, Wright Patterson Air Force Base, OH: AMRL Technical Report 69–26.

GARRETT, J., 1971, The adult human hand: some anthropometric and biomechanical considerations, *Human Factors*, **13**, 117–131.

GIANOLA, S.V. and REINS, D.A., 1976, *Low Temperature Handwear with Improved Dexterity*, Report No. 117, Natick, MA: Navy Clothing and Textile Research Unit.

GOEL, V.K. and RIM, K., 1987, Role of gloves in reducing vibration: an analysis for pneumatic chipping hammer, *American Industrial Hygiene Association Journal*, **48**, 9–14.

GRANT, K.A. and HABES, D.J., 1993, Effectiveness of a handle flange for reducing manual effort during hand tool use, *International Journal of Industrial Ergonomics*, **12**, 199–207.

GREENBERG, L. and CHAFFIN, D.B., 1977, *Workers and Their Tools*, Midland, MI: Pendell.

GRIEVE, D. and PHEASANT, S., 1982, Biomechanics, in Singleton, W.T. (Ed.), *The Body at Work*, Cambridge: Cambridge University Press, pp. 142–150.

GURRAM, R., GOUW, G.J. and RAKHJA, S., 1993, Grip pressure distribution under static and dynamic loading, *Experimental Mechanics*, **33**, 169–173.

GURRAM, R., RAKHEJA, S., SOUW, S. and GERARD, J., 1994, Vibration transmission characteristics of the human hand–arm and gloves, *International Journal of Industrial Ergonomics*, **13**, 217–234.

HAMMER, A., 1934, Tenosynovitis, *Medical Record*, 353–355.

HAMMERSKJOELD, E., HARMS-RINGDAHL, K., EKHOLM, J. and SAMUELSON, B., 1991, Effect of short-time vibration exposure on work movements with carpenters' hand tools, *International Journal of Industrial Ergonomics*, **8**, 125–134.

HERTZBERG, H., 1973, Engineering anthropometry, in Van Cott, H. and Kinkade, R. (Eds), *Human Engineering Guide to Equipment Design*, Washington, DC: US Government Printing Office.

HUNT, L., 1934, A study of screwdrivers for small assembly work, *The Human Factor*, **9**, 70–73.

IWATA, H., MATSUDA, A., TAKAHASHI, H. and WATABE, S., 1971, Roentgenographic findings in elbows of rock drill workers, *Acta Scholae Medicine of University of Gifu*, **19**, 393–404.

JENKINS, W.L., 1958, The superiority of gloved operation of small control knobs, *Journal of Applied Psychology*, **42**, 97–98.

JOHNSON, S.L. and CHILDRESS, L.J., 1988, Powered screwdriver design and use: tool, task, and operator effects, *International Journal of Industrial Ergonomics*, **2**, 183–191.

JONSSON, B., LEWIN, T., TOMSIC, P., GARDE, G. and FORSSBLAD, P., 1977, *Handen som arbetsredskap (The hand as a work-tool)*, Stockholm, Sweden: Arbetarskyddsstyrelsen.

KAO, H., 1976, An analysis of user preference toward hand writing instruments, *Perceptual and Motor Skills*, **43**, 522.

KARLQVIST, L., 1984, Cutting operation at canning bench – a case study of hand tool design, in *Proceedings of the 1984 International Conference on Occupational Ergonomics*, Rexdale, Ontario: Human Factors Association of Canada, pp. 452–456.

KELLOR, M., KONDRASUK, R., IVERSON, I., FROST, J., SILBERBERG, N. and HOGLUND, M., 1971, *Hand Strengths and Dexterity Tests*, Manual 721, Minneapolis, MN: Sister Kenny Institute.

KIHLBERG, S., KJELLBERG, A. and LINDBECK, L., 1993, Pneumatic tool torque reaction: reaction forces, displacement, muscle activity and discomfort in the hand-arm system, *Applied Ergonomics*, **24**, 165–173.

KILBOM, A. and EKHOLM, J., 1991, *Handgreppsstyrka (Hand grip strength, Swedish with English Summary)*, Stockholm, Sweden: Stockholm MUSIC study group.

KILBOM, A., MAKARAINEN, M., SPERLING, L., KADEFORS, R. and LIEDBERG, L., 1993, Tool design, user characteristics and performance: a case study on plate-shears, *Applied Ergonomics*, **24**, 221–230.

KIM, J.Y., YUN, M.H. and LEE, M.W., 1996, Design of optimum grip and control area for one-handed manual control devices, *Computers and Industrial Engineering*, **31**, 661–664.

KONZ, S., 1974, Design of hand tools, in *Proceedings of the Human Factors Society 18th Annual Meeting*, Santa Monica, CA: Human Factors Society, pp. 292–300.

KONZ, S., 1986, Bent handle hammers, *Human Factors*, **28**, 317–323.

KONZ, S., 1990, *Work Design: Industrial Ergonomics*, Worthington, OH: Publishing Horizons, Inc.

KONZ, S. and WARRAICH, M., 1985, Performance differences between the preferred and non-preferred hand when using various tools, in Brown, I.D., Goldsmith, R., Coombes, K. and Sinclair, M.A. (Eds), *Ergonomics International 85*, London: Taylor and Francis, pp. 451–453.

KRIEFELDT, J.G. and HILL, P.K., 1975, Towards a theory of man-tool system design applications to the consumer product area, in *Proceedings of the Human Factors Society 19th Annual Meeting*, Santa Monica, CA: Human Factors Society, pp. 301–309.

KUORINKA, I. and KOSKINEN, P., 1979, Occupational rheumatic diseases and upper limb strain in manual jobs in a light mechanical industry, *Scandinavian Journal of Work, Environment and Health*, **5**(Suppl. 3), 39–47.

KURPPA, K., WARRIS, P. and KOKKANEN, P., 1979, Tennis elbow, *Scandinavian Journal of Work, Environment and Health*, **5**(Suppl. 3), 15–18.

LAVESON, J.I. and MEYER, R.P., 1976, Left out 'lefties' in design, in *Proceedings of the Human Factors Society 20th Annual Meeting*, Santa Monica, CA: Human Factors Society, pp. 122–125.

LEAKY, L.S.B., 1960, Finding the world's earliest man, *National Geographic*, **118**, 420–435.

LEE, Y.-H. and CHENG, S.-L., 1995, Triggering force and measurement of maximal finger flexion force, *International Journal of Industrial Ergonomics*, **15**, 167–177.

LINDSTROM, F.E., 1973, *Modern Pliers*, Enkoping, Sweden: BAHCO Vertyg.

LUNDSTROM, R. and JOHANSSON, R.S., 1986, Acute impairment of the sensitivity of skin mechanoreceptive units caused by vibration exposure of the hand, *Ergonomics*, **29**, 687–698.

LUOPAJARVI, T., KUORINKA, I., VIROLAINEN, M. and HOLMBERG, M., 1979, Prevalence of tenosynovitis and other injuries of the upper extremities in repetitive work, *Scandinavian Journal of Work, Environment and Health*, **5**(Suppl. 3), 48–55.

LYMAN, J., 1957, The effects of equipment design on manual performance, in Fisher, R. (Ed.), *Production and Functioning of the Hands in Cold Climates*, Washington, DC: National Academy of Sciences, National Research Council, pp. 86–101.

LYMAN, J. and GROTH, H., 1958, Prehension forces as a measure of psychomotor skill for bare and gloved hands, *Journal of Applied Psychology*, **42**, 18–21.

MARRAS, W.S. and ROCKWELL, T.H., 1986, An experimental evaluation of method and tool effects in spike maul use, *Human Factors*, **28**, 267–281.

MCGINNIS, J.M., BENSEL, C.K. and LOCKHAR, J.M., 1973, *Dexterity Afforded by CB Protective Gloves*, Report No. 73–35-PR, Natick, MA: US Army Natick Laboratories.

MEAGHER, S., 1991, Vibration: causation of repetitive trauma disorders, in Karwowski, W. and Yates, J.W. (Eds), *Trends in Ergonomics/Human Factors*, London: Taylor and Francis, pp. 69–74.

MILLER, G.D., 1981, Significance of Dominant Hand Grip Strengths in Hand Tools, unpublished MS thesis, Pennsylvania State University, University Park, Pennsylvania, USA.

MILNER, N.P., 1985, Modeling Fatigue and Recovery in Static Postural Exercise, PhD Thesis, University of Nottingham, Nottingham, UK.

MITAL, A., 1986, Effect of body posture and common hand tools on peak torque exertion capabilities, *Applied Ergonomics*, **17**, 87–96.

MITAL, A., 1991, Hand tools: injuries, illnesses, design and usage, in Mital, A. and Karwowski, W. (Eds), *Workspace, Equipment and Tool Design*, Amsterdam, The Netherlands: Elsevier Science Publishers, pp. 219–256.

MITAL, A., 1996, *Recognition of Musculoskeletal Injury Hazards for the Upper Extremity and Lower Back*, Report No. CDC-94071VID, Cincinnati, OH: National Institute of Occupational Safety and Health.

MITAL, A. and CHANNAVEERAIAH, C., 1988, Peak volitional torques for wrenches and screwdrivers, *International Journal of Industrial Ergonomics*, **3**, 41–64.

MITAL, A. and SANGHAVI, N., 1986, Comparison of maximum volitional torque exertion capabilities of males and females using common hand tools, *Human Factors*, **28**, 283–294.

MITAL, A., KUO, T. and FAARD, H.F., 1994, Quantitative evaluation of gloves used with non-powered hand tools in routine maintenance tasks, *Ergonomics*, **37**, 333–343.

NAPIER, J., 1956, The prehensile movements of the human hand, *Journal of Bone and Joint Surgery*, **38B**, 902–913.

NIOSH (National Institute for Occupational Safety and Health), 1983, *Current Intelligence Bulletin 38: Vibration Syndrome*, Cincinnati, OH.

NOLAN, R.W. and CATTROLL, S.W., 1977, *Evaluation of British and Canadian Conductive Rubber Heating Elements for Handwear: Preliminary Report*, Report No. 77–24, Ottawa, Ontario: Canadian Defense Research Establishment.

OBOLENSKAJA, A.J. and GOLJANITZKI, I., 1927, Die serose Tendovainitis in der Klinik und im Experiment, *Deutsches Z. Chir.*, **201**, 388–399.

OERTENGREN, R., CEDERQVIST, T., LINDBERG, M. and MAGNUSSON, B., 1991, Workload in lower arm and shoulder when using manual and powered screwdrivers at different working heights, *International Journal of Industrial Ergonomics*, **8**, 225–235.

PHEASANT, S. and O'NEILL, D., 1975, Performance in gripping and turning – a study in hand/handle effectiveness, *Applied Ergonomics*, **6**, 205–208.

PLUMMER, R., STOBBE, T., RONK, R., MYERS, W., KIM, H. and JARAIEDI, M., 1985, Manual dexterity evaluation of gloves used in handling hazardous materials, in *Proceedings of the Human Factors Society 29th Annual Meeting*, Santa Monica, CA: Human Factors and Ergonomics Society, pp. 819–823.

POETH, D.F. and FREIVALDS, A., 1996, Design of a zero-force switch for use in industrial soldering guns, *International Journal of Industrial Engineering – Applications & Practice*, **3**, 126–130.

PUTZ-ANDERSON, V., 1988, *Cumulative Trauma Disorders: A Manual for Musculoskeletal Diseases of the Upper Limbs*, London: Taylor and Francis.

RADONJIC, D. and LONG, C., 1971, Kinesiology of the wrist, *American Journal of Physical Medicine*, **50**, 57–71.

RILEY, M., COCHRAN, D. and SCHANBACHER, C., 1985, Force capability differences due to gloves, *Ergonomics*, **28**, 441–447.

ROHMERT, W., 1973, Problems of determination of rest allowances, Part II: Determining rest allowances in different tasks, *Applied Ergonomics*, **24**, 158–162.

RUBARTH, B., 1928, Untersuchung zur Bestgestaltung von Handheften fur Schraubenzieher und Ahnliche Werkzeuge (Investigations concerning the best shape for handles for screwdrivers and similar tools), *Industrielle Psychotechnik*, **5**, 129–142.

SARAN, C., 1973, Biomechanical evaluation of T-handles for a pronation supination task, *Journal of Occupational Medicine*, **15**, 712–716.

SCHOENMARKLIN, R.W. and MARRAS, W.S., 1989a, Effects of handle angle and work orientation on hammering; Part I: Wrist motion and hammering performance, *Human Factors*, **30**, 397–411.

SCHOENMARKLIN, R.W. and MARRAS, W.S., 1989b, Effects of handle angle and work orientation on hammering; Part II: Muscle fatigue and subjective ratings of body discomfort, *Human Factors*, **30**, 413–420.

SHIH, Y.-C. and WANG, M.-J., 1996, Hand/tool interface effects on human torque capacity, *International Journal of Industrial Ergonomics*, **18**, 205–213.

SHOCK, N., 1962, The physiology of aging, *Scientific American*, **206**, 100–110.

SILVERSTEIN, B.A., FINE, L.J. and ARMSTRONG, T.J., 1987a, Occupational factors and carpal tunnel syndrome, *American Journal of Industrial Medicine*, **11**, 343–358.

SILVERSTEIN, B.A., FINE, L.J. and ARMSTRONG, T.J., 1987b, Hand wrist cumulative trauma disorders in industry, *British Journal of Industrial Medicine*, **43**, 779–794.

SPERLING, L., 1980, *Test Program for Work Gloves, Research Report No. 1980: 18*, Umea, Sweden: Department of Occupational Safety, Division for Occupational Medicine, Labor Physiology Unit.

SPERLING, L., 1986, *Work with Hand Tools: Development of Force, Exertion and Discomfort in Work with Different Grips and Grip Dimensions*, Report in Swedish with English summary Arbetarskyddsstyrelsen, Undersokninsrapport, 25.

SPERLING, L., DAHLMAN, S., WIKSTROM, L., KADEFORS, R. and KILBOM, A., 1991, Tools and hand function: the cube model – a method for analysis of the handling of hand tools, presentation at the 11th International Ergonomics Association Congress, Paris, France.

SUDHAKAR, L.R., SCHOENMARKLIN, R.W., LAVENDER, S.A. and MARRAS, W.S., 1988, The effects of gloves on grip strength and muscle activity, in *Proceedings of the Human Factors Society 30th Annual Meeting*, Santa Monica, CA: Human Factors and Ergonomics Society, pp. 647–650.

SWANSON, A., MATEV, I. and GROOT, G., 1970, The strength of the hand, *Bulletin of Prosthetics Research*, 145–153.

TAYLOR, W., 1988a, Hand-arm vibration syndrome: a new clinical classification and an updated British standard guide for hand transmitted vibration, *British Journal of Industrial Medicine*, **45**, 281–282.

TAYLOR, W., 1988b, Biological effects of the hand-arm vibration syndrome – historical perspective and current research, *Journal of the Acoustical Society of America*, **83**, 415–422.

TECHNICAL RESEARCH CENTRE OF FINLAND, 1988, *Evaluating and Choosing Pneumatic Screwdrivers and Nut Runners*, Tampere, Finland: Occupational Safety Engineering Laboratory.

TERRELL, R. and PURSWELL, J., 1976, The influence of forearm and wrist orientation on static grip strength as a design criterion for hand tools, in *Proceedings of the Human Factors Society 20th Annual Meeting*, Santa Monica, CA: Human Factors Society, pp. 28–32.

TICHAUER, E.R., 1966a, Some aspects of stress on forearm and hand in industry, *Journal of Occupational Medicine*, **8**, 63–71.

TICHAUER, E.R., 1966b, *Gilbreth Revisited*, Publication No. 66-WA/BHF, American Society of Mechanical Engineers.

TICHAUER, E.R., 1976, Biomechanics sustains occupational safety and health, *Industrial Engineering*, February, 46–56.

TICHAUER, E.R. and GAGE, H., 1977, Ergonomic principles basic to hand tool design, *American Industrial Hygiene Association Journal*, **38**, 622–634.

WASHBURN, S., 1960, Tools and human evolution, *Scientific American*, **203**, 3–15.

WASSERMAN, D.E. and BADGER, D.W., 1973, *Vibration and the Worker's Health and Safety*, Technical Report No. 77, Washington, DC: National Institute for Occupational Safety and Health, US Government Printing Office.

WEIDMAN, B., 1970, *Effect of Safety Gloves on Simulated Work Tasks, AD 738981*, Springfield, VA: National Technical Information Service.

WU, Y., 1975, Material properties criteria for thermal safety, *Journal of Materials*, **7**, 575–579.

YAKAO, T., YAMAMOTO, K., KOYAMA, M. and HYODO, K., 1996, Sensory evaluation of grip using cylindrical objects, *Nippon Kikai Gakkai Ronbunshu*, **62**, 3999–4004.

YODER, T.A., LUCAS, R.L. and BOTZUM, C.D., 1973, The marriage of human factors and safety in industry, *Human Factors*, **15**, 197–205.

CHAPTER NINE

Work and activity-related musculoskeletal disorders of the upper extremity

RICHARD WELLS AND PETER KEIR

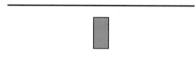

INTRODUCTION

One of the goals of the ergonomic process is to design or modify people's work and other activities to be within their capabilities and limitations. One possible outcome of a poor harmonisation is disorders of the musculoskeletal system known as repetitive strain injuries (RSI), cumulative trauma disorders (CTD) or, as they are termed here, activity and work-related musculoskeletal disorders (WMSD).

The relationship between human activity and WMSD can be investigated from a number of disciplines using many methodological approaches. Most evidence is available from the relationship between work and WMSD; however in this chapter other activities will be mentioned where appropriate. The epidemiological research addressing the relationship between work exposure and WMSD will not be addressed here as it has been extensively reviewed in Hagberg *et al.* (1995) and NIOSH (1997). These reviews found strong and consistent relationships between many types of WMSD and workplace exposures. Modification of these risk factors, both physical and psychosocial, is therefore a reasonable strategy for both primary and secondary prevention. Biomechanics offers one approach to analysing and understanding the mechanical function of the musculoskeletal system and thus the relationships between work activity and the loads on the tissues. Coupling this understanding with a knowledge of the response of tissues to loading can help support the biological plausibility of epidemiological investigations and suggest ways in which the work environment can be changed.

The distal arm will be used in this chapter to illustrate the role of biomechanics in understanding the injury potential of manual activity. Although the anatomy of the region is unique, other regions can be studied using similar approaches. The relationships between work and WMSD will be described for the major types of tissue involved: tendon, nerve and muscle. It is acknowledged that clinically, patients may present with more complex symptoms. These are the result of complex interactions between the many sub-systems.

Biomechanics can make its best contributions at the tissue load level. Biomechanics does this by helping us understand the effects of the many interacting physical stressors that act on the hand, wrist and forearm during work.

BIOMECHANICAL APPROACHES AND WMSD POTENTIAL IN TENDON DISORDERS

Aetiology of tendon disorders due to mechanical factors

Aetiologically, reduced lubrication between tendons and tendon sheaths due to excess relative movement has been suggested in tenosynovitis (Moore *et al.*, 1991; Rowe, 1987), whilst high peak loads and cumulative strain have been suggested for tendinitis (Abrahams, 1967; Goldstein, 1981). Mechanical stresses due to impingement are also of importance.

In-vivo animal experiments under high load, high frequency movement conditions have created tendon damage in rabbits from high frequency movements (Backman *et al.*, 1990). High frequency, low load conditions produced with electrical stimulation did not however produce any tendon damage in monkeys' finger flexor tendon or sheath (Smutz *et al.*, 1995). More recently Archambault *et al.* (1997) have supported the findings of Backhouse and colleagues but at more realistic movement rates. Damage was found in the paratenon, the outer covering of the tendon. It is suggested that this is consistent with frictional damage due to the long term sliding of the tendon under load.

Biomechanical models of tendon disorders

Norman and Wells (1990) have proposed a model for understanding the origin of hand wrist tenosynovitis in which the frictional work done by the tendon sliding through its sheath is proposed as an important risk factor for WMSD. Frictional work is present due to a 'belt–pulley' interaction when the wrist deviates from a straight position. Armstrong and Chaffin (1978) originally estimated the radius of curvature of the flexor tendons in the carpal tunnel from wrist angle changes and tendon displacement. More recently Keir (1995) measured the tendon positions using MRI scanning techniques on living subjects exerting known forces in a variety of functional posture. Using mathematical differentiation, the instantaneous radii of curvature were calculated throughout the length of the carpal tunnel. It was observed that tendon tension reduced the radius of curvature of the flexor tendons as they traversed the carpal tunnel (Figure 9.1).

The magnitude of the transmitted (normal) tendon forces is dependent on the tendon axial load and the radius of curvature. Any tendon load will create a frictional resistance to sliding and, if the wrist and/or fingers move, frictional work will be done at the tendon–sheath interface (Figure 9.2). It is also suggested that a non-negligible resistance to movement be present to move the tendons through the carpal tunnel even in the straight position. Estimates extrapolated from the work of Goldstein (1981), put this resistance at around 5N in the neutral position in humans; however values of the order 0.5N have been measured (Smutz, P., personal communication). Recent efforts have been made to examine the friction in the A2 pulley of the finger in cadaveric tendons (Coert *et al.*, 1995; Uchiyama *et al.*, 1995). Under a 4.9N load the frictional force was found to range from 0.12 to 0.2N for angles of 20–60 degrees (Uchiyama *et al.*, 1995); from this the mean coefficient of friction was 0.04 to 0.14. When the tendon was cut and rejoined using a running suture the friction increased to 0.146 to 0.432N for angles from 20 to 60 degrees.

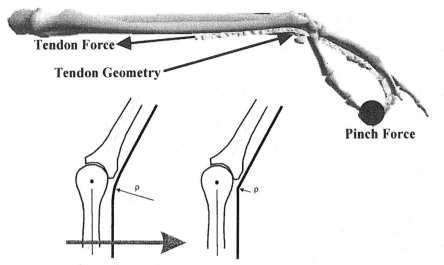

Figure 9.1 The effect of tendon load on tendon radius of curvature through the carpal tunnel. Loading the tendon with 10N force decreased the radius of curvature (Keir, 1995).

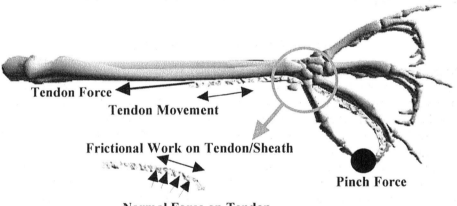

Figure 9.2 Combined effect of gripping, with time varying postures. The gripping requires tendon tension. The time varying wrist posture creates sliding of the digital flexor (and extensor) tendons. The combined effect is friction and energy input to the tissues. Finger motion will likewise create tendon sliding.

Summary and usage

Excursion of the tendons at the wrist (caused by finger and wrist movement) in both straight and deviated postures (especially when the tendons are under tension) creates an energy input, possibly beyond the recovery capability of the tissue. This is in keeping with injury and accident theory where 'energy' is the source of injury (e.g. Haddon, 1980).

Moore *et al.* (1991) calculated a wide range of biomechanical exposure measures during four kinds of simulated manual work in the laboratory. These measures were based upon peak and cumulative external measures and estimated internal loads. Of these, frictional work best matched the injury risk in a large epidemiological study by Silverstein *et al.* (1986, 1987). More recently tendon excursion has been calculated to characterise typing on different keyboards (Flannery *et al.*, 1995).

BIOMECHANICAL APPROACHES AND WMSD POTENTIAL IN NERVE DISORDERS

Aetiology of nerve disorders due to mechanical factors

Mechanical insult to the nerve can be due to increased hydrostatic pressures in the carpal canal, direct mechanical insult (contact stresses) upon the nerve by overlying tendon(s) or impingement (pinched nerve) and stretch (Wall *et al.*, 1992). All have been suggested as likely mechanisms of work-related nerve disorders. Nerve, or more properly its blood supply, is sensitive to the hydrostatic pressure. Lundborg *et al.* (1982) induced pressures in the carpal tunnel and concluded that '. . . there is a critical pressure level between 30 and 60 mmHg where nerve fibre viability is acutely jeopardised'. They also note that the effects in their experiments were due to ischaemia rather than mechanical compression. Rydevik and Lundborg (1977) noted however that mechanical trauma increases susceptibility to ischaemia. Szabo and Sharkey (1993) developed a method studying the response of nerve to sinusoidally varying pressures. They reported that the changes in conduction were related to the mean pressure rather than the peak but the choice of pressure waveforms requires expanding to examine better the impact of different work conditions (Rempel, 1995).

Direct mechanical compression of nerves can be seen at many sites: in the wrist between the flexor retinaculum and the flexor tendons (Smith *et al.*, 1977), in the lumbar spine between adjacent spinal motion units or due to extruded nuclear material (Rydevik *et al.*, 1990) or in the neck between scalene muscles or against the upper ribs. Direct compression inducing pressures of 10–50 mmHg produce effects such as reduced blood flow, and increased permeability of blood vessels with oedema. Direct compression of the nerve at low levels of 20–30 mmHg (Rydevik *et al.*, 1981) affects local blood flow as well as impairing axonal transport at 30 mmHg (Dahlin *et al.*, 1987). It is noteworthy that compression does not cause pain in all cases; however the presence of inflammation and compression does appear to be painful (Rydevik *et al.*, 1990).

Stretch of nerves has been suggested as a possible cause of non-specific nerve disorders. It has been shown in a rabbit model that stretch of the order 6 per cent gives rise to changes in conduction behaviour (Wall *et al.*, 1992). It has also been demonstrated that nerves slide over their course from the spinal cord to their destination to accommodate motion at the intervening joints; for example, McLellan and Swash (1976) demonstrated sliding of nerves at the shoulder level due to wrist movement. Szabo *et al.* (1994) found that the median nerve excursion with flexion–extension of the fingers is 43 per cent of the excursion experienced by the flexor tendons. The differences between specimens was significant but the difference before and after sectioning the TCL was not. It has been found that there is reduced sliding of the median nerve in patients with CTS (Nakamichi and Tachibana, 1995; Valls-Soli *et al.*, 1995), indicating that there may be increased frictional forces or adhesions in the diseased arm. If sliding is restricted at some level, perhaps by adhesions, the excursion of the nerve due to joint motion will increase the stretch in the segments adjacent to the restriction with possible chronic effects. This is the basis for a provocative test such as straight leg raising in sciatica.

Biomechanical models of carpal canal hydrostatic pressure

Hydrostatic pressure exists in anatomical compartments. Compartment syndromes demonstrating elevated pressure have been described in many parts of the body. The elevated pressure may be due to processes after trauma when acute damage can result or be due to processes occurring as a result of activity. A nerve that passes through a compartment under elevated pressure is subject to possible damage, depending on the pressure and length of exposure. Despite the carpal canal having the appearance of an open ended tube, it behaves like a compartment (Szabo and Chidgey, 1989). Compartment (hydrostatic) pressures are measured using invasive techniques; however recent *in-vivo* and *in-vitro* testing allows estimates of carpal tunnel pressure from postural and force data.

Rempel (1995) reported on a series of *in-vivo* measures of carpal tunnel pressures during a wide variety of manual activities in many participants. It appears that wrist and finger posture as well as the force exerted affect the carpal canal pressure. It appears also that many work activities exceed the benchmark 30 mmHg pressure and many exceed the 60 mmHg level. Rempel *et al.* (1997) found that the effects of fingertip force on carpal tunnel pressure were independent of and greater than those due to wrist posture during a finger pressing task. Keir *et al.* (1998) determined that at the same fingertip force magnitude, a pinch grip created twice the carpal tunnel pressure than a simple finger press. This latter finding supports the epidemiological evidence that pinch grip activities are highly correlated to findings of CTS and tendinitis in the forearm. Full supination has also been shown to increase CTP (Rempel *et al.*, 1998). Previously, Rempel *et al.* (1994) determined the effects of wearing a flexible splint on carpal tunnel pressure during a simulated supermarket checker/bagger task and found that the splints did not reduce pressures.

In order to determine better the multiple effects of posture and force exertion, Keir *et al.* (1997) used a cadaver preparation to examine these same effects. Cadaver arms were instrumented for wrist posture in flexion/extension and ulnar/radial deviation and the tendons for index and middle finger flexors as well flexor pollicis longus and palmaris longus were connected to wires so that known forces could be applied. A two finger pinch grip was simulated. The responses to wrist angle changes are seen in Figure 9.3 whilst Figure 9.4 shows the effects of adding load to the flexor tendons. Rempel (1995), who measured responses in volunteers, found very similar responses in the unloaded condition.

Biomechanical models of direct nerve compression

Mechanical stress to the median nerve can be predicted by modified belt-pulley models of the wrist. As was described in the section on tendon disorders, when the tendon is under tension and must change direction, a force at right angles to the tendon (normal force) must be present. If the wrist is in flexion this force will be directed against the median nerve. Moore *et al.* (1991) used existing data to predict loading of the median nerve during manual work. More recently, Keir (1995) estimated the tendon radius of curvature from MRI (and thus the resulting contact pressure) at a range of wrist angles (Figure 9.1).

Measurements, *in-vitro*, of the pressure in a balloon transducer which has replaced the median nerve are available (Keir *et al.*, 1997) (Figure 9.4). The belt-pulley models predict loading of the median nerve only in flexion whereas the experimental data of Smith *et al.* (1977) and Keir *et al.* (1997) show loads in both flexion and extension wrist postures. Instrumented measures of local contact stress are needed for clarification.

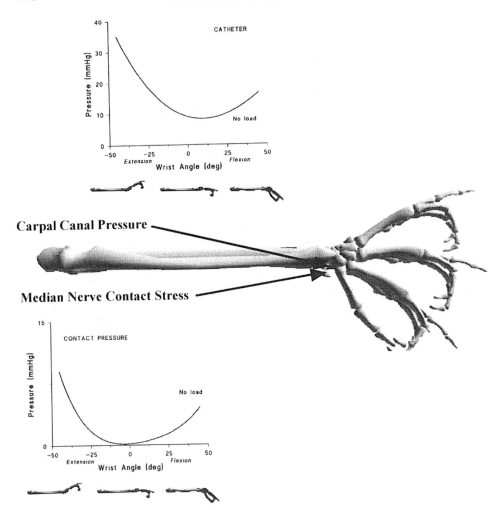

Figure 9.3 The effect of wrist posture on carpal tunnel pressure and median nerve contact stress. Hydrostatic pressure was measured by catheter and contact stress by a tubular rubber transducer replacing the excised median nerve (Keir *et al.*, 1997)

Summary and usage

There exist models of contact stress as well hydrostatic pressure in the carpal canal. There are few data on nerve stretch during work or other activities. Drury (1987) calculated an exposure parameter (which he termed daily damaging wrist motions) when wrist flexion and force exertion coincided. Moore *et al.* (1991) calculated median nerve contact stress and its time integral during four kinds of simulated manual work in the laboratory. Under 'natural' conditions participants elected to work with the wrist in extension as they squeezed the tool. Even under 'forced' conditions where the work was configured to require flexed wrist postures, wrist postures varied close to straight and little loading on the median nerve by the tendons was predicted.

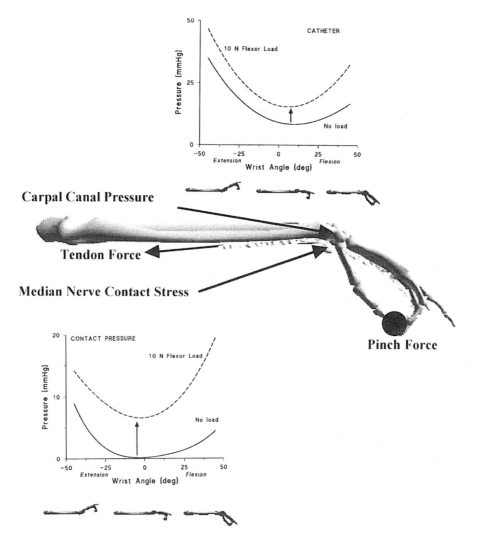

Figure 9.4   The effect of tendon tension on carpal tunnel pressure and median nerve contact stress. Flexor tendons loaded with 10N force. Hydrostatic pressure was measured by catheter and contact stress by a tubular rubber transducer replacing the excised median nerve (Keir *et al.*, 1997)

BIOMECHANICAL APPROACHES AND WMSD POTENTIAL IN MUSCLE DISORDERS

Aetiology of muscle disorders due to mechanical factors

Muscular loading during upper limb intensive work has been linked to the development of chronic muscle problems in the shoulder and neck (Veiersted *et al.*, 1993). Recent clinical findings have suggested that forearm muscle pain may be an overlooked problem in studying work-related chronic musculoskeletal disorders (Ranney *et al.*, 1995). While work-related muscle pain is well accepted in the shoulder area, pain in the forearm is usually attributed to tendinitis or epicondylitis. Suggested mechanisms for muscle pain include fatigue induced hypoxia leading to metabolic changes as a result of low level continuous activation, increased intracompartmental pressure and physical disruption of the muscle with high force (especially eccentric) contractions.

The major approaches to determining potential for development of muscle work-related disorders have been electromyography (Jonsson, 1982), biomechanical models (McGill and Norman, 1986) and fatigue/recovery type curves (Rohmert, 1973). This review will touch on recent findings using electromyography.

Electromyography has been extensively used in the trapezius and other shoulder and neck musculature although more work is now seen in the distal arm. Furthermore, the extensors of the wrist and fingers appear to be a critical area to consider (Hägg and Milerad, 1997). Their importance in manual activity is highlighted by the relationship of gripping to high extensor activity (Snijders *et al.*, 1987).

Appropriate processing of the electromyographic signal can serve as a link between the work done and the muscle usage required. Jonsson (1982) described a technique in which the frequency of occurrence of any particular level of EMG occurring is calculated. From this, an amplitude probability distribution function (APDF) curve is developed. The static level of this curve describes the ability of the muscle to rest at least 10 per cent of the time and appears important in the development of chronic work-related muscle problems. If the value is greater than zero the muscle is not given a chance to completely rest at least 10 per cent of the time during a task.

Static muscle loading, even at low levels, has been linked to muscle fatigue, pain and myalgia (e.g. Larsson *et al.*, 1988). Examination of the muscle fibres has revealed that in chronically statically loaded muscles there exist increased numbers of type I (slow twitch) fibres and what are termed 'ragged red' fibres (Henriksson, 1988; Larsson *et al.*, 1988; Lindman *et al.*, 1991). Ragged red fibres have damaged mitochondria and are likely indicative of present or past ischaemia. These findings and an understanding of motor recruitment (order of motor unit recruitment (Henneman *et al.*, 1965)) have led to the hypothesis termed the 'Cinderella motor unit' (Hägg, 1991).

While a knowledge of the APDF is a useful method of quantifying muscle usage throughout the duration of a task, it gives no indication of the duration of each rest pause, i.e. whether the rests came as numerous pauses or one big pause. Veiersted *et al.* (1990, 1993) addressed this by using a 'gaps' analysis. This analysis looks at the number of times the muscle is turned off (less than 0.5 per cent MVC) and it appeared that people with pain had fewer numbers of gaps. More recently Mathiassen and Winkel (1991) have proposed a measure, exposure variability assessment (EVA), which combines elements of both these approaches.

Summary and usage

Veiersted *et al.* (1990, 1993) addressed the relationship between work exposure, quantified by trapezius activation using a 'gaps' analysis. It appeared that people with pain had fewer numbers of gaps and workers with fewer gaps were more likely to develop trapezius myalgia. This is in accordance with the notion that muscle fibres need a 'rest' for recovery. Figure 9.5 illustrates the patterns of muscular activity currently believed to create high and low risk of muscle pain.

Keir and Wells (1994) used a biomechanical model to assess the demands on the extensors of the wrist during typing. The biomechanical model took account of gravitational and passive forces and related this to the capacity of the musculature. This agreed with the demand evidenced by electromyography (Rose, 1991).

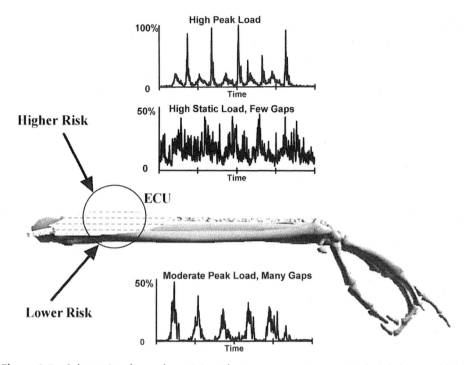

Figure 9.5 Schematic of muscle activity (electromyograms) associated with low and high risk of developing myalgia. Electromyograms are rectified and normalised to a maximum voluntary effort (MVE) and represent a period of about a minute.

DISCUSSION AND CONCLUSIONS

In the introduction we noted the ability of biomechanics to elucidate the relationships between work activity and the loads on the tissues. Moving from this understanding of *load* to one of *injury* is not so simple. Our knowledge of acute tissue response is improving, but data on the response of tissues to low loads extending over time periods of the order of weeks or months is almost non-existent.

Work and other activities are inherently dynamic, albeit interspersed with quasi-static postures; a single static analysis is usually not sufficient for most jobs although the 'peak' loading remains important. As a result some investigators are moving to continuous recording in the field for periods counted in hours, This has two results: it challenges data collection but also raises questions concerning how to analyse long records of forces or posture. To provide biomechanical load estimates over industrially useful time periods using most current measurement systems results in very tedious collection and analysis. Electromyography has a clear advantage in this respect.

However, once these records have been collected one must then make decisions regarding summarising the data. There is a concern that at least information concerning the intensity of the exposure variable, its time variation and the duration of exposure be described (Winkel and Mathiassen, 1994). There is no consensus on which variables to record nor how to report them in forms useful in understanding the development of activity and work-related musculoskeletal disorders (Marras *et al.*, 1993; Hansson *et al.*, 1996). Moore *et al.* (1991) proposed a possible framework utilising both peak and time integrated measures for upper limb risk assessment (Table 9.1).

Table 9.1 WMSD injury mechanisms and modelled risk factors.

Disorder	Proposed pathophysiology	Possible biomechanically modelled risk factors
Nerve e.g. Carpal tunnel syndrome[a]	Force of tendons on median nerve	Peak force against flexor retinaculum and median nerve Time integrated force against flexor retinaculum and median nerve
	Hydrostatic pressure in carpal canal	Hydrostatic pressure predicted based upon *in-vivo* and *in-vitro* experimentation
	Contact stress on median nerve	Contact stress predicted from *in-vitro* experimentation and belt-pulley models
Tendon e.g. Tenosynovitis	Bearing loads on sheath Movement of tendon with respect to the sheath	Time integrated force against sheath Cumulative tendon excursion
	Friction between tendon and tendon sheath	Frictional work[b]
e.g. Tendinitis	Strain and cumulative strain in tendon	Peak tendon tension Time integrated tendon force
Muscle Myalgia = pain and disorders	Static or uninterrupted activation	'Static' muscle load (10th percentile APDF) EMG 'gaps'
	Dynamic muscle use	EMG (50 and 90th percentile APDF) Exposure variation assessment (EVA)

[a] Carpal tunnel syndrome may also be secondary to tenosynovitis and other causes.
[b] Variable which showed good match to Silverstein *et al.* (1986) injury risk in laboratory tests (Moore *et al.*, 1991).

This chapter has reviewed how biomechanics offers an approach to analysing and understanding the mechanical function of the musculoskeletal system and thus the relationships between work activity and the loads on the tissues. The interpretation of tissue load poses many challenges. There are precious few acute tolerance data available for most parts of the musculoskeletal system. There are even fewer chronic data available. A possible way around this difficulty is to use biomechanics to estimate tissue loads in epidemiological studies and use the health outcomes to set high and low risk tissue loads. Recently, Wells *et al.* (1997) proposed and successfully used (Norman *et al.*, 1998) such an approach in a study of risk factors for low back pain.

References

ABRAHAMS, M., 1967, Mechanical behaviour of tendon in vitro, *Medical and Biological Engineering*, **5**, 433–443.
ARCHAMBAULT, J.M., HERZOG, W. and HART, D., 1997, The effect of load history in an experimental model of tendon repetitive motion disorders, in Rempel, D. and Armstrong, T.J. (Eds), *Marconi Research Conference*, San Francisco, 1997.

ARMSTRONG, T.J. and CHAFFIN, D.B., 1978, An investigation of the relationship between displacements of the finger and wrist joints and the extrinsic flexor tendons, *Journal of Biomechanics*, **11**, 119–128.

BACKMAN, C., BOQUIST, L., FRIDÉN, J., LORENTZON, R. and TOOLANEN, G., 1990, Chronic Achilles paratenonitis: an experimental model in the rabbit, *Journal of Orthopaedic Research*, **8**, 541–547.

COERT, J.H., UCHIYAMA, S., AMADIO, P.C., BERGLUND, L.J. and AN, K.N., 1995, Flexor tendon-pulley interaction after tendon repair. A biomechanical study, *J Hand Surg*, **20B**(5), 573–577.

DAHLIN, L.B., NORDBORG, C. and LUNDBORG, G., 1987, Morphologic changes in nerve cell bodies induced by experimental graded compression, *Exp Neurol*, **95**, 611–621.

DRURY, C.G., 1987, A biomechanical evaluation of the repetitive motion injury potential of industrial jobs, *Seminars in Occupational Medicine*, **2**(1), 41–49.

FLANNERY, M.M., ROBERTSON, R.N. and COOPER, R.A., 1995, Quantification of tendon excursion through kinematic analysis of typing movements on alternative keyboard layouts, in *Proceedings of the 19th Annual Meeting of the American Society of Biomechanics*, Stanford, US, pp. 195–196.

GOLDSTEIN, S.A., 1981, Biomechanical Aspects of Cumulative Trauma to Tendons and Tendon Sheaths, PhD Thesis, Ann Arbor, University of Michigan.

HADDON, W., 1980, The basic strategies of reducing damage from hazards of all kinds, *Hazard Prevention*, **16**, 8–11.

HAGBERG, M., SILVERSTEIN, B., WELLS, R., SMITH, R., CARAYON, HENDRICK, H.P., *et al.* (Eds), 1995, *Work-related Musculoskeletal Disorders (WMSD): A Handbook for Prevention*, London: Taylor and Francis.

HÄGG, G.M., 1991, Static work loads and occupational myalgia – a new explanation model, in Anderson, P.A., Hobart, D.J. and Danoff, J.V. (Eds), *Electromyographical Kinesiology*, Amsterdam: Elsevier Science Publishers, pp. 141–144.

HÄGG, G.M. and MILERAD, E., 1997, Forearm extensor and flexor exertion during simulated gripping work – an electromyographic study, *Clinical Biomechanics*, **12**(1), 39–43.

HANSSON, G.-A., BALOGH, I., OHLSSON, K., RYLANDER, L. and SKERFVING, S., 1996, Goniometer measurement and computer analysis of wrist angles and movements applied to occupational repetitive work, *Journal of Electromyography and Kinesiology*, **6**(1), 23–35.

HENNEMAN, E., SOMJEN, G. and CARPENTER, D.O., 1965, Functional significance of cell size in spinal motoneurons, *J Neurophys*, **28**, 560–580.

HENRIKSSON, K.G., 1988, Muscle pain in neuromuscular disorders and primary fibromyalgia, *Eur J Appl Physiol*, **57**, 348–352.

JONSSON, B., 1982, Measurement and evaluation of local muscular strain in the shoulder during constrained work, *Journal of Human Ergology*, **11**, 73–88.

KEIR, P., 1995, Functional Implications of the Musculoskeletal Anatomy and Tissue Properties of the Forearm, Unpublished PhD Thesis, Department of Kinesiology, University of Waterloo, Waterloo.

KEIR, P. and WELLS, R., 1994, The effect of typing posture on wrist extensor loading, *Proceedings of the Canadian Society for Biomechanics*, pp. 268–269.

KEIR, P.J., WELLS, R., RANNEY, D. and LAVERY, W., 1997, The effects of tendon load and posture on carpal tunnel pressure, *Journal of Hand Surgery*, **22A**, 628–634.

KEIR, P.J., BACH, J.M. and REMPEL, D.M., 1998, Fingertip loading and carpal tunnel pressure: differences between a pinching and pressing task, *Journal of Orthopedic Research*, **16**(1), 112–115.

LARSSON, S.E., BENGTSSON, A., BODEGÅRD, L., HENRIKSSON, K.G. and LARSSON, J., 1988, Muscle changes in work related chronic myalgia, *Acta Orthop Scand*, **59**(5), 552–556.

LINDMAN, R., HAGBERG, M., DNGQVIST, K., SVDERLUND, K., HULTMAN, E. and THORNELL, L., 1991, Changes in muscle morphology in chronic trapezius myalgia, *Scand J Work Environ Health*, **17**, 347–355.

LUNDBORG, G., GELBERMAN, R.H., MINTEER-CONVERY, M., LEE, Y.H. and HARGENS, A.R., 1982, Median nerve compression in the carpal tunnel: functional response to experimentally induced controlled pressure, *Journal of Hand Surgery*, **7**(3), 252–259.

MARRAS, W.S., LAVENDER, S.A., LEURGANS, S.E., RAJULU, S.L., ALLREAD, W.G., FATHALLAH, F.A. and FERGUSON, S.A., 1993, The role of dynamic three-dimensional trunk motion in occupational-related low back disorders: the effects of workplace factors trunk position and trunk motion characteristics on risk of injury, *Spine*, **18**, 617–628.

MATHIASSEN, S.-E. and WINKEL, J., 1991, Quantifying variation in physical load using exposure-vs-time data, *Ergonomics*, **34**, 1455–1468.

McGILL, S.M. and NORMAN, R.W., 1986, Partitioning of the L4/L5 dynamic moment into disc, ligamentous and muscular components during lifting, *Spine*, **11**(7), 666–678.

McLELLAN, D.L. and SWASH, M., 1976, Longitudinal sliding of the median nerve during movements of the upper limb, *Journal of Neurology, Neurosurgury and Psychiatry*, **39**, 566–570.

MOORE, A., WELLS, R. and RANNEY, D., 1991, Quantifying exposure in occupational manual tasks with cumulative trauma disorder potential, *Ergonomics*, **34**(12), 1433–1453.

NAKAMICHI, K. and TACHIBANA, S., 1995, Restricted motion of the median nerve in carpal tunnel syndrome, *J Hand Surg*, **20B**(4), 460–464.

NIOSH, 1997, *A Critical Review of Epidemiological Evidence for Work-related Musculoskeletal Disorders of the Neck, Upper Extremity, and Low Back*, US Department of Health and Human Services, National Institute of Occupational Safety and Health, 1997.

NORMAN, R. and WELLS, R., 1990, Biomechanical aspects of occupational injury, in *Proceedings of the 23rd Annual Congress of the Human Factors Association of Canada*, pp. 109–118.

NORMAN, R., WELLS, R., NEUMANN, P., FRANK, J., SHANNON, H. and KERR, M., 1998, A comparison of peak vs cumulative physical loading factors for reported low back pain in the automobile industry, *Clinical Biomechanics*, **13**(8), 561–573.

RANNEY, D., WELLS, R. and MOORE, A., 1995, The anatomical location of work-related chronic musculoskeletal disorders in selected industries characterised by repetitive upper limb activity, *Ergonomics*, **38**(7), 1408–1423.

REMPEL, D., 1995, Musculoskeletal loading and carpal tunnel pressure, in Gordon, S., Blair, S. and Fine, L. (Eds), *Repetitive Motion Disorders of the Upper Extremity*, Rosemont, IL: American Academy of Orthopaedic Surgeons, pp. 123–133.

REMPEL, D., MANOJLOVIC, R., LEVINSOHN, D.G., BLOOM, T. and GORDON, L., 1994, The effect of wearing a flexible wrist splint on carpal tunnel pressure during repetitive hand activity, *Journal of Hand and Surgery*, **19A**, 106–110.

REMPEL, D., KEIR, P.J., SMUTZ, W.P. and HARGENS, A.R., 1997, The effects of static fingertip loading on carpal tunnel pressure, *Journal of Orthopedic Research*, **15**(3), 422–426.

REMPEL, D.M., BACH, J., GORDON, L. and SO, Y., 1998, Effects of forearm pronation/supination and metacarpophanangeal flexion on carpal tunnel pressure, *Journal of Hand Surgery*, **23A**, 38–42.

ROHMERT, W., 1973, Problems of determination of rest allowances, part 2: determining rest allowances in different human tasks, *Applied Ergonomics*, **4**(3), 158–162.

ROSE, M.J., 1991, Keyboard operating posture and actuation force: implications for muscle over-use, *Applied Ergonomics*, **22**, 198–203.

ROWE, M., 1987, The diagnosis of tendon and tendon sheath injuries, *Seminars in Occupational Medicine*, **2**(1), 1–6.

RYDEVIK, B. and LUNDBORG, G., 1977, Permeability of intraneural microvessels and perineurium following acute, graded experimental nerve compression, *Scand J Plast Reconstr Surg*, **11**, 179–187.

RYDEVIK, B., LUNDBORG, G. and BAGGE, U., 1981, Effects of graded compression on intraneural blood flow. An in vivo study on rabbit tibial nerve, *J Hand Surg*, **6**(1), 3–12.

RYDEVIK, B.L., PEDOWITZ, R.A., HARGENS, A.R., SWENSON, M.R., MYERS, R.R. and GARFIN, S.R., 1990, Effects of acute, graded compression on spinal nerve root function and structure, *Spine* **16**, 487–493.

SILVERSTEIN, B.A., FINE, L.J. and ARMSTRONG, T.J., 1986, Hand wrist cumulative trauma disorders in industry, *British Journal of Industrial Medicine*, **42**, 779–784.

SILVERSTEIN, B.A., FINE, L.J. and ARMSTRONG, T.J., 1987, Occupational factors and the carpal tunnel syndrome, *American Journal of Industrial Medicine*, **11**, 343–358.

SMITH, E.M., SONSTEGARD, D. and ANDERSON, W., 1977, Carpal tunnel syndrome: contribution of the flexor tendons, *Archives of Physical Medicine and Rehabilitation*, **58**, 379–385.

SMUTZ, W.P., BISHOP, A., NIBLOCK, H. and DREXLER, M., 1995, Measurement of creep strain in flexor tendons during low-force, high-frequency activities such as computer keyboard use, *Clinical Biomechanics*, **10**(2), 67.

SNIJDERS, C., VOLKERS, K. and VLEEMING, A., 1987, Provocation of epicondylalgia (tennis elbow) by power grip or pinching, *Medicine and Science in Sports and Exercise*, **19**(5), 518–523.

SZABO, R.M. and CHIDGEY, L.K., 1989, Stress carpal tunnel pressures in patients with carpal tunnel syndrome and normal patients, *Journal of Hand Surgery*, **14A**(4), 624–627.

SZABO, R.M. and SHARKEY, N.A., 1993, Response of peripheral nerve to cyclic compression in a laboratory rat model, *J orthop Res*, **11**(6), 828–833.

SZABO, R.M., BAY, B.K., SHARKEY, N.A. and GAUT, C., 1994, Median nerve displacement through the carpal canal, *J Hand Surg*, **19A**, 901–906.

UCHIYAMA, S., COERT, J.H., BERGLUND, L., AMADIO, P.C. and AN, K., 1995, Method for the measurement of friction between tendon and pulley, *J Orthop Res*, **13**, 83–89.

VALLS-SOLI, J., ALVAREZ, R. and NUNEZ, M., 1995, Limited longitudinal sliding of the median nerve in patients with carpal tunnel syndrome, *Muscle & Nerve*, **18**, 761–767.

VEIERSTED, K., WESTGAARD, R. and ANDERSEN, P., 1990, Pattern of muscle activity during stereotyped work and its relation to muscle pain, *Int Arch Occup Environ Health*, **62**, 31–41.

VEIERSTED, K.B., WESTGAARD, R.H. and ANDERSEN, P., 1993, Electromyographic evaluation of muscular work pattern as a predictor of trapezius myalgia, *Scandinavian Journal Work Environment and Health*, **19**, 284–290.

WALL, E., MASSIE, J., KWAN, M., RYDEVIK, B., MYERS, R. and GARFIN, S., 1992, Experimental stretch neuropathy, *Journal of Bone and Joint Surgery*, **74B**(1), 126–129.

WELLS, R., NORMAN, R., NEUMANN, P., ANDREWS, D., FRANK, J., SHANNON, H. and KERR, M., 1997, Assessment of physical work load in epidemiologic studies: common measurement metrics for exposure, *Ergonomics*, **40**(1), 51–62.

WINKEL, J. and MATHIASSEN, S.E., 1994, Assessment of physical work load in epidemiologic studies: concepts, issues and operational considerations, *Ergonomics*, **37**(6), 979–989.

CHAPTER TEN

Biomechanical models of the hand, wrist and elbow in ergonomics

RICHARD E. HUGHES AND KAI-NAN AN

INTRODUCTION

Although practicing ergonomists rarely use sophisticated biomechanical models of the hand, wrist, and elbow in conducting job analysis or equipment design, knowledge gained from biomechanical models has had a great influence on the practice of ergonomics. Static models of elbow flexion are used in ergonomics training and teaching to illustrate how large tissue stresses can arise from small loads applied to the hands. Models of the wrist are used to explain the effect of wrist posture on stresses acting on the contents of the carpal tunnel. The purpose of this chapter is to provide an overview of biomechanical models of the hand, wrist, and elbow that may be of use to ergonomists. It will identify impediments to widespread use of upper extremity models in ergonomics practice, and recent work to overcome these barriers will be reviewed.

ELBOW

Biomechanical models of elbow flexion/extension are commonly encountered in ergonomics textbooks and training manuals because they clearly illustrate the principles of levers in occupational ergonomics. Figure 10.1 illustrates a free body analysis of the forearm that forms the basis of a static single muscle biomechanical model of forearm flexion while holding a ball in the hand. Gravity acts on the mass of the ball and centre of mass of the forearm, which produces downward forces having magnitudes of W and G, respectively. Each force acts through a moment arm (15 cm and 30 cm, respectively) to generate clockwise moments. An upward force of magnitude B is generated by the active contraction of the biceps muscle, and it acts at a distance of 3 cm from the elbow flexion/extension axis. To maintain static equilibrium, the net flexion/extension moment at the elbow joint must be zero, which produces the moment equilibrium condition:

$$(G \times 15 \text{ cm}) + (W \times 30 \text{ cm}) - (B \times 3 \text{ cm}) = 0 \qquad (10.1)$$

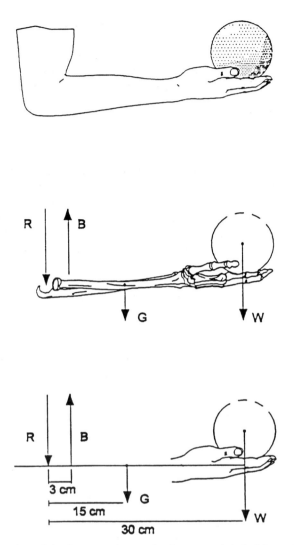

Figure 10.1   Illustration of the forces acting on the forearm while holding a ball weighing W in the hand. The biceps muscle force, B, acts upward on the ulna. The joint reaction force, R, and weight of the forearm, G, act downward. The vector sum of these forces must be zero to maintain static equilibrium. Similarly, the net moment about the joint centre must also be zero. These two conditions can be written algebraically as Equations 10.1 and 10.2.

If the forearm and ball weigh 15N and 20N, respectively, the biceps must generate B = 275N to maintain a static posture. Force equilibrium conditions require that the sum of all forces acting on the forearm in the vertical direction be zero to maintain static equilibrium:

$$B - G - W - R = 0 \tag{10.2}$$

Therefore, the reaction force acting on the trochlear notch of the ulna is 240N. This type of example is widely used in ergonomics training and teaching, because it illustrates how mechanical forces acting on biological tissues (biceps force B and joint reaction force R) can be much greater than the magnitude of externally applied forces. A similar free body analysis can be conducted with forearm rotation to develop a dynamic biomechanical model (Chaffin and Andersson, 1984).

Suppose that an additional muscle is added to the example in Figure 10.1 at a distance of 2 cm from the centre of rotation, and it produces a force acting parallel to the biceps. Then the moment equilibrium and vertical force equilibrium conditions, respectively, are:

$$(G \times 15 \text{ cm}) + (W \times 30 \text{ cm}) - (B \times 3 \text{ cm}) - (H \times 2 \text{ cm }) = 0 \tag{10.3}$$

$$H + B - G - W - R = 0 \tag{10.4}$$

Now there are three unknowns (B, H, and R) but only two equations. Note force equilibrium in the horizontal direction is trivial since all forces in this example are vertical. It is common for biomechanical models to have more muscles than mechanical equilibrium conditions, which is known as 'static indeterminacy'. Mathematically, static indeterminacy means that there is an infinite number of muscle force combinations that can satisfy the equilibrium conditions. Two approaches are typically used to rationally select muscle forces from the potentially infinite set: optimisation and electromyographic (EMG) recordings.

Muscle force prediction using optimisation

It is intuitively reasonable that the central nervous system (CNS) might select muscle forces to optimise some quantity, such as minimising energy expenditure or maximising endurance. It is possible to use static equilibrium condition 10.3 as the foundation for a mathematical optimisation problem that can be solved numerically:

Minimise $\Theta(H,B)$

such that the following conditions hold:

$$(G \times 15 \text{ cm}) + (W \times 30 \text{ cm}) - (B \times 3 \text{ cm}) - (H \times 2 \text{ cm}) = 0 \tag{10.5}$$

$$H \geq 0, B \geq 0 \tag{10.6}$$

The function $\Theta(H,B)$ is the 'objective' or 'criterion' function to be minimised. If it is a convex function, it is easy to find a global minimum for this problem. Note the muscle forces are required to be non-negative (Equation 10.6), because a muscle cannot generate compressive forces. Elbow models in the literature have used a variety of objective functions: sum of muscle forces (Yeo, 1976); sum of muscle stresses (Crowninshield, 1978); maximum muscle stress (An et al., 1984); maximum muscle neural activation (An et al., 1989); and sum of weighted muscle forces raised to integer powers, e.g. $H^n + B^n$ (Raikova, 1996). Gonzales et al. (1996) have formulated a dynamic elbow model using optimal control theory which minimises movement time. However, there is considerable controversy about whether the CNS really does select muscle force activations to minimise a quantitatively definable criterion, and if it does, what the criterion should be.

Muscle force prediction using EMG-driven models

An alternative to the optimisation approach is to estimate muscle forces from EMG recordings. This method requires developing a 'muscle model' that relates measured EMGs to muscle force. Woldstad (1989) developed an EMG-driven model for predicting biceps and triceps muscle forces during rapid elbow flexion and extension movements. The elbow moment at time t, $M(t)$, was modelled as:

$$M(t) = c_B * E_B(t) * MA_B(\theta(t)) * LC_B(\theta(t)) * VC_B\left(\theta(t), \frac{d\theta(t)}{dt}\right)$$

$$+ c_T * E_T(t) * MA_T(\theta(t)) * LC_T(\theta(t)) * VC_T\left(\theta(t), \frac{d\theta(t)}{dt}\right) \tag{10.7}$$

where c was a coefficient that relates EMG, $E(t)$, to muscle force under isometric conditions, and $\theta(t)$ was the included elbow angle at time t (note the subscript, T or B, denotes triceps and biceps, respectively). MA represented the muscle moment arm, which was derived from a simple geometric model of the upper arm. LC was a quadratic polynomial used to incorporate the length–tension property of muscle physiology, and VC was an exponential function used to compensate for the speed of muscle shortening. Parameters for this model were estimated from isometric and isokinetic elbow exertions. Note the basis of this model was a multiple regression relating EMG and net joint moment measured under isometric, anisotonic conditions:

$$M(t) = c_B * (E_B(t) * MA_B(\theta(t))) + c_T * (E_T(t) * MA_T(\theta(t))) + \varepsilon(t) \tag{10.8}$$

The independent variables in the regression model were the product of the EMG and moment arm, so the regression coefficients, c_B and c_T, were the relationships between EMG magnitudes and muscle forces.

From Equation 10.7 it is clear that the forces generated by the biceps and triceps muscles were predicted to be:

$$F_B(t) = c_B * E_B(t) * LC_B(\theta(t)) * VC_B\left(\theta(t), \frac{d\theta(t)}{dt}\right) \tag{10.9}$$

and

$$F_T(t) = c_T * E_T(t) * LC_T(\theta(t)) * VC_T\left(\theta(t), \frac{d\theta(t)}{dt}\right) \tag{10.10}$$

The data requirements for an EMG-driven model are substantial, including EMG recordings of all relevant muscles and elbow angle. Although Woldstad (1989) used joint angle as a surrogate for muscle length, the reported agreement between model predictions and laboratory measurements were high.

Flexion and extension of the forearm is not the only motion of the elbow to model. Baildon and Chapman (1983) and Caldwell and Chapman (1989, 1991) have used EMG recordings to estimate muscle forces during supination in a laboratory setting. Cnockaert et al. (1975) used an EMG model to analyse flexion and supination moments at the elbow. Unfortunately, no applications of EMG-driven models of the elbow to field situations have been reported, probably due to the complex instrumentation required.

Strength prediction models

Since muscle moment arms and lengths change through the joint range of motion, maximal isometric strength depends on joint angle. Biomechanical models of elbow flexion strength have been developed (Hutchins et al., 1993; Ismail and Ranatunga, 1978; van Zuylen et al., 1988; Winters and Kleweno, 1993). Elbow extension strength has also been modeled by Hatze (1981). Prediction of maximum isometric strength through the range of motion is one method for estimating parameters in the length–tension relationship of muscle (An et al., 1989; Hatze, 1981).

WRIST

Carpal tunnel syndrome (CTS) is an important occupational health problem that has both psychosocial and biomechanical risk factors. Epicondylitis of the elbow is also prevalent in many workplaces. Biomechanical models have been proposed for estimating forces in the prime wrist flexors, some of which are involved in epicondylitis, and for predicting stresses in the tissues passing through the carpal tunnel.

Muscle force prediction using optimisation

The optimisation approach to predicting muscle forces from net intersegmental joint moments has been applied to the wrist (Buchanan and Shreeve, 1996; McLaughlin and Miller, 1980; Penrod et al., 1974). In a detailed laboratory study of the forearm and wrist, Buchanan and Shreeve (1996) evaluated the effects of the mechanical representation of the system (number of degrees of freedom, DOF) and objective function selection. The wrist was modelled with two DOF (flexion/extension and radial/ulnar deviation), but simulations were conducted with a variety of elbow representations (one, two, and three DOF). Objective functions considered included sum of squared forces, sum of squared stresses, sum of cubed stresses, and a minimum fatigue criterion proposed by Dul et al. (1984). That study reported that the results strongly depended on the mechanical description of the system used, and that none of the model formulations studied produced muscle force predictions that agreed well with measured EMGs.

Muscle force prediction using EMG-driven models

Several EMG-driven models of the wrist have been outlined (Buchanan et al., 1993; Laurie, 1995; Schoenmarklin and Marras, 1992), but only Buchanan et al. (1993) have described experimental results. Buchanan et al. (1993) assumed a linear relationship between muscle tension and EMG recordings, and a least squares minimisation technique was used to estimate model parameters. Subjects performed isometric contractions at prescribed combinations of flexion/extension and radial/ulnar deviation moments. A Monte Carlo simulation was performed to assess the sensitivity of model parameters to noise in the EMG signal, and they were found to be very stable.

Belt–pulley models

A biomechanical model that has had wide impact on industrial ergonomics is the pulley model of the carpal tunnel developed by Armstrong and Chaffin (1979). In that model the extrinsic finger flexor tendons (flexor digitorum profundus, flexor digitorum superficialis, and flexor pollicis longus) were conceptualised as belts wrapping around a pulley (Figure 10.2). In a flexed wrist posture, the flexor retinaculum acts as a pulley; in extension, the carpal bones are the pulley. The model relates tendon force, which can be estimated using hand models (see later), to normal forces acting between the extrinsic tendons and surrounding tissues. One anatomic structure near these tendons, the median nerve, is of particular interest to occupational ergonomics because of its role in carpal tunnel syndrome. Armstrong and Chaffin (1979) argued that compression of the median nerve in the

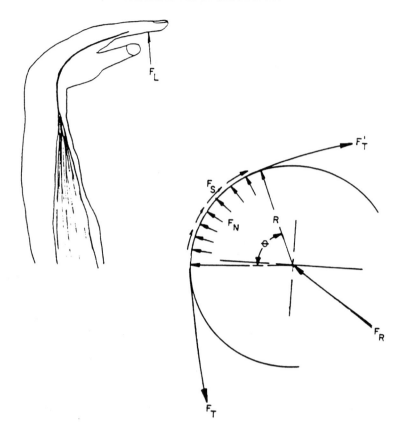

Figure 10.2   The tendons of the extrinsic finger flexor muscles can be conceptualised as belts wrapping around a pulley. The tension in the tendon, F_T' and F_T, are different because of frictional forces acting on the belt by the pulley. Normal forces acting on the belt by the pulley, F_N, are required to maintain equilibrium (reprinted from Chaffin and Andersson, 1984, by permission of John Wiley and Sons, Inc.).

carpal tunnel by adjacent tendons is an aetiological factor in carpal tunnel syndrome. The normal force acting between the belt and pulley, F_N, is (per unit length):

$$F_N = \frac{F_T e^{\mu\theta}}{R} \qquad\qquad (10.11)$$

where F_N is the tension in the belt, μ is the coefficient of friction between belt and pulley, θ is the included angle of belt–pulley contact, and R is the radius of curvature of the pulley (LeVeau, 1977). Because of the lubrication of the tendons by synovial fluid, ignoring frictional forces gives:

$$F_N = \frac{F_T}{R} \qquad\qquad (10.12)$$

This relation was used by Armstrong and Chaffin (1979) to evaluate the effects of wrist posture and gender-related wrist anthropometry on tendon stresses, based on wrist radii measurements made on cadavers (Armstrong and Chaffin, 1978). According to the model, wrist size affects the normal forces acting between the tendons and surrounding tissues (Figure 10.3).

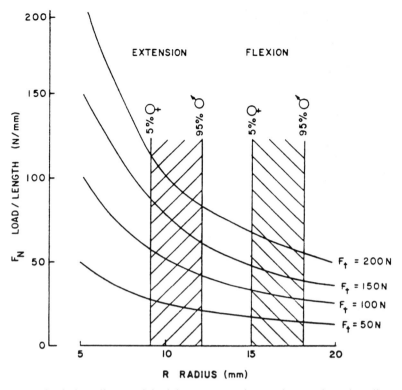

Figure 10.3 The belt–pulley model of the wrist can be used to analyse the effect of wrist size and posture on the normal force, F_N, acting on the contents of the carpal tunnel. A small wrist (5 per cent female) has larger normal force than a large wrist (95 per cent male) because the radius of curvature is smaller. Forces with the wrist in extension are larger than forces with the wrist in flexion because the radius of curvature in extension is smaller than in flexion (reprinted from Armstrong and Chaffin, 1979, with kind permission from Elsevier Sciences Ltd, UK).

The total normal force acting between the tendon and surrounding tissues is:

$$F_R = 2F_T Sin\frac{\theta}{2} \tag{10.13}$$

where F_R is the total reaction force acting on the tendon. This indicates that wrist angle is a critical determinant of forces acting to support the extrinsic finger flexors. Figure 10.4, which is based on Equation 10.13, illustrates that larger wrist angles lead to more reaction force on the tendon. This observation provides a basis for 'neutral wrist posture' guidelines in the prevention of carpal tunnel syndrome.

Because some parameters were virtually impossible to determine *in vivo* at the time, Armstrong and Chaffin (1979) did not use their model to analyse jobs quantitatively. However, the model has had a wide influence on ergonomic practice by highlighting the importance of non-neutral wrist postures in the development of carpal tunnel syndrome.

Other researchers have worked to estimate parameters in the model. Albin (1987) used the pulley model to estimate the *in vivo* coefficient of friction for the extrinsic finger flexor tendons to be 0.12. Keir and Wells (1992) used magnetic resonance imaging (MRI) to estimate the radius of curvature of the flexor digitorum profundus and flexor digitorum

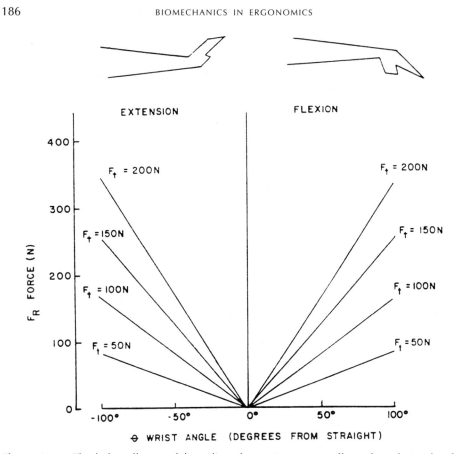

Figure 10.4 The belt–pulley model predicts that wrist posture affects the relationship be-tween tendon tension, F_T, and the reaction force, F_R. This observation supports the widely used ergonomic principle that neutral wrist postures reduce stress on the tissues in the carpal tunnel (reprinted from Armstrong and Chaffin, 1979, with kind permission from Elsevier Sciences Ltd, UK).

superficialis tendons *in vivo* under loaded and unloaded finger conditions. Extended (20°), neutral, and flexed (20° and 45°) wrist postures were tested. Radii of curvature for the flexor digitorum profundus ranged from 8.6 mm in 45° flexion to 57.6 mm in neutral under loaded conditions. More importantly, the study found that the tendons did not have constant radius of curvature throughout the length of the carpal tunnel. In fact, there is a smaller radius at the distal end of the tunnel when in a flexed posture. Tensile force in the tendon also appeared to affect the radii of curvature.

The pulley model described by Armstrong and Chaffin (1979) was – like most bio-mechanical models – deterministic, even though there is significant anatomical and physiological variability within a population. Miller and Freivalds (1995) used the pulley model of the extrinsic finger flexor tendons passing through the carpal tunnel as the basis for a stochastic model of extrinsic finger flexor tendon trauma. The material properties and mechanical loading on the tendons were considered to be random variables, and the probability of injury was derived.

The belt–pulley model of the wrist has also been incorporated into a sophisticated method for assessing exposures in epidemiological studies of upper extremity cumulative trauma disorders. In contrast to most exposure assessment methods that focus on job checklists or simple EMG techniques, Moore *et al.* (1991) used a belt–pulley model to estimate internal mechanical stresses on the extrinsic finger flexor tendons from EMG and electrogoniometer data. The belt–pulley model was used to estimate forces on the tissues surrounding the tendons, tendon excursion, and the frictional work done by the tendons on the surrounding tissues. In a laboratory study of simulated jobs, the frictional work measure was closest to the estimates of risk identified in the cross sectional epidemiological study of cumulative trauma disorders (Silverstein *et al.*, 1986) and carpal tunnel syndrome (Silverstein *et al.*, 1987). More importantly, this model-based exposure assessment system has been used to identify a relationship between exposure to physical risk factors and risk of cumulative trauma disorders (Wells *et al.*, 1992). The modeling approach has also been used to evaluate alternative job rotation systems for cumulative trauma disorder potential (Wells *et al.*, 1995).

Strength prediction models

Loren *et al.* (1996) have developed a biomechanical model for predicting wrist flexion and extension strength throughout the flexion/extension range of motion. The model includes both mechanical and physiological factors, including the effects of wrist posture on tendon moment arms and muscle fibre lengths. Moreover, the model incorporates the effect of tendon compliance on muscle fibre length, which has the effect of changing the length–tension curve of the musculotendinous unit.

HAND

The high incidence and economic cost associated with cumulative trauma disorders of the hand and wrist has generated a significant amount of research on the biomechanics of the hand. Even musculoskeletal disorders occurring in the wrist and forearm are affected by hand mechanics, because forces applied to the fingers affect the extrinsic flexor and extensor muscle forces.

Muscle force prediction models

Biomechanical models similar to that described in Equations 10.5 and 10.6 can be developed for fingers. Force and moment equilibrium conditions for the articulations of the hand can be formulated under static conditions (An *et al.*, 1985; Chao and An, 1978a, 1978b; Chao *et al.*, 1976). Figure 10.5 illustrates a model of the finger in which the interphalangeal joints are assumed to be revolute joints having only flexion/extension motion; the carpometacarpal and metacarpophalangeal joints are modelled as universal joints (flexion/extension and abduction/adduction motions). The geometry of the finger segments must be specified, which can be done by specifying the rotation between coordinate systems fixed to each bone in the finger. Maximum muscle forces can be modelled as being proportional to the physiological cross sectional area of each muscle. Due to the interconnectedness of the tendons of the finger extensor mechanism, additional constraints are added to the allowable forces in the intrinsic muscles and the extensor digitorum communis muscle (An *et al.*, 1985). Since the mechanical description of the finger is statically indeterminate, the optimisation approach can be used to solve for the muscle

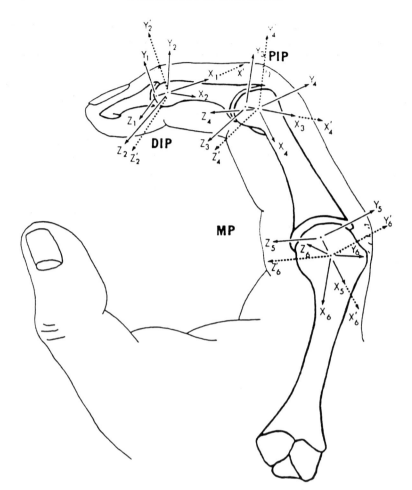

Figure 10.5 Sagittal plane view of a finger model. Finger posture is described by defining the orientations of coordinate systems fixed to each bone relative to each other. Moment and force equilibrium conditions are formulated at each joint of the finger.

forces, given a specified externally applied force at the fingertip. An *et al.* (1985) solved this model using several objective functions, including combinations of muscle forces, joint reaction forces, joint moments, and maximum muscle stress. Table 10.1 shows the range of muscle forces predicted, normalised to external force magnitude for several types of grips (Figure 10.6) and tasks. Force generated by the flexor digitorum profundus muscle during tip pinch was between 1.93 and 2.08 times the magnitude of the force applied to the fingertip, depending on the objective function used in the optimisation. For the lateral key pinch, the ratio was 3.17 to 3.47. Given the uncertainty about what objective function is to be minimised, how realistic are the model predictions?

Due to the long, slender morphology of extrinsic hand tendons, it is possible to measure tendon tension directly *in vivo* using a miniature S-shaped force transducer (An *et al.*, 1990). Schuind *et al.* (1992) used such a force transducer to measure tension intraoperatively in the flexor digitorum profundus, flexor digitorum superficialis, and flexor pollicis longus muscles in five patients undergoing carpal tunnel surgery. Since the operations were conducted using local anaesthesia, subjects could actively perform grip-

Table 10.1 Finger muscle forces predicted by optimisation (expressed as a ratio of tendon tension to externally applied force) using a variety of objective functions.

Function	FDP	FDS	RI	LU	UI	LE
Tip pinch	1.93–2.08	1.75–2.16	0.0–0.99	0.0–0.72	0.21–0.65	–
Pulp pinch	2.53–3.14	0.32–1.32	0.0–1.61	0.0–1.17	0.62–1.19	–
Lateral pinch	1.37–5.95	–	1.01–7.04	0.0–6.10	–	7.45–15.94
Grasp	3.17–3.47	1.51–2.14	0.0–1.19	0.0–0.91	0.0–0.49	–
Briefcase grip	0.0–0.02	1.70–1.78	0.0–0.45	0.0–0.33	0.11–0.27	–
Holding glass	2.77–2.99	1.29–1.57	–	0.48–0.53	0.28–0.38	–
Opening jar	3.50–5.49	–	4.2–4.53	0.0–1.15	0.0–1.0	9.48–16.23

Ranges indicate the range of force predictions that can be generated by minimising different objective functions (An *et al.*, 1985). Muscles listed are the flexor digitorum profundus (FDP), flexor digitorum superficialis (FDS), extrinsic extensor (LE), lumbrical (LU), radial interosseus (RI), and ulnar interosseus (UI).

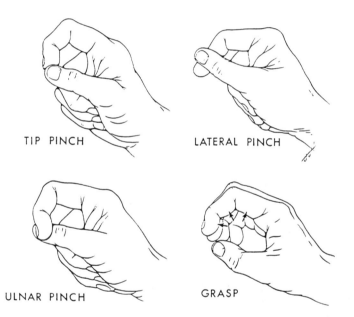

Figure 10.6 Grip postures analysed by An *et al.* (1985). Summary results for these postures are presented in Table 10.1.

ping tasks while the tension in their tendons were being recorded. Table 10.2 provides the measured forces and ranges of forces predicted by models (An *et al.*, 1985; Chao *et al.*, 1989; and Cooney and Chao, 1977). Although measurements of forces during tip pinch were outside the range of model predictions, lateral pinch measurements agreed well. The *in vivo* measurements do confirm model predictions that tendon forces are greater than the applied force, sometimes by a significant amount.

An optimisation model of the finger similar to that of Chao and An (1978a, 1978b) and An *et al.* (1985) was implemented in a system specifically designed for ergonomic analysis of hand tools (Yun and Freivalds, 1995). Force sensing resistors were used to

Table 10.2 Comparison of *in vivo* measurements and predicted tendon forces during pinch (expressed as a ratio of tendon tension to external pinch force).

Tendon	Measurements	Predictions
Tip pinch		
FPL	3.60 (4.62)	2.28–3.52
FDP	7.92 (6.33)	1.93–2.08
FDS	1.73 (1.51)	1.75–2.16
Lateral pinch		
FPL	3.05 (3.04)	2.47–3.84
FDP	2.90 (2.61)	1.37–5.95
FDS	0.71 (0.69)	–

Tendon forces were measured using an S-shaped buckle transducer placed around the tendon, and predictions were made using models (An *et al.*, 1985; Chao *et al.*, 1989; Cooney and Chao, 1977). FPL is the flexor pollicis longus, FDP is the flexor digitorum profundus, and FDS is the flexor digitorum superficialis. Means (and standard deviations) are presented for the forces measured *in vivo*; ranges are given for model predictions using different objective functions.

measure hand contact forces, and a Cyberglove (Virtual Technologies) was used to measure finger geometry. This instrumentation system provided data for the biomechanical model, which produced muscle forces estimates.

Unlike hand tool use, where static gripping is common, keyboarding and piano playing are fast enough to require dynamic biomechanical models of the fingers. Harding *et al.* (1989, 1993) developed an optimisation type sagittal plane finger model for use in analysing piano playing. Tendon tensions between 0.7 and 3.2 times the applied fingertip force were predicted. Harding *et al.* (1989) reported using an optimisation model of the finger for determining finger positions for piano playing that would minimise internal tissue loads. Wolf *et al.* (1993) used the model of Harding *et al.* (1989) to analyse the biomechanics of the index finger while playing Mendelssohn's *Song Without Words* (op. 19, no. 2) and identify potential risk factors for the development of cumulative trauma disorders in pianists. Dynamic finger models have also been developed by Brook *et al.* (1995) and Buchner *et al.* (1985).

Compared to the finger, few models of the thumb have been developed. Planar (Hirsch *et al.*, 1974) and three-dimensional (Cooney and Chao, 1977; Toft and Berme, 1980) models of the thumb have been used to estimate tendon and joint contact forces. These models solved the problem of static indeterminacy by assuming only agonist muscles were active and lumping functionally similar muscles together, which reduced the number of unknowns to the number of equilibrium conditions. Cooney and Chao (1977) predicted that for each Newton of force applied to the thumb during lateral pinch, the flexor pollicis longus tension was between 2.28 and 3.52N. Similarly, lateral pinches produced flexor pollicis longus forces 2.47 to 3.84 times the magnitude of the externally applied force. The authors concluded that the compression force at the carpometacarpal joint, which is often involved in arthritis of the hand, could range between 837 and 1609N during a strong grasp. An EMG-driven model of thumb flexion/extension was developed based on an assumed polynomial relationship between muscle tension and EMG (An *et al.*, 1983). The EMG-driven model predicted flexor and extensor pollicis longus muscle forces similar to those reported in Cooney and Chao (1977).

Fingertip pulp models

Fingertip pulp is comprised of the skin and underlying fatty tissue on the ventral surface of the distal phalanx of each digit. Forces applied to the skin by contact with the environment may not be the same as the forces applied to the skeleton, because the pulp of the fingertips may affect the temporal and spatial distribution of the forces. A biomechanical model of the fingertip pulp is needed to bridge the gap between the external force applied to the skin and the forces acting on the phalanges of the digits. Serina (1996) developed a quasi-static mechanical model of fingertip pulp for use in analysing keyboarding tasks. It used an axisymmetric, ellipsoidally shaped membrane with a uniform internal pressure to model the finger pulp. The membrane was assumed to extend infinitely between two parallel, rigid plates. The subcutaneous tissue was modelled as an incompressible, inviscid fluid; the skin was modelled as an isotropic, elastic, incompressible continuum undergoing finite deformations. Model predictions were compared to *in vivo* measurements of pulp displacement under a variety of loading conditions. Although that model assists in understanding finger pulp mechanics quasi-statically, a fully dynamic model is necessary for use in analysing the rapid finger movements associated with keyboard use or piano playing.

Geometric contact models

The ergonomics of using hand tools depends on the contact between the palm, thumb, fingers and the tool itself. Models have been developed for predicting hand kinematics as it wraps around various types of objects. Buchholz and Armstrong (1992) developed a kinematic model of the hand based on modelling each segment of the fingers as a three-dimensional ellipse. They used it to predict hand geometry during power grips. Models for predicting hand kinematics have also been implemented in computer-aided design (CAD) software (Davidoff and Freivalds, 1990, 1993) and custom software (Buford and Thompson, 1987). Gourret *et al.* (1989) developed a finite element model for predicting the behaviour of the soft tissues of the hand when grasping soft objects.

Strength prediction models

Models have been developed for predicting maximum finger flexion strength (An *et al.*, 1985; Chao and An, 1978b; Lee and Kroemer, 1993; Lee and Rim, 1990; Valero-Cuevas *et al.*, 1996). These models maximise force generated by the finger against an object subject to mechanical equilibrium conditions and maximum muscle force limits.

Belt–pulley models

Tendons wrap around connective tissue structures in the fingers, just as they do in the carpal tunnel. Uchiyama *et al.* (1995) modelled the interaction of the flexor digitorum profundus tendon and the fibrous bands restraining it in the finger as a belt and pulley. The model was used to estimate the coefficient of friction between tendon and pulley in the index finger, which ranged from 0.03 to 0.05.

MULTIPLE SEGMENT ARM MODELS

While most published models have focused on isolated joints or joint complexes, some biomechanical models of the upper extremity have included the shoulder, elbow, and wrist. Raikova (1992) formulated an optimisation model for predicting muscle forces in the upper extremity that included the glenohumeral, elbow (flexion/extension and supination/pronation), and wrist (radial/ulnar deviation and flexion/extension) joints. Lemay and Crago (1996) developed a model to simulate forearm and wrist movements using a sophisticated muscle modelling approach. Hogan (1985) has proposed biomechanical models of the upper extremity based on joint stiffness considerations. Buchner *et al.* (1985) formulated a sagittal five-link model that included the forearm and multi-segment finger representation and analysed it for controllability. Detailed models of the whole arm have not been extensively used in ergonomics, but whole body models that include arms are used in ergonomics practice and applied research.

WHOLE BODY BIOMECHANICAL MODELS

The most widely used biomechanical models of the upper extremity are whole body biomechanical models used primarily for assessing stresses on the low back, such as the Two-Dimensional Static Strength Prediction Model (2DSSPP) and Three-Dimensional Static Strength Prediction Model (3DSSPP) developed by the University of Michigan. These models predict maximal strength capabilities and estimate internal mechanical forces on the lumbar spine. The biomechanical models implemented in the 2DSSPP (Chaffin and Andersson, 1984) and 3DSSPP (Chaffin and Erig, 1991; Garg and Chaffin, 1975) contain a single DOF elbow joint but no wrist or hand joints. It computes net intersegmental elbow flexion/extension moment and compares it to normative strength values, but it does not compute internal muscle forces at the elbow. Nor does it model supination/pronation torque on the forearm. It is unclear how the simplified representation of the upper extremity in these models affects their results. However, Al-Eisawi *et al.* (1994) reported experimental observations that wrist strength is not a limiting factor for whole body exertions, except when the wrist is in an extended posture and the task requires wrist flexion strength.

Whole body biomechanical models are being incorporated into computer-aided design (CAD) programs to augment the traditional anthropometry assessments of workstation design. An AutoCAD system called ergoSHAPE (Launis and Lehtel, 1992) computes elbow joint moments and compares them to estimated maximum strengths (no detailed wrist or hand is included in the model). Models of the upper extremity can also be used to solve the 'inverse kinematics' problem that arises in these applications for determining joint angles required to reach specific targets (Jung *et al.*, 1995; Lenarcic and Umek, 1994; Lepoutre, 1993).

Whole body biomechanical models are also used for computing net intersegmental moments in field and laboratory research studies. Some models include the elbow but not the hand or wrist (Chaffin and Andersson, 1984; Kromodihardjo and Mital, 1986), but others include a wrist joint (Cheng and Kumar, 1991; Khalil and Ramadan, 1988; McGill and Norman, 1985).

Ergonomics researchers and practitioners should be aware of how the upper extremity is represented in whole body biomechanical models, because they are so commonly used in ergonomics practice.

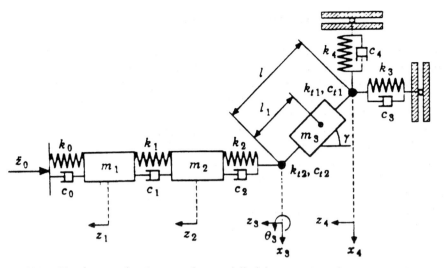

Figure 10.7 Hand–arm vibration can be modelled by a series of masses, springs, and dashpots. An external acceleration can be placed on the distal element of the model, and the resulting mass displacements can be simulated. Energy dissipation by model elements can also be computed (reprinted from Thomas *et al.*, 1996, with kind permission from Academic Press, London, UK).

HAND–ARM VIBRATION MODELS

Numerous biomechanical models have been developed for studying the effect of vibration on the upper extremity, especially vibration occurring as the result of using vibrating hand tools. These models provide insight into what anatomic structures absorb the vibrational energy applied to the hand. The models can be used to simulate a variety of engineering controls for reducing the effect of vibration on the body, especially those parts of the body known to respond unfavourably to hand–arm vibration.

The models are based on sets of spring–mass–dashpot systems connected in series, each representing a part of the arm. The mechanical system is mathematically represented by systems of second order differential equations. Figure 10.7 illustrates a five DOF model of the arm (Thomas *et al.*, 1996). Masses m_1, m_2, and m_3 can be loosely thought of as representing the masses of the hand, forearm, and upper arm, respectively. The mechanical properties of the skin, muscles, bones, ligaments and other tissues are represented by linear springs and dashpots. Accelerations, Z_o, are applied to the end of the system. Energy dissipation in model elements, which correspond to anatomic regions, can be computed.

The distinguishing characteristic of these models is the number of DOF they contain. Many models contain two (Gurram *et al.*, 1994), three (Gurram *et al.*, 1994, 1995; Rakheja *et al.*, 1993; Reynolds and Jokel, 1974; Reynolds and Falkenberg, 1984), four (Rakheja *et al.*, 1993; Reynolds and Falkenberg, 1984) or five DOFs (Thomas *et al.*, 1996). The differences arise from how the arm is represented. For example, Gurram *et al.* (1994) analysed a two DOF model containing hand and forearm masses and a three DOF model that contained an additional mass corresponding to a glove on the hand. Similarly, some authors choose to model the tissues of the hand in more detail (Reynolds and Falkenberg, 1984; Reynolds and Keith, 1977) while others choose a more aggregate approach with finger, hand, and arm elements (Reynolds and Falkenberg, 1984; Suggs and Mishoe, 1977; Wood and Suggs, 1977).

Model parameters are determined experimentally. Subjects hold a vibrating handle which has an accelerometer attached to it. The driving point impedance, which is the ratio of the excitation force to driving point response velocity, is computed. Model parameters are chosen so that model predictions match the magnitude and phase of the measured data. Earlier authors used trial and error methods (Mishoe and Suggs, 1977; Reynolds and Falkenberg, 1984); model parameters can also be estimated by solving a numerical optimisation problem in which the objective function is the square of the difference between model predictions and measurements (Gurram *et al.*, 1994; Rakheja *et al.*, 1993). Many authors have noted that model parameters depend on grip strength, which affects the coupling between the vibration source and hand.

SUMMARY

Although biomechanical models of the upper extremity have not been widely used for analyses by ergonomics practitioners, they are commonly used to develop insight into the biomechanical basis of ergonomics. Elbow flexion models illustrate that internal muscle forces can be much greater than the actual hand loads being lifted. Similarly, biomechanical models illustrate that tension in the extrinsic hand tendons can be much greater than fingertip loads, and they illustrate the effect of grip type on tendon loading.

Large data requirements for hand models are a major impediment to their widespread use by ergonomics practitioners. Improvements in sensors for measuring forces acting on the hand have occurred (Bishu *et al.*, 1993; Fellows and Freivalds, 1989; Jensen *et al.*, 1991; Rempel *et al.*, 1994), but the development of low cost data collection equipment and data analysis software is necessary for biomechanical models of the hand, wrist, and elbow to become part of the ergonomist's armamentarium.

Recent emphasis on ergonomic interventions for the prevention of carpal tunnel syndrome has highlighted the importance of understanding the forces acting on the median nerve as it passes through the carpal tunnel. Biomechanical models have illustrated the effects of grip type on the extrinsic finger flexor tendons, and the pulley model explains how wrist flexion and extension modifies the relationship between tendon tension and the normal force acting between the tendons and surrounding tissues in the carpal tunnel.

Hand–arm vibration models have provided insight into which tissues of the upper extremity absorb vibrational energy. Vibration models have contributed to the development of vibration standards, which has a direct impact on ergonomics practice. Moreover, hand–arm vibration models can be used to modify tool design to change their frequency characteristics.

References

ALBIN, T.J., 1987, In vivo estimation of the coefficient of friction between extrinsic flexor tendons and surrounding structures in the carpal tunnel. *Proceedings of the Human Factors Society 31st Annual Meeting*, Vol. 1, pp. 323–324, New York, NY, October 19–23.

AL-EISAWI, K.W., KERK, C.J. and CONGLETON, J.J., 1994, Limitations of wrist strength to manual exertion capability in 2D biomechanical modeling, *Proceedings of the Human Factors and Ergonomics Society 38th Annual Meeting,* Vol. 1, pp. 559–563.

AMIS, A.A., DOWSON, D. and WRIGHT, V., 1979, Muscle strengths and musculo-skeletal geometry of the upper limb, *Engineering in Medicine,* **8**, 41–48.

AN, K.N., COONEY, W.P., CHAO, E.Y., ASKEW, L.J. and DAUBE, J.R., 1983, Determination of forces in extensor pollicis longus and flexor pollicis longus of the thumb, *Journal of Applied Physiology*, **54**, 714–719.

AN, K.N., KWAK, B.M., CHAO, E.Y. and MORREY, B.F., 1984, Determination of muscle and joint forces: a new technique to solve the indeterminate problem, *Journal of Biomechanical Engineering*, **106**, 364–367.

AN, K.N., CHAO, E.Y., COONEY, W.P. and LINSCHEID, R.L., 1985, Forces in the normal and abnormal hand, *Journal of Orthopaedic Research*, **3**, 202–211.

AN, K.N., KAUFMAN, K.R. and CHAO, E.Y.S., 1989, Physiological considerations of muscle force through the elbow joint, *Journal of Biomechanics*, **22**, 1249–1256.

AN, K.-N., BERGLUND, L., COONEY, W.P., CHAO, E.Y.S. and KOVACEVIC, N., 1990, Direct in vivo tendon force measurement system, *Journal of Biomechanics*, **23**, 1269–1271.

ARMSTRONG, T.J. and CHAFFIN, D.B., 1978, An investigation of the relationship between displacements of the finger and wrist joints and the extrinsic finger flexor tendons, *Journal of Biomechanics*, **11**, 119–128.

ARMSTRONG, T.J. and CHAFFIN, D.B., 1979, Some biomechanical aspects of the carpal tunnel, *Journal of Biomechanics*, **12**, 567–570.

BAILDON, R.W.A. and CHAPMAN, A.E., 1983, Mechanical properties of a single equivalent muscle producing forearm supination, *Journal of Biomechanics*, **16**, 811–819.

BISHU, R.R., WANG, W. and CHIN, A., 1993, Force distribution at the container hand/handle interface using force-sensing resistors, *International Journal of Industrial Ergonomics*, **11**, 225–231.

BROOK, N., MIZRAHI, J., SHOHAM, M. and DAYAN, J., 1995, A biomechanical model of index finger dynamics, *Medical Engineering and Physics*, **17**, 54–63.

BUCHANAN, T.S. and SHREEVE, D.A., 1996, An evaluation of optimization techniques for the prediction of muscle activation patterns during isometric tasks, *Journal of Biomechanical Engineering*, **118**, 565–574.

BUCHANAN, T.S., MONIZ, M.J., DEWALD, J.P.A. and RYMER, W.Z., 1993, Estimation of muscle forces about the wrist joint during isometric tasks using an EMG coefficient method, *Journal of Biomechanics*, **26**, 547–560.

BUCHHOLZ, B. and ARMSTRONG, T.J., 1992, A kinematic model of the human hand to evaluate its prehensile capabilities, *Journal of Biomechanics*, **25**, 149–162.

BUCHNER, H.J., HINES, M.J. and HEMAMI, H., 1985, A mechanism for touch control of a sagittal five-link finger-hand, *IEEE Transactions on Systems, Man, and Cybernetics*, **SMC-15**, 69–77.

BUFORD, W.L. and THOMPSON, D.E., 1987, A system for three-dimensional interactive simulation of hand biomechanics, *IEEE Transactions on Biomedical Engineering*, **BME-34**, 444–453.

CALDWELL, G.E. and CHAPMAN, A.E., 1989, Applied muscle modelling: implementation of muscle-specific models, *Computers in Biology and Medicine*, **19**, 417–434.

CALDWELL, G.E. and CHAPMAN, A.E., 1991, The general distribution problem: a physiological solution which includes antagonism, *Human Movement Science*, **10**, 355–392.

CHAFFIN, D.B. and ANDERSSON, G.B.J., 1984, *Occupational Biomechanics*, New York: John Wiley and Sons.

CHAFFIN, D.B. and ERIG, M., 1991, Three-dimensional biomechanical static strength prediction model sensitivity to postural and anthropometric inaccuracies, *IIE Transactions*, **23**, 215–227.

CHAO, E.Y. and AN, K.N., 1978a, Determination of internal hand forces in human hand, *Journal of Engineering Mechanics Division*, Div. ASCE, **104**, 255–272.

CHAO, E.Y. and AN, K.N., 1978b, Graphical interpretation of the solution to the redundant problem in biomechanics, *Journal of Biomechanical Engineering*, **100**, 159–167.

CHAO, E.Y., OPGRANDE, J.D. and AXMEAR, F.E., 1976, Three-dimensional force analysis of finger joints in selected isometric hand functions, *Journal of Biomechanics*, **9**, 387–396.

CHAO, E.Y.S., AN, K.N., COONEY, W.P. and LINSCHEID, R.L., 1989, *Biomechanics of the Hand: A Basic Research Study*. Singapore: World Scientific, 1989.

CHENG, C. and KUMAR, S., 1991, A three-dimensional static torso model for the six human lumbar joints, *International Journal of Industrial Ergonomcs*, **7**, 327–339.

CNOCKAERT, J.C., LENSEL, G. and PERTUZON, E., 1975, Relative contribution of individual muscles to the isometric contraction of a muscular group, *Journal of Biomechanics*, **8**, 191–197.

COONEY, W.P. and CHAO, E.Y.S., 1977, Biomechanical analysis of static forces in the thumb during hand function, *Journal of Bone and Joint Surgery*, **59-A**, 27–36.

CROWNINSHIELD, R.D., 1978, Use of optimization techniques to predict muscle forces, *Journal of Biomechanical Engineering*, **100**, 88–92.

DAVIDOFF, N. and FREIVALDS, A., 1990, Computer-aided design modeling of the human hand, in Lovesey, E.J. (Ed.), *Contemporary Ergonomics*, London: Taylor and Francis, pp. 181–186.

DAVIDOFF, N.A. and FREIVALDS, A., 1993, A graphic model of the human hand using CATIA, *International Journal of Industrial Ergonomics*, **12**, 255–264.

DUL, J., JOHNSON, G.E., SHIAVI, R. and TOWNSEND, M.A., 1984, Muscular synergism – II. A minimum-fatigue criterion for load sharing between synergistic muscles, *Journal of Biomechanics*, **17**, 675–684.

FELLOWS, G.L. and FREIVALDS, A., 1989, The use of force sensing resistors in ergonomic tool design, *Proceedings of the Human Factors Society 33rd Annual Meeting*, Denver, CO, October 16–20, pp. 713–717.

GARG, A. and CHAFFIN, D.B., 1975, A biomechanical computerised simulation of human strength, *AIIE Transactions*, **7**, 1–15.

GONZALES, R.V., HUTCHINS, E.L., BARR, R.E. and ABRAHAM, L.D., 1996, Development and evaluation of a musculoskeletal model of the elbow joint complex, *Journal of Biomechanical Engineering*, **118**, 32–40.

GOURRET, J.-P., THALMANN, N.M. and THALMANN, D., 1989, Simulation of object and human skin deformations in a grasping task, *Computer Graphics*, **23**, 21–30.

GURRAM, R., RAKHEJA, S. and GOUW, G.J., 1994, Vibration transmission characteristics of the human hand-arm and gloves, *International Journal of Industrial Ergonomics*, **13**, 217–234.

GURRAM, R., RAKHEJA, S. and GOUW, G.J., 1995, Mechanical impedance of the human hand-arm system subject to sinusoidal and stochastic excitations, *International Journal of Industrial Ergonomics*, **16**, 135–145.

HARDING, D.C., BRANDT, K.D. and HILBERRY, B.M., 1989, Minimization of finger joint forces and tendon tensions in pianists, *Medical Problems of Performing Artists*, **4**, 103–113.

HARDING, D.C., BRAND, K.D. and HILLBERRY, B.M., 1993, Finger joint force minimization in pianists using optimization techniques, *Journal of Biomechanics*, **26**, 1403–1412.

HATZE, H., 1981, Estimation of myodynamic parameter values from observations on isometrically contracting muscle groups, *European Journal of Applied Physiology*, **46**, 325–338.

HIRSCH, D., PAGE, D., MILLER, D., DUMBLETON, J.H. and MILLER, E.H., 1974, A biomechanical analysis of the metacarpophalangeal joint of the thumb, *Journal of Biomechanics*, **7**, 343–348.

HOGAN, N., 1985, The mechanics of multi-joint posture and movement control, *Biological Cybernetics*, **52**, 315–331.

HUTCHINS, E.L., GONZALES, R.V. and BARR, R.E., 1993, Comparison of experimental and analytical torque-angle relationships of the human elbow joint complex, *Biomedical Sciences Instrumentation*, **29**, 17–24.

ISMAIL, H.M. and RANATUNGA, K.W., 1978, Isometric tension development in a human skeletal muscle in relation to its working range of movement: the length-tension relation of biceps brachii muscle, *Experimental Neurology*, **62**, 595–604.

JENSEN, T.R., RADWIN, R.G. and WEBSTER, J.G., 1991, A conductive polymer sensor for measuring external finger forces, *Journal of Biomechanics*, **24**, 851–858.

JUNG, E.S., KEE, D. and CHUNG, M.K., 1995, Upper body reach posture prediction for ergonomic evaluation models, *International Journal of Industrial Ergonomics*, **16**, 95–107.

KEIR, P.J. and WELLS, R.P., 1992, MRI of the carpal tunnel. Implications for carpal tunnel syndrome, in Kumar, S. (Ed.), *Advances in Industrial Ergonomics and Safety IV*, Philadelphia: Taylor and Francis, pp. 753–760.

KHALIL, T.M. and RAMADAN, M.Z., 1988, Biomechanical evaluation of lifting tasks: a microcomputer-based model, *Computers in Industrial Engineering*, **14**, 153–160.

KROMODIHARDJO, S. and MITAL, A., 1986, Kinetic analysis of manual lifting activities: Part I – Development of a three-dimensional computer model, *International Journal of Industrial Ergonomics*, **1**, 77–90.

LAUNIS, M. and LEHTEL, J., 1992, ergoSHAPE – a design oriented ergonomic tool for AutoCAD, in Mattila, M. and Karwowski, W. (Eds), *Computer Applications in Ergonomics, Occupational Safety and Health*, New York: Elsevier, pp. 121–128.

LAURIE, N.E., 1995, A proposed model which uses physiological properties of muscles as constraints for predicting muscle forces during industrial tasks, in Bittner, A.C. and Champney, P.C. (Eds), *Advances in Industrial Ergonomics and Safety VII*, New York: Taylor and Francis, pp. 51–58.

LEE, K.-H. and KROEMER, K.H.E., 1993, A finger model with constant tendon moment arms, *Proceedings of the Human Factors and Ergonomics Society 37th Annual Meeting*, Vol. 2, pp. 719–714, Seattle, WA, October 11–15, 1993.

LEE, J.W. and RIM, K., 1990, Maximum finger force prediction using a planar simulation of the middle finger, *Proceedings of the Insitute of Mechanical Engineers Part H: Journal of Engineering in Medicine*, **204**, 169–178.

LEMAY, M.A. and CRAGO, P.E., 1996, A dynamic model for simulating movements of the elbow, forearm, and wrist, *Journal of Biomechanics*, **29**, 1319–1330.

LENARCIC, J. and UMEK, A., 1994, Simple model of human arm reachable workspace, *IEEE Transactions on Systems, Man, and Cybernetics*, **24**, 1239–1246.

LEPOUTRE, F.X., 1993, Human posture modelisation as a problem of inverse kinematic of redundant robots, *Robotica*, **11**, 339–343.

LEVEAU, B., 1977, *Williams and Lissner: Biomechanics of Human Motion*, Philadelphia: Saunders.

LOREN, G.J., SCHOEMAKER, S.D., BURKHOLDER, T.J., JACOBSON, M.D., FRIDEN, J. and LIEBER, R.L., 1996, Human wrist motors: biomechanical design and application to tendon transfers, *Journal of Biomechanics*, **29**, 331–342.

MCGILL, S.M. and NORMAN, R.W., 1985, Dynamically and statically determined low back moments during lifting, *Journal of Biomechanics*, **18**, 877–885.

MCLAUGHLIN, T.M. and MILLER, N.R., 1980, Techniques for evaluation of loads on the forearm prior to impact in tennis strokes, *Journal of Mechanical Design*, **102**, 701–710.

MILLER, S.A. and FREIVALDS, A., 1995, A stress-strength interference model for predicting CTD probabilities, *International Journal of Industrial Ergonomics*, **15**, 447–457.

MISHOE, J.W. and SUGGS, C.W., 1977, Hand arm vibration – Part II: vibrational responses of the human hand, *Journal of Sound and Vibration*, **53**, 545–558.

MOORE, A., WELLS, R. and RANNEY, D., 1991, Quantifying exposure in occupational manual tasks with cumulative trauma disorder potential, *Ergonomics*, **34**, 1433–1453.

PENROD, D.D., DAVY, D.T. and SINGH, D.P., 1974, An optimization approach to tendon force analysis, *Journal of Biomechanics*, **7**, 123–129.

RAIKOVA, R., 1992, A general approach for modelling and mathematical investigation of the human upper limb, *Journal of Biomechanics*, **25**, 857–867.

RAIKOVA, R., 1996, A model of the flexion-extension motion in the elbow joint – some problems concerning muscle forces modelling and computation, *Journal of Biomechanics*, **29**, 763–772.

RAKHEJA, S., GURRAM, R. and GOUW, G.J., 1993, Development of linear and nonlinear hand-arm vibration models using optimization and linearization techniques, *Journal of Biomechanics*, **26**, 1253–1260.

REMPEL, D., DENNERLEIN, J., MOTE, C.D. and ARMSTRONG, T., 1994, A method of measuring fingertip loading during keyboard use, *Journal of Biomechanics*, **27**, 1101–1104.

REYNOLDS, D.D. and FALKENBERG, R.J., 1984, A study of hand vibration on chipping and grinding operators. Part II: Four-degree-of-freedom lumped parameter model of the vibration response of the human hand, *Journal of Sound and Vibration*, **95**, 499–514.

REYNOLDS, D.D. and JOKEL, C., 1974, Hand-arm vibration – an engineering approach, *American Industrial Hygiene Association Journal*, **35**, 613–622.

REYNOLDS, D.P. and KEITH, R.H., 1977, Hand arm vibration. Part I. Analytical model of the vibration response characteristics of the hand, *Journal of Sound and Vibration*, **51**, 237–253.

SCHOENMARKLIN, R.W. and MARRAS, 1992, An EMG-assisted biomechanical model of the wrist joint, in Kumar, S. (Ed.), *Advances in Industrial Ergonomics and Safety IV*, Philadelphia, PA: Taylor and Francis, pp. 777–781.

SCHUIND, F., GARCIA-ELIAS, M., COONEY, W.P. III and AN, K.-N., 1992, Flexor tendon forces: in vivo measurements, *Journal of Hand Surgery*, **17A**, 291–298.

SERINA, E.R., 1996, *Characterization and Modeling of the Fingertip Pulp under Repeated Loading*, PhD Dissertation, University of California, Berkeley, CA.

SILVERSTEIN, B.A., FINE, L.J. and ARMSTRONG, T.J., 1986, Hand-wrist cumulative trauma disorders in industry, *British Journal of Industrial Medicine*, **43**, 779–784.

SILVERSTEIN, B.A., FINE, L.J. and ARMSTRONG, T.J., 1987, Occupational factors and carpal tunnel syndrome, *American Journal of Industrial Medicine*, **11**, 343–358.

SUGGS, C.W. and MISHOE, J.W., 1977, Hand-arm vibration: implications drawn from lumped parameter models, in Wasserman, D.E., Taylor, W. and Curry, M.G. (Eds), *Proceedings of the International Occupational Hand Arm Vibration Conference*, NIOSH, Cincinnati, OH, DHEW Pub. No. 77–170, pp. 136–141.

THOMAS, C., RAKHEJA, S., BHAT, R.B. and STIHARU, I., 1996, A study of the modal behavior of the human hand-arm system, *Journal of Sound and Vibration*, **191**, 171–176.

TOFT, R. and BERME, N., 1980, A biomechanical analysis of the joints of the thumb, *Journal of Biomechanics*, **13**, 353–360.

UCHIYAMA, S., COERT, J.H., BERGLUND, L., AMADIO, P.C. and AN, K.N., 1995, Method for the measurement of friction between tendon and pulley, *Journal of Orthopaedic Research*, **13**, 83–89.

VALERO-CUEVAS, F.J., BURGAR, C., ZAJAC, F.E., HENTZ, V.R., McGILL, V.R. and AN, K.N., 1996, Index finger muscle coordination during ad-abduction forces may be explained by three degrees of freedom at MCP joint, in Fyhrie, D. and Gregor, R. (Eds), *Proceedings of the Twentieth Annual Meeting of the American Society of Biomechanics*.

VAN ZUYLEN, E.J., VAN VELZEN, A., DENIER VAN DER GON, J.J., 1988, A biomechanical model for flexion torques of human arm muscles as a function of elbow angle, *Journal of Biomechanics*, **21**, 183–190.

WELLS, R.P., RANNEY, D., MOORE, A.E. and GENTLEMAN, R., 1992, Relationship between chronic musculoskeletal disorders and work exposures: results from repetitive manual tasks, in Hagberg, M. and Kilbom, A. (Eds), *International Scientific Conference on Prevention of Work-related Musculoskeletal Disorders (PREMUS) Book of Abstracts*, Stockholm, Sweden: National Institute of Occupational Health, pp. 324–325.

WELLS, R.P., KEIR, P.J. and MOORE, A.E., 1995, Application of biomechanical hand and wrist models to work-related musculoskeletal disorders of the upper extremity, in Gordon, S.L., Blair, S.J. and Fine, L.J. (Eds), *Repetitive Motion Disorders of the Upper Extremity*, Rosemont, II: American Academy of Orthopedic Surgeons, pp. 111–121.

WINTERS, J.M. and KLEWENO, D.G., 1993, Effect of initial upper-limb alignment on muscle contributions to isometric strength curves, *Journal of Biomechanics*, **26**, 143–153.

WOLDSTAD, J.C., 1989, *Electromyographic Analysis of Rapid Elbow Movements*, PhD Thesis, Department of Industrial and Operations Engineering, University of Michigan-Ann Arbor, MI, USA.

WOLF, F.G., KEANE, M.S., BRANDT, K.D. and HILBERRY, B.M., 1993, An investigation of finger joint and tendon forces in experienced pianists, *Medical Problems of Performing Artists*, **8**, 84–95.

WOOD, L.A. and SUGGS, C.W., 1977, Distributed parameter dynamic model of the human forearm, in Wasserman, D.E., Taylor, W. and Curry, M.G. (Eds), *Proceedings of the International Occupational Hand Arm Vibration Conference*, NIOSH, Cincinnati, OH, DHEW Pub. No. 77–170, pp. 142–145.

YEO, B.P., 1976, Investigations concerning the principle of minimal total muscle force, *Journal of Biomechanics*, **9**, 413–416.

YUN, M.H. and FREIVALDS, A., 1995, Analysis of hand tool grips, *Proceedings of the Human Factors and Ergonomics Society 39th Annual Meeting*, pp. 553–557, San Diego, CA, October 9–13, 1995.

PART THREE

Shoulder and Neck

CHAPTER ELEVEN

Shoulder and neck

CHRIS JENSEN, BJARNE LAURSEN AND GISELA SJØGAARD

INTRODUCTION

Work tasks impose specific demands on the worker, who for instance has to carry loads of specific weights or reach for objects at a specific distance from the body and move these at a specific speed and in a specific direction. The work requirements correspond to the occupational exposure (Armstrong *et al.*, 1993). A complete description of the exposure includes not only the demands of the work tasks imposed by the design of the work place and tools, but also demands imposed by the organisation of the work (i.e., how much time is spent on different tasks). Thus, conceptually demands of a mental character are also to be included; for instance, a certain number of objects have to be counted, working under time pressure, or conflicts with colleagues or employer. The total exposure will result in physiological responses within the worker, such as changes in muscle and nerve activity, tension in tendons, cardiovascular and respiratory responses, etc. The extent or magnitude of these physiological responses depend on the job demands but additionally on the worker's physical work capacity, work technique and psychological factors. Work-related musculoskeletal disorders may be caused by an acute overload beyond the tolerance limit of the tissues or by an accumulation of submaximal loads and mediated through the concomitant physiological responses (Sjøgaard *et al.*, 1995). In order to identify acceptable exposures as well as risk factors the work requirements and the physiological responses must be quantified together with the physical capacity of the worker. This chapter focuses primarily on the biomechanics of the shoulder.

ANATOMY OF THE SHOULDER

The shoulder represents one of the most complicated biomechanical structures in humans and detailed biomechanical modelling of this joint is still scarce. It is composed of the shoulder girdle complex and the glenohumeral joint. The latter is made up of the articulation of the glenoid fossa of the scapula and the head of the humerus. The glenoid fossa is a shallow socket which at any arm posture covers less than half of the spherical head of the humerus. The shoulder girdle includes the bony structures of the clavicula and the scapula as well as the additional articulations: acromioclavicular, sternoclavicular, and coracoclavicular. Further, the scapulocostal, costosternal, and costovertebral articulations extend shoulder motion. For more detailed information the reader is referred to the literature (Kreighbaum and Barthels, 1996; Rockwood and Matsen, 1990). This anatomical arrangement provides a large amount of mobility for the arm on the account of stability. The structures maintaining the shoulder in place include the joint capsule, numerous ligaments and muscles. The connective tissues, however, are rather loose in their structure to allow for motion and therefore the muscles play an important role for shoulder stability. A classical subdivision of shoulder muscle function is: stabilisers and predominantly movers (Figure 11.1). However, as discussed below, such a strict division may not be relevant in most occupational settings, where all shoulder muscles in synergy contribute to performing the task. The significance of muscles for joint stability is by far most pronounced for the shoulder joint. Of note is that some shoulder muscles connect to the joints of the neck, and therefore the neck will be included to some extent in this chapter when relevant. A large number of occupational tasks rely on stability in the shoulder and neck, which act as punctum fixum for hand and eyes, respectively, during a variety of tasks ranging from heavy manual handling to light precision work. When reviewing the mechanics of the shoulder and neck, the main emphasis is on the muscle activity and the role the muscles play, both in the stabilisation and movement of the joint.

MUSCLE FORCES AND PHYSIOLOGICAL RESPONSES

In the living human, muscle forces cannot be measured directly but have to be measured indirectly from the electrical muscle activity. A positive relationship exists between electromyography (EMG) and muscle force or tension, which, in the unfatigued state, may be almost linear for some muscles. However, detailed force/EMG calibration is necessary in most cases since more complex relationships are common (further details are described below). EMG recordings are truly physiological responses, and as such also play a decisive role in identifying risk factors for the development of occupational musculoskeletal disorders. The evaluation of acceptable EMG patterns relies on basic knowledge regarding simultaneous responses of intramuscular pressure, blood flow, metabolism, and electrolyte balance, etc. A detailed analysis of the cascading events that may lead to muscle dysfunction has been presented recently (Sjøgaard and Jensen, 1997). Here it should only be pointed out that a positive linear relationship exists between EMG and intramuscular pressure in a given location of a muscle. However, the slope of this relationship may vary considerably and depends on muscle structure, muscle location (deep versus superficial), and the surrounding anatomy (Sjøgaard, 1997). The electrical events elicit active force development in combination with increased muscle ATP breakdown and subsequent metabolic reactions. The chemical energy (substrate) for this energy turnover is in part stored in the muscle fibre but additionally delivered to the muscle by the blood flow. The magnitude of the muscle blood flow increases with increased arterial blood pressure, but decreases with increased intramuscular tissue pressure. Thus, intramuscular pressure plays a crucial role, since on the one hand it increases with increased muscle force and on the other hand it impedes the blood supply for the increased muscle energy turnover, which is necessary for the increased force output. Prolonged insufficient blood supply is considered a risk factor which may cause malfunction in all tissues.

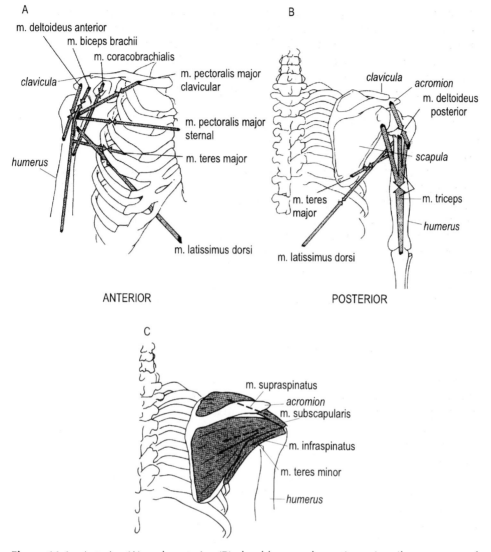

A

m. deltoideus anterior
m. biceps brachii
m. coracobrachialis
clavicula
m. pectoralis major clavicular
m. pectoralis major sternal
humerus
m. teres major
m. latissimus dorsi

ANTERIOR

B

clavicula
acromion
m. deltoideus posterior
scapula
m. teres major
m. triceps
humerus
m. latissimus dorsi

POSTERIOR

C

m. supraspinatus
acromion
m. subscapularis
m. infraspinatus
m. teres minor
humerus

Figure 11.1 Anterior **(A)** and posterior **(B)** shoulder muscles acting primarily as movers of the shoulder joint and **(C)** rotator cuff muscles acting primarily as stabilisers (redrawn from (Kreighbaum and Barthels, 1996).

MUSCLE ACTIVITY DURING WORK

Surface EMG recordings are often used in occupational studies to measure muscle activity. The process of EMG signal analysis usually consists of filtering, rectification, averaging or taking the root mean square (RMS) of the signal over a given time period (e.g. 0.2 sec). The amplitude of the EMG signal is often used as a measure of the exposure *level*, illustrated by the RMS amplitudes shown in Figure 11.2A. The calculations are based on a 10 sec EMG registration from the upper trapezius muscle during computer work, a registration which was selected for illustrative purposes; usually a representative recording for a given work task is longer, i.e. several minutes. Thereafter, the 'static', 'median' and 'peak' levels of EMG activity may be calculated based on the amplitude probability distribution function (APDF) (Jonsson, 1978, 1982). Figure 11.2B illustrates the APDF curve for the full 10 sec recording period corresponding to the RMS amplitudes shown in Figure 11.2A. Recently, methods for signal analysis which quantify variables related to repetitiveness or variation in the muscle activity pattern have been developed. One method is the quantification of gaps, defined as the number of silent periods (EMG level below 0.5 per cent EMG_{max}) which exceed 0.2 sec in the EMG activity pattern (Veiersted et al., 1990). In the example shown in Figure 11.1A one gap with a duration of 0.6 sec was recorded about 1.5 sec after the start of the recording. Another method which quantifies both exposure level (or amplitude) and repetitiveness is the exposure variation analysis (EVA) method (Mathiassen and Winkel, 1991). By separating both exposure level and time into intervals, the EVA method provides information about the levels of exposure and the duration for which the EMG activity is recorded within each exposure level (Figure 11.2C).

Normalisation of the EMG activity is necessary to compare results between subjects and studies, but no consensus exists on the normalisation procedure for the different shoulder muscles, mainly because it is not possible to measure the force produced by individual muscles. This may be exemplified with EMG recordings of the upper trapezius muscle. The recordings have often been normalised against the force recorded during a maximal isometric shoulder elevation with the point of force application on the acromion; the results are subsequently expressed in terms of relative force values (percentage MVC, maximal voluntary contraction). During this contraction the force is produced by muscles which elevate and rotate the scapular and clavicular bones, whereas no force is produced across the glenohumeral joint. However, when a glenohumeral joint moment is added to a submaximal shoulder elevation the EMG activity increases and when the arm posture is altered (e.g. from abduction to flexion) the EMG activity changes even when the glenohumeral torque is kept constant (Mathiassen and Winkel, 1990). This limits the interpretation of EMG activity into exerted force. Therefore, for some purposes it may be preferable to use EMG recordings directly as a measure of upper trapezius muscle activity and express results in terms of relative EMG amplitude (per cent EMG_{max}). Submaximal test contractions are also commonly used to normalise EMG data. Such procedures may aim at expressing EMG levels relative to forces, which are commonly experienced during work, such as lifting the arms or holding hand tools (Mathiassen et al., 1995).

Table 11.1 shows a number of work place studies where EMG activity levels have been measured on workers while performing their normal work tasks. Although differences in the prevalence rates of shoulder–neck disorders exist between the occupations, it should be emphasised that such disorders are common problems among workers from all of the jobs listed. One year prevalences of symptoms in the shoulder–neck region of around 50 per cent have been reported in several of these studies.

High levels of shoulder muscle activity have been recorded during work tasks such as floor cleaning and work with hand tools (e.g. drilling work), which require considerable force. Thus, the median EMG activity levels were above 20 per cent Max, where 'Max' refers to 'MVC' or 'EMG_{max}'. More moderate EMG levels are found in different types of industrial assembly work, sewing machine work and during manual letter sorting, where the median EMG levels were between 10 per cent Max and 20 per cent Max. These work tasks are characterised by repetitive handling of light materials, often at a high work pace in awkward postures. The lowest levels of muscle activity occur during office work, VDU work and during light manual material handling, e.g. during chocolate bar packing

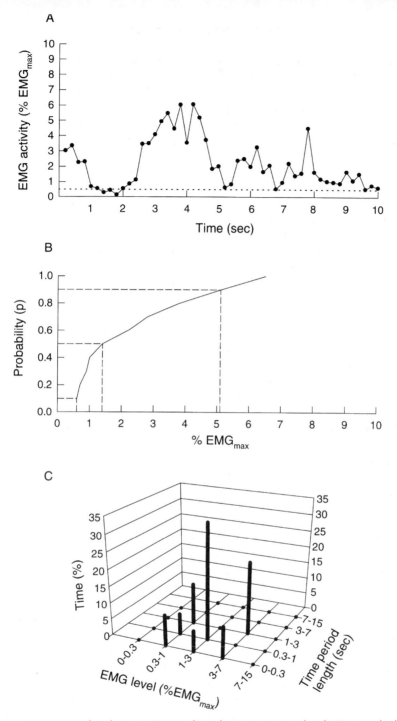

Figure 11.2 An example of an EMG recording during 10 seconds of VDU work showing principles of signal analysis. **(A)** The EMG signals were RMS converted in 0.2 sec windows and normalised in relation to the EMG amplitude recorded during a maximal isometric contraction. The broken line indicates the 0.5 per cent EMG_{max} level used for detection of EMG gaps. **(B)** An amplitude probability distribution function analysis was performed on the RMS amplitudes shown in (A) and the static (p = 0.1), median (p = 0.5) and peak (p = 0.9) levels are indicated with broken lines. **(C)** An exposure variation analysis of the RMS amplitudes shown in (A) is shown in a three-dimensional graph. Here, the time spent within the indicated exposure levels and time period lengths are indicated.

Table 11.1   Mean EMG activity levels in different occupations.

Work task	Muscles	Static level (% Max)	Median level (% Max)	Peak level (% Max)	Reference
Floor cleaning	Upper trapezius	10	25	54	(Søgaard et al., 1996)
Drilling work	Deltoideus	11	20	47	(Christensen, 1986b)
	Infraspinatus	8.5	17.5	45.5	
	Upper trapezius	20.5	29	48.5	
Electronic assembly work	Deltoideus	6.6	13*	28*	(Christensen, 1986a)
	Infraspinatus	13.2	19.9	33*	
	Upper trapezius	7.4	14.9	27*	
Assembly work (telephone exchanges)	Upper trapezius	4.3	–	–	(Aarås, 1994)
Sewing machine work	Upper trapezius	9	15	23	(Jensen et al., 1993a)
Letter sorting	Deltoideus	5.3	13.8	27.4	(Jørgensen et al., 1989)
	Infraspinatus	5.0	10.4	16.4	
	Upper trapezius	5.0	9.8	19*	
Chocolate packing	Upper trapezius	2.1	5.3	–	(Jensen et al., 1993b)
Light manual material handling	Upper trapezius	0.7	3.4	11.1	(Vasseljen and Westgaard, 1995)
VDU work, data entry/dialogue	Upper trapezius	2.7	–	–	(Aarås, 1994)
Office work	Upper trapezius	1.2	4.1	–	(Jensen et al., 1993b)
Office work	Upper trapezius	1.1	4.6	8.0	(Vasseljen and Westgaard, 1995)
Computer-aided design work (PC-mouse work)	Upper trapezius	2.0	4.6	9.0	(Jensen et al., 1997)

The term % Max is used no matter whether the original study expressed results in relation to EMG_{max} or MVC.
* Estimated from graphs.

at an assembly line where the median EMG activity levels were about 5 per cent Max and the static levels were 1–2 per cent EMG_{max}.

Work tasks which require high force levels may be improved by changes which reduce the exposure level; however, an evaluation of such interventions requires more detailed biomechanical analyses. For example, the forces required when using two specific floor cleaning tools, a mop and a scrub, have been compared (Søgaard et al., 1998). Hand force registrations and video recordings were used to describe three-dimensional external forces and movements (Figure 11.3). By applying inverse dynamics and a 3-D linked-segment model glenohumeral torques were calculated. The highest mean moments of force were registered in shoulder flexion and they were similar for mopping and scrubbing (11 per cent and 11 per cent MVC, respectively for one shoulder, 13 per cent and 9 per cent MVC for the other shoulder). However, bilateral EMG measurements on m. deltoideus, m. trapezius and m. infraspinatus showed higher peak EMG levels on m. deltoideus of one shoulder and on m. infraspinatus of the other shoulder during scrubbing as compared to mopping. Inspite of this the authors concluded that the exposure level could not be sufficiently changed by changing the cleaning method because similar peak EMG levels from four muscles, similar static EMG levels on all six muscles and similar moments of force were recorded.

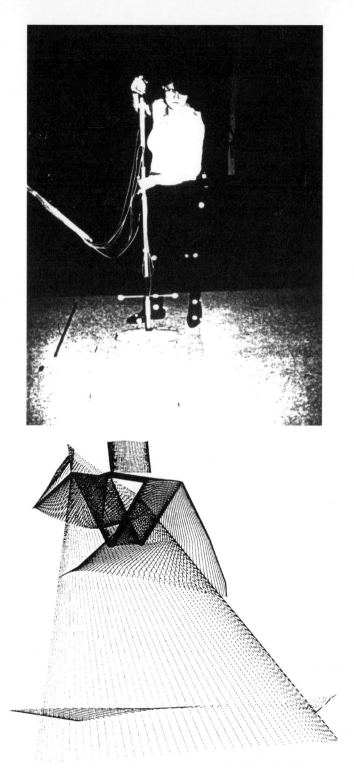

Figure 11.3 A picture of a cleaning person with markers is shown at the top. After video-recording the body markers were digitalised and the corresponding stickdiagrams at the bottom are depicted repeatedly during one half cycle of a mopping task. The long stick is the mop and the small horizontal stick at the bottom was used to record twisting of the mop.

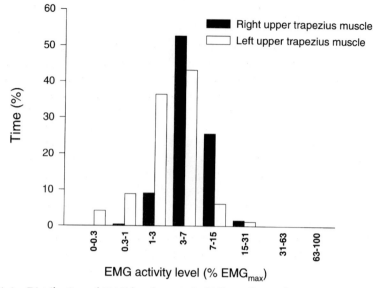

Figure 11.4   Distribution of EMG levels recorded bilaterally on the upper trapezius muscles during the performance of computer-aided-design work with a mouse. The percentage time is shown, where the EMG level was recorded within level classes according to the exposure variation analysis (EVA).

During the performance of low-level work tasks the difference between the static and peak EMG levels are often small due to relatively sustained muscle activity patterns. Improvements of such work tasks may not be achieved through reductions in exposure levels and focus should rather be directed towards the number of rest pauses and the variation in the exposure pattern which may be quantified by gap or EVA analyses of EMG signals. For instance, EVA analyses of the EMG recording from the left and right upper trapezius muscles of a computer-aided design worker showed no periods of muscular rest on the right side, which almost continuously operated a computer mouse (Jensen et al., 1997) (see Figure 11.4). On the left side, which performed occasional keyboard operations, periods of very low or no activity at all (< 1 per cent EMG_{max}) were recorded for about 13 per cent of the recording time. Similarly, gap analyses showed 0.1 gaps/min in the recordings from the right m. trapezius and 7.3 gaps/min in the recordings from the left m. trapezius.

POSTURE AND EXTERNAL FORCES

Working posture and external forces are the most important factors determining the shoulder load. When the arm is vertical or supported, ligament forces, passive muscle forces, and bone contact forces are sufficient to counteract the effect of gravity, and active muscle forces are not needed. When the arm is elevated and unsupported, gravity creates a shoulder moment, which must be counteracted by the shoulder muscles. For a straight arm loaded only by the gravity of the mass of the arm the moment M_{GH} at the glenohumeral joint is:

$$M_{GH} = m \cdot d_{CM} \cdot g \cdot \sin(\alpha)$$

where m is the mass of the arm (approximately 5 per cent of the body mass), d_{CM} is the distance from the glenohumeral joint to the centre of mass of the arm, about 0.3 m for a straight arm, g is the gravity acceleration (9.8 ms^{-2}), and α is the elevation angle of the upper arm. According to pure mechanics, the magnitude of the moment is independent of the direction of the arm elevation (abduction, flexion, etc.), and is highest at 90° elevation, according to the sinus function. However, muscle moment arms depend on the direction of arm elevation. Different studies present different magnitudes for the moment arms (Karlsson, 1992; Liu et al., 1997; Otis et al., 1994; Wood et al., 1989b) and it has been shown that muscle moment arm magnitudes remain constant or may increase with elevation angle at least for the muscles responsible for performing an abduction, especially m. deltoideus (Poppen and Walker, 1978). Therefore, the required muscle force may have a maximum for abduction angles somewhat below 90°. However, the muscle length influences the ability to produce force and most muscles responsible for abduction are substantially shortened when the arm is abducted. Therefore, their maximum force is reduced, and the relative muscle load is increased, especially for arm elevation above 90°. Based on anatomy, muscles contributing to abduction are mainly the anterior and middle parts of m. deltoideus, m. supraspinatus, and probably the upper part of m. subscapularis. A flexion moment can mainly be produced by the anterior part of m. deltoideus, m. supraspinatus, m. biceps brachii and m. pectoralis major. If the elbow is flexed, the distance to the CM of the arm is smaller, while there may also be a moment of outward or inward rotation in the shoulder.

Actual activation patterns of some shoulder–neck muscles in response to postures and external forces have been reported in a number of studies, especially in settings involving static contractions (Table 11.2). Regarding arm postures, the three parts of the deltoid muscle, the upper trapezius and infraspinatus muscles show considerably higher activity when the upper arm is flexed or abducted as compared to hanging vertically downward (Sigholm et al., 1984). An exception is the posterior part of the deltoid muscle during arm flexion. Supraspinatus muscle activity increases mostly during the first part of arm elevation from 0° to 45° and less so from 45° to 90°. Similarly, the intramuscular pressure in the supraspinatus muscle increases when the arm is elevated from 0° to 30° and 60°, but almost no pressure increase occurs from 60° to 90° (Järvholm et al., 1988). Due to the low compliance of the supraspinatus muscle compartment, the intramuscular pressures may exceed 50 mmHg already at 30° of arm abduction, which impedes blood flow (Jensen et al., 1995). For the middle part of the deltoid, the upper trapezius and the supraspinatus muscles, arm abduction requires higher muscle force than arm flexion at comparable angles of arm elevation. Also the intramuscular pressure in the supraspinatus muscle is higher in abduction compared to flexion (Jensen et al., 1995; Järvholm et al., 1988). Arm rotation and elbow flexion angle has little or no effect on shoulder muscle activity (Sigholm et al., 1984).

External forces applied to the hands, e.g. by carrying tools or weights, require increased activity in the shoulder muscles. The relative increase seems larger in rotator-cuff muscles than in the deltoid muscle (Table 11.2). For the muscles listed in Table 11.2 the relative increases in EMG activity ranged from about 10 per cent to 40 per cent per kg lifted with the hand. In the supraspinatus muscle the pressure may easily increase by more than 50 mmHg when adding a 2 kg hand load (Järvholm et al., 1988).

In work situations, shoulder moments are needed to elevate the arm as well as to perform external forces, often in quasi-static conditions. These situations were simulated

Table 11.2   The effect of posture and hand loads on shoulder muscle EMG activity.

	Arm posture			
	Flexion 0° vs 45°	Flexion 0° vs 90°	Abduction 0° vs 45°	Abduction 0° vs 90°
Deltoideus, anterior	100%	185%	67%	122%
Deltoideus, medial	175%	433%	329%	775%
Deltoideus, posterior	NS	NS	64%	273%
Upper trapezius	51%	100%	109%	154%
Infraspinatus	92%	196%	118%	172%
Supraspinatus	98%	106%	135%	169%

	Hand load	
	Flexion 1 kg increase	Abduction 1 kg increase
Deltoideus, anterior	21%	16%
Deltoideus, medial	17%	9%
Deltoideus, posterior	14%	17%
Upper trapezius	15%	17%
Infraspinatus	35%	41%
Supraspinatus	22%	20%

Table reproduced from Sigholm *et al.* (1984). The mean difference in EMG amplitude when two situations were compared is shown as the percentage increase (%) between the two situations. Positive values indicate that the latter situation was associated with higher EMG amplitudes than the former situation.

in a study where forces were applied to a fixed handle (Laursen, 1996). EMG activity was recorded from 13 shoulder muscles while the subjects performed static contractions with forces varying from 0 per cent to approximately 20 per cent MVC in different directions. The hand forces were performed in different directions in the horizontal plane, in a fixed position with a vertical straight arm. The shoulder muscles were found to be activated at different levels, but for all force directions several shoulder muscles were activated while others were silent (Figure 11.5). When pushing or pulling in the arm direction, most muscles were less activated, because no moment was required in the glenohumeral joint, and only muscle activity for stabilisation of the shoulder was needed.

Varying the sitting posture may also affect muscle activity. Several shoulder and neck muscles were reported to show the lowest activity with a slightly backward inclined, straight back and vertical neck during light arm/hand work (Schüldt *et al.*, 1987). EMG activity recorded on the upper trapezius muscle decreased with 7 per cent EMG_{max} due to a change in thoraco-lumbar spine posture from vertical to backward inclined, whereas EMG activity recorded on the levator scapula and sternocleidomastoideus muscles was less affected.

Arm support can be used to reduce the force required to perform hand/arm work in several muscles, but the change in EMG activity in different muscles when comparing hand/arm work with and without the use of arm support also depends on the sitting posture (Schüldt *et al.*, 1987). If the sitting posture is associated with low EMG activity,

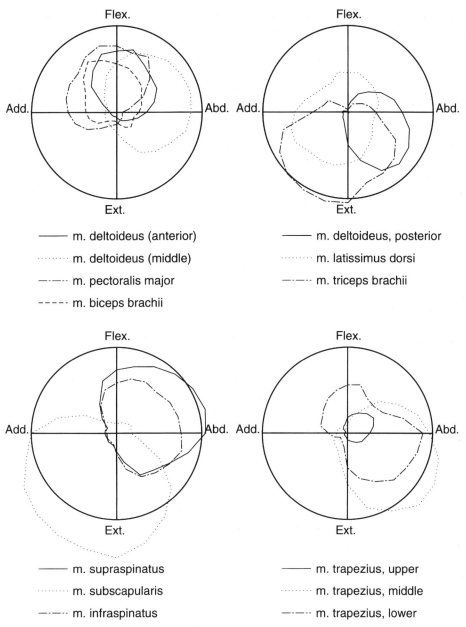

Figure 11.5 Example of muscle activation patterns for one female subject performing forces in a vertical arm position. The curves show the EMG level for 13 shoulder muscles when performing a 10 N force in different directions in the horizontal plane (representing attempted abduction, flexion, adduction, and extension). The 10 N force corresponded to approximately 14 per cent MVC for all force directions. The circles represent a level of 10 per cent EMG_{max}.

the effect of using arm support is small (1–2 per cent EMG_{max}). Other sitting postures may be associated with differences corresponding to 5–10 per cent EMG_{max}, when comparing work with and without the use of arm support. Thus, also the intramuscular pressure in the supraspinatus muscle may be reduced by using arm support. During simulated assembly work and welding without arm support the intramuscular pressure was 35 mmHg (7 per cent MVC) and 65 mmHg (12 per cent MVC), respectively. This was significantly reduced by using arm suspension to 23 mmHg and 51 mmHg (Järvholm *et al.*, 1991).

In the glenohumeral joint a torque due to arm elevation depends strongly on shoulder muscle forces as discussed above. Concerning the neck one study has reported that an increase in neck flexion resulting in an increase in joint extension moment from 32 per cent to 45 per cent of the maximal extension moment was performed with an unchanged mean splenius EMG activity level of 9 per cent EMG_{max} (Finsen, 1998). Thus, when the neck is flexed the torque in the seventh cervical–first thoracal joint is less dependent on muscle force and relatively more dependent on counteracting forces produced by passive structures such as ligaments.

BIOMECHANICAL MODELLING

The recording of working postures and external forces allows for the application of inverse dynamics for the calculation of net forces and moments. These forces and moments should be produced by the combined action of muscle, ligament and bone forces. Since there are far more muscles and muscle parts which can be independently activated than force and moment constraints, the number of possible muscle force combinations is infinite. To determine which muscle force patterns can be used for a given external shoulder load, modelling is needed. Most biomechanical modelling is based on optimisation principles by choosing the set of muscle forces which minimise a certain cost function (Högfors *et al.*, 1995; Niemi *et al.*, 1996; van der Helm, 1994). By using such optimisation principles only one force distribution is found for each load condition. A different approach is to use EMG for the determination of the voluntary muscle activation patterns and based on this to assess the muscle force distribution which actually is used. However, as mentioned above, EMG may provide good information on muscle activation while muscle force estimation from EMG is difficult. One reason is that many shoulder muscles are involved when performing external forces or sustaining a force-demanding posture. Therefore, the combined action of the shoulder muscles should be considered.

For the glenohumeral joint, the net moment produced by the muscles is:

$$M_{net,\ muscles} = \Sigma_{muscles\ i}\ a_i \cdot F_i$$

where a_i is the moment arm magnitude of muscle i, F_i is the force from muscle i, which for static muscle contractions may be estimated as:

$$F_i = \sigma \cdot PCSA_i \cdot EMG_i \cdot c_i$$

where σ is the specific tension of muscle tissue for maximum muscle activation, $PCSA_i$ is the physiological cross-sectional area of muscle i, EMG_i is the EMG for muscle i, normalised to maximum voluntary contraction, and c_i is a factor for transforming relative EMG into relative muscle force. For a linear EMG/force relationship, this factor is 1.

The constants may be determined by using information regarding muscle cross-sectional areas from cadaver studies (Table 11.3), and recording of EMG and force during maximum voluntary contractions (MVC) in different directions. Except for the contributions from ligament forces, the model can be validated by comparing $M_{net,\ muscles}$ to the moment calculated from the external forces. Reasonable agreement has been found for static submaximal contractions, and the general result from using the model is a consistency in muscle activation patterns between subjects (Laursen *et al.*, 1998a). Further,

Table 11.3 Literature values on physiological cross-sectional areas of some shoulder muscles. Values are in cm².

	Poppen and Walker (1978)[1]	Bassett et al. (1990)	Howell et al. (1986)	Wood et al. (1989a)[2]	Veeger et al. (1991)	Keating et al. (1993)	Karlsson (1992)	Laursen (1996)
No. of cadavers	2+6	7	5	1	7	5	3	1
m. deltoideus, ant.	9.9		8.12	5.2			5.30	7.11
m. deltoideus, middle	14.8	18.17[3]	8.66	13.5	25.904[4]		6.95	15.26
m. deltoideus, post.	13.0	5.00	9.94	4.5			6.43	6.00
m. latissimus dorsi	7.4	12.00		12.9	8.64		7.11	
m. pectoralis major		13.34		13.5	13.65		8.93	
m. subscapularis	13.8	16.30	16.0	9.7	13.51	13.5	12.13	20.00
m. supraspinatus	6.2	5.72		4.5	5.21	4.0	4.73	5.72
m. infraspinatus	11.4	13.74[5]	17.57	5.8	9.51	5.9	9.78	13.15
m. teres minor				2.6	2.92	2.6	2.33	4.63
m. teres major		8.77		5.8	10.02		5.53	
m. biceps brachii		4.12		3.2	6.29		4.98	
m. triceps brachii (long head)		3.96		3.9	6.84		10.95	
m. trapezius (whole)				23.2	15.99		14.88	13.93

[1] In combination with data from Fick (six specimens).
[2] PCSA calculated as volume/muscle length.
[3] Anterior and middle part of m. deltoideus.
[4] PCSA for all parts of m. deltoideus.
[5] m. infraspinatus + m. teres minor.

the results show that most shoulder muscles are activated for the force direction, for which they are generally consided as prime movers (Figure 11.5). When comparing a biomechanical optimisation model with voluntary muscle activation patterns based on EMG, there is a general agreement in the results for most muscle forces. However, for some muscles, especially m. deltoideus, anterior part and m. subscapularis, the EMG-based model predicts higher muscle forces for a wider range of performed external forces than predicted by the optimisation model (Laursen et al., 1997). Thus, optimisation models may underestimate the voluntary involvement of shoulder muscles during occupational tasks.

PRECISION, PACE AND MENTAL DEMANDS

Our knowledge of the biomechanical effects of other than static, mechanical exposure factors is less comprehensive although muscular responses to precision demands, work pace and mental demands have been studied. In general, a higher work pace increases muscle activity and so does an increased precision demand if the work speed is not reduced (Arndt, 1987; Laursen et al., 1998b; Mathiassen and Winkel, 1996). Both work speed and precision demands affect the activity in all shoulder muscles (Laursen et al., 1998b). In the latter study, the strongest effect of precision demands was found in a situation with a combination of high working speed and high precision demands at the same time. If the work speed is freely chosen, increased precision demands result in a decreased working speed, and the muscle activity may decrease.

The effect of the increased precision demand on EMG activity may be caused by the requirement of increased joint stiffness since an increased muscle tension is an important way to increase joint stiffness. However, increased precision demands may also require a change in movement pattern towards more time for the precision demanding part of the work task and higher movement velocities and accelerations in between (more jerky movements). Such change in acceleration may also require higher muscle activity.

Some work-related psychosocial exposures can also induce activation of shoulder and neck muscles, especially cognitive loads (Lundberg et al., 1994; Westgaard and Bjørklund, 1987). Not all muscles are equally responsive to such exposures, but the upper trapezius muscle may respond with higher and more prolonged activation than most others (Wærsted and Westgaard, 1996). Interestingly, reaction times of eye movements decrease when the upper trapezius muscle is activated up to 30 per cent MVC (Kunita and Fujiwara, 1996). The muscular response to mental effort varies greatly between subjects and is partly dependent on emotional factors, e.g. a subject's motivation (Wærsted et al., 1994). The relationship to colleagues and superiors may also have an indirect effect on muscle tension by a similar mechanism. Increased muscle activity due to mental loads serves no biomechanical purpose, since muscular forces are not required to perform mental operations. However, the peripheral mechanisms of muscle activation are probably not different from those that are due to physical exposures. As the activation of motor units in a muscle or at least within a motor neuron pool occurs in a predictable order, mental loads may cause prolonged or repeated activation of the same low-threshold motor units (Wærsted et al., 1996).

In real work situations it may be impossible to distinguish which factors provoke a given muscular response. For instance in VDU work involving computer mouse use the muscular response may be the result of a combination of cognitive loads, visual demands and precision hand work. High visual demands require stabilisation of the neck, precision work requires stabilisation of the shoulder, and the cognitive load may further increase or prolong the activation of shoulder–neck muscles. The physiological responses to psychosocial exposures are of course not confined to muscular responses, but here it should be realised that muscular forces are not only generated for movements and stabilising actions, and that it may be particularly important to be aware of psychosocial exposures in ergonomic assessments of shoulder muscle loads.

MOTOR CONTROL

Coordination of muscular forces operates at several levels. Each muscle is controlled as an independent unit. However, different parts of the same muscle may also be independently activated to achieve finer control of movements, e.g. the trapezius muscle is composed of at least three parts, the upper, the middle and the lower part (Figure 11.6). Furthermore, within the upper part of m. trapezius the muscle fibres have different lines of action (Johnson *et al.*, 1994) and different regions within this part may be activated independently (Jensen and Westgaard, 1995, 1997; Mathiassen and Winkel, 1990; Schüldt and Harms-Ringdahl, 1988; Sundelin and Hagberg, 1992). In the study of Jensen and Westgaard (1995) an eight-channel multielectrode was used to record the EMG activity above the upper trapezius muscle at electrode positions stretching from the clavicula to spina scapula. During the performance of isometric shoulder elevation at increasing force the EMG amplitude increased differently at different electrode positions (Figure 11.7). For instance, at a mean amplitude of 20 per cent EMG_{max} at electrode position D, the difference between the mean normalised amplitudes at positions B and F was 6.6 per cent EMG_{max}. EMG studies of m. subscapularis (Kadaba *et al.*, 1992), m. biceps brachii (Brown *et al.*, 1993) and m. pectoralis major (Paton and Brown, 1994) indicated that they also are subdivided in compartments and dissection studies have shown that the

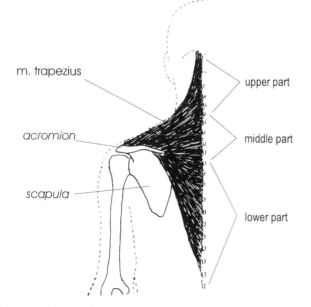

Figure 11.6 The trapezius muscle.

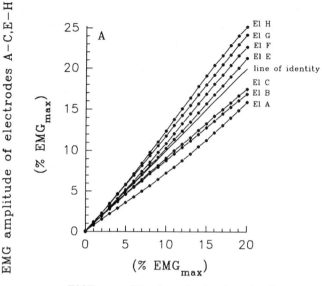

EMG amplitude of electrode D

Figure 11.7 Mean EMG amplitudes of 22 subjects recorded at different positions (1 cm distance between electrode positions) across the upper trapezius from near the clavicle (El.A) to near the scapula (El.H) during an isometric shoulder elevation with increasing force (acromion as the point of force application). The EMG amplitudes were plotted against the amplitude recorded at position D corresponding to the standard position approximately halfway between the clavicle and spina scapula (reproduced from Jensen and Westgaard, 1995).

supraspinatus muscle is divided in a superficial and a deep part (Jensen *et al.*, 1995). Thus, some muscles consist of several compartments, which in most of the above mentioned studies has been suggested to be of functional significance, if fibres in different compartments have different lines of action.

Although it remains controversial, another principle of motor unit regulation may exist. The phenomenon is termed motor unit rotation, i.e., newly recruited motor units replace previously active units, possibly to avoid or postpone signs of fatigue. Indications of motor unit rotation have been obtained during prolonged isometric contractions of the biceps brachii at 10 per cent MVC, whereas the phenomenon was not observed at 40 per cent MVC (Fallentin *et al.*, 1993). Motor unit rotation may not only depend on the required force level; other demands which lead to activation of more motor units such as an increased demand of precision, mental demands, etc. may also reduce the potential for motor unit rotation. Continous long-term activation of even a few motor units in a muscle may be causally related to the development of muscle disorders (Hägg, 1991).

ERGONOMIC SIGNIFICANCE

Detailed understanding of organ mechanics under various occupational exposures is essential for the assessment of specific tissue loadings imposed on the worker in the work place. For the shoulder/neck region it has been demonstrated that especially loadings of muscles, i.e. the muscle forces, constitute an important variable for ergonomic risk assessment. Muscle force development implies a large number of cascading physiological responses which acutely or more prolonged over time may overload the tissues. Based on a knowledge of organ mechanics exposures can be identified which imply a risk for the development of musculoskeletal disorders due to either acute high forces or prolonged low forces in individual muscles. Thus, peak muscle forces of around 50 per cent of maximum strength in the shoulder region have been reported during, for example, drilling work and floor cleaning, which acutely may cause muscle fatigue.

Whenever high muscle forces (peak level around 50 per cent max) have to be developed for performing the work, the ergonomic advice will be first to identify the specific tasks, which require these high forces. Secondly, interventions should be scheduled by redesign of tools and/or work technique. Thirdly, the redesigned work must be tested using knowledge of organ mechanics to validate whether peak tissue forces have actually been reduced, and if this is not the case further intervention strategies must be tested. Finally, the new work task with less muscle force demands is implemented in the workplace.

When low level forces have to be developed (static level less than 5 per cent max) over prolonged periods of time a quite different ergonomic strategy is recommended. In such a case it should be realised that it is the level of exposure in combination with the duration which must be evaluated. Reduction in exposure time may therefore be recommended. However, the variation of exposures is another important issue to address in ergonomy. In a study of the effect of daily working hours on the occurrence of sick-leave due to shoulder–neck disorders full-time sewing machine operators initially had more sick-leave than part-time workers (Wærsted and Westgaard, 1991). Their work tasks were described as strenuous with a static load level on the trapezius muscle of about 5 per cent of max. However, although the development of disorders was postponed for part-time workers compared to full-time workers no lasting effect was observed. Thus, only the introduction of different work tasks may efficiently reduce the risk for the sewing machine operators, that is by reducing the repetitiveness of the work. Actually, the repetitiveness of muscle contractions as well as sustained contractions at any level of muscular activation for prolonged time present risk factors for the development of disorders. The general guidelines for ergonomic interventions must for every individual muscle consider the following issues:

(1)   reduce high peak forces;

(2)   limit time for sustained contractions;

(3)   minimise repetitions of the same movements; and

(4)   optimise variation, i.e. include rest as well as moderately high work intensity.

References

AARÅS, A., 1994, Relationship between trapezius load and the incidence of musculoskeletal illness in the neck and shoulder, *Int J Ind Erg*, **14**, 341–348.

ARMSTRONG, T.J., BUCKLE, P., FINE, L.J., HAGBERG, M., JONSSON, B., KILBOM, Å., *et al.*, 1993, A conceptual model for work-related neck and upper-limb musculoskeletal disorders, *Scand J Work Environ Health*, **19**(2), 73–84.

ARNDT, R., 1987, Work pace, stress, and cumulative trauma disorders, *J Hand Surg*, **12A**(2 pt 2), 866–869.

BASSETT, R.W., BROWNE, A.O., MORREY, B.F. and AN, K.N., 1990, Glenohumeral muscle force and moment mechanics in a position of shoulder instability, *J Biomech*, **23**(5), 405–415.

BROWN, J.M.M., SOLOMON, C. and PATON, M., 1993, Further evidence of functional differentiation within biceps brachii, *Electromyogr Clin Neurophysiol*, **33**, 301–309.

CHRISTENSEN, H., 1986a, Muscle activity and fatigue in the shoulder muscles of assembly-plant employees, *Scand J Work Environ Health*, **12**(6), 582–587.

CHRISTENSEN, H., 1986b, Muscle activity and fatigue in the shoulder muscles during repetitive work. An electromyographic study, *Eur J Appl Physiol*, **54**, 596–601.

FALLENTIN, N., JØRGENSEN, K. and SIMONSEN, E.B., 1993, Motor unit recruitment during prolonged isometric contractions, *Eur J Appl Physiol*, **67**, 335–341.

FINSEN, L., 1999, Biomechanical aspects of occupational neck postures during dental work. *Int J Ind Erg*, **23**, 397–406.

HÄGG, G.M., 1991, Static work loads and occupational myalgia – a new explanation model, in Anderson, P.A., Hobart, D.J. and Danoff, J.V. (Eds), *Electromyographical Kinesiology*, Elsevier Science Publishers, pp. 141–144.

HÖGFORS, C., KARLSSON, D. and PETERSON, B., 1995, Structure and internal consistency of a shoulder model, *J Biomech*, **28**, 767–777.

HOWELL, S.M., IMOBERSTEG, A.M., SEGER, D.H. and MARONE, P.J., 1986, Clarification of the role of the supraspinatus muscle in shoulder function, *Bone Joint Surg (Am)*, **68-A**(3), 398–404.

JÄRVHOLM, U., PALMERUD, G., STYF, J., HERBERTS, P. and KADEFORS, R., 1988, Intramuscular pressure in the supraspinatus muscle, *J Orthop Res*, **6**(2), 230–238.

JÄRVHOLM, U., PALMERUD, G., KADEFORS, R. and HERBERTS, P., 1991, The effect of arm support on the supraspinatus muscle during simulated assembly work and welding, *Ergonomics*, **34**(1), 57–66.

JENSEN, C. and WESTGAARD, R.H., 1995, Functional subdivision of the upper trapezius muscle during maximal isometric contractions, *J Electromyogr Kinesiol*, **5**, 227–237.

JENSEN, C. and WESTGAARD, R., 1997, Functional subdivision of the upper trapezius muscle during low-level activation, *Eur J Appl Physiol*, **76**, 335–339.

JENSEN, B.R., SCHIBYE, B., SØGAARD, K., SIMONSEN, E.B. and SJØGAARD, G., 1993a, Shoulder muscle load and muscle fatigue among industrial sewing-machine operators, *Eur J Appl Physiol*, **67**, 467–475.

JENSEN, C., NILSEN, K., HANSEN, K. and WESTGAARD, R.H., 1993b, Trapezius muscle load as a risk indicator for occupational shoulder-neck complaints, *Int Arch Occup Environ Health*, **64**, 415–423.

JENSEN, B.R., JØRGENSEN, K., HUIJING, P.A. and SJØGAARD, G., 1995, Soft tissue architecture and intramuscular pressure in the shoulder region, *Eur J Morphol*, **33**(3), 205–220.

JENSEN, C., FINSEN, L., OLSEN, H.B., JUUL-KRISTENSEN, B., HANSEN, K. and CHRISTENSEN, H., 1997, CAD-work: physical exposure and musculoskeketal troubles, in Seppälä, P., Luopajärvi, T., Nygård, C.-H., Mattila, M., Kulha, K. and Hänninen, E. (Eds), *From Experience to Innovation. IEA '97. Proceedings of the 13th Triennial Congress of the International Ergonomics Association, Tampere, Finland 1997*, Helsinki: Finnish Institute of Occupational Health, pp. 413–415.

JOHNSON, G., BOGDUK, N., NOWITZKE, A. and HOUSE, D., 1994, Anatomy and actions of the trapezius muscle, *Clin Biomech*, **9**, 44–50.

JONSSON, B., 1978, Kinesiology. With special reference to electromyographic kinesiology, in Cobb, W.A. and Van Duijn, H. (Eds), *Contemporary Clinical Neurophysiology, EEG*, Suppl. 34, Amsterdam: Elsevier Scientific Publishing Company, pp. 417–428.

JONSSON, B., 1982, Measurement and evaluation of local muscular strain in the shoulder during constrained work, *J Hum Ergol*, **11**, 73–88.

JØRGENSEN, K., FALLENTIN, N. and SIDENIUS, B., 1989, The strain on the shoulder and neck muscles during letter sorting, *Int J Ind Erg*, **3**, 243–248.

KADABA, M.P., COLE, A., WOOTTEN, M.E., McCANN, P., REID, M., MULFORD, G., et al., 1992, Intramuscular wire electromyography of the subscapularis, *J Orthop Res*, **10**, 394–397.

KARLSSON, D., 1992, *Force Distribution in the Human Shoulder*, Göteborg: Chalmers University of Technology.

KEATING, J.F., WATERWORTH, P., SHAW-DUNN, J. and CROSSAN, J., 1993, The relative strengths of the rotator cuff muscles, *J Bone Joint Surg (Br)*, **75-B**, 137–140.

KREIGHBAUM, E. and BARTHELS, K.M., 1996, *Biomechanics. A Qualitative Approach for Studying Human Movement*, 4th edn, Boston: Allyn and Bacon.

KUNITA, K. and FUJIWARA, K., 1996, Relationship between reaction time of eye movement and activity of the neck extensors, *Eur J Appl Physiol*, **74**, 553–557.

LAURSEN, B., 1996, *Shoulder Muscle Forces During Work. EMG-based Biomechanical Models, PhD thesis*, Copenhagen: National Institute of Occupational Health and Technical University of Denmark.

LAURSEN, B., JENSEN, B.R. and SJØGAARD, G., 1997, Shoulder muscle force predictions – comparison of two models, in Veeger, H.E.J., Van der Helm, F.C.T. and Rozing, P.M. (Eds), *Proceedings of the First Conference of the International Shoulder Group*, Maastricht: Shaker Publishing, pp. 71–75.

LAURSEN, B., JENSEN, B.R., NÉMETH, G. and SJØGAARD, G., 1998a, A model predicting individual shoulder muscle forces based on relationship between electromyographic and 3D external forces in static position, *J Biomech*, **31**, 731–739.

LAURSEN, B., JENSEN, B.R. and SJØGAARD, G., 1998b, Effect of speed and precisio demands on human shoulder muscle electromyography during a repetitive task, *Eur J Appl Physiol*, **78**, 544–548.

LIU, J., HUGHES, R.E., SMUTZ, W.P., NIEBUR, G. and NAN-AN, K., 1997, Roles of deltoid and rotator cuff muscles in shoulder elevation. *Clin Biomech*, **12**, 32–38.

LUNDBERG, U., KADEFORS, R., MELIN, B., PALMERUD, G., HASSMÉN, P., ENGSTRÖM, M. and DOHNS, I.E., 1994, Psychophysiological stress and EMG activity of the trapezius muscle, *International Journal of Behavioral Medicine*, **1**, 354–370.

MATHIASSEN, S.E. and WINKEL, J., 1990, Electromyographic activity in the shoulder-neck region according to arm position and glenohumeral torque, *Eur J Appl Physiol*, **61**, 370–379.

MATHIASSEN, S.E. and WINKEL, J., 1991, Quantifying variation in physical load using exposure-vs-time data, *Ergonomics*, **34**(12), 1455–1468.

MATHIASSEN, S.E. and WINKEL, J., 1996, Physiological comparison of three interventions in light assembly work: reduced work pace, increased break allowance and shortened working days, *Int Arch Occup Environ Health*, **68**, 94–108.

MATHIASSEN, S.E., WINKEL, J. and HÄGG, G.M., 1995, Normalization of surface EMG amplitude from the upper trapezius muscle in ergonomic studies – a review, *J Electromyogr Kinesiol*, **5**(4), 197–226.

NIEMI, J., NIEMINEN, H., TAKALA, E.P. and VIIKARI-JUNTURA, E., 1996, A static model based on a time dependent criterion for load sharing between synergistic muscles, *J Biomech*, **29**, 451–460.

OTIS, J.C., JIANG, C., WICKIEWICZ, T.L., PETERSON, M.G.E., WARREN, R.F. and SANTNER, T.J., 1994, Changes in the moment arms of the rotator cuff and deltoid muscles with abduction and rotation, *J Bone Joint Surg (Am)*, **76-A**, 667–676.

PATON, M.E. and BROWN, J.M.M., 1994, An electromyographic analysis of functional differentiation in human pectoralis major muscle, *J Electromyogr Kinesiol*, **4**, 161–169.

POPPEN, N.K. and WALKER, P.S., 1978, Forces at the glenohumeral joint in abduction, *Clin Orthop*, **135**, 165–170.

ROCKWOOD, C.A. and MATSEN, F.A., 1990, *The Shoulder. Volume 1*, Philadelphia: W.B. Saunders Company.

SCHÜLDT, K. and HARMS-RINGDAHL, K., 1988, Activity levels during isometric test contractions of neck and shoulder muscles, *Scand J Rehabil Med*, **20**, 117–127.

SCHÜLDT, K., HARMS-RINGDAHL, K., ARBORELIUS, U.P. and NEMETH, G., 1987, Influence of sitting postures on neck and shoulder E.M.G. during arm-hand work movements, *Clin Biomech*, **2**, 126–139.

SIGHOLM, G., HERBERTS, P., ALMSTRÖM, C. and KADEFORS, R., 1984, Electromyographic analysis of shoulder muscle load, *J Orthop Res*, **1**(4), 379–386.

SJØGAARD, G., 1997, Intramuscular pressure may prevent delayed onset muscular soreness. Theoretical considerations based on de novo biomechanical modelling, in Capodaglio, P. and

Bazzini, G. (Eds), *Advances in Occupational Medicine and Rehabilitation. Activities of the Upper Limbs: Aspects of Occupational and Rehabilitation Medicine*, Pavia, Italy: Le Collane della Fondazione Salvatore Maugeri, pp. 37–44.

SJØGAARD, G. and JENSEN, B.R., 1997, Muscle pathology with overuse, in Ranney, D. (Ed.), *Chronic Musculoskeletal Injuries in the Workplace*, Philadelphia: W.B. Saunders Company, pp. 17–40.

SJØGAARD, G., SEJERSTED, O.M., WINKEL, J., SMOLANDER, J., JØRGENSEN, K. and WESTGAARD, R., 1995, Exposure assessment and mechanisms of pathogenesis in work-related musculoskeletal disorders: significant aspects in the documentation of risk factors, in Svane, O. and Johansen, C. (Eds), *Work and Health. Scientific Basis of Progress in the Working Environment*. Luxembourg: European Commission, Directorate-General V, pp. 75–87.

SØGAARD, K., FALLENTIN, N. and NIELSEN, J., 1996, Work load during floor cleaning. The effect of cleaning methods and work technique, *Eur J Appl Physiol*, **73**, 73–81.

SØGAARD, K., LAURSEN, B., JENSEN, B.R. and SJØGAARD, G., 1998, 3-D dynamic calculations of the loads on the upper extremities during two different floor cleaning methods. *J Clin Biomech* (Submitted).

SUNDELIN, G. and HAGBERG, M., 1992, Electromyographic signs of shoulder muscle fatigue in repetitive arm work paced by the methods-time measurement system, *Scand J Work Environ Health*, **18**, 262–268.

VAN DER HELM, F.C.T., 1994, A finite element musculoskeletal model of the shoulder mechanism, *J Biomech*, **27**, 551–569.

VASSELJEN, O. and WESTGAARD, R.H., 1995, A case-control study of trapezius muscle activity in office and manual workers with shoulder and neck pain and symptom-free controls, *Int Arch Occup Environ Health*, **67**, 11–18.

VEEGER, H.E.J., VAN DER HELM, F.C.T., VAN DER WOUDE, L.H.V., PRONK, G.M. and ROZENDAL, R.H., 1991, Inertia and muscle contraction parameters for musculoskeletal modelling of the shoulder mechanism, *J Biomech*, **24**, 615–629.

VEIERSTED, K.B., WESTGAARD, R.H. and ANDERSEN, P., 1990, Pattern of muscle activity during steroptyped work and its relation to muscle pain, *Int Arch Occup Environ Health*, **62**, 31–41.

WÆRSTED, M. and WESTGAARD, R.H., 1991, Working hours as a risk factor in the development of musculoskeletal complaints. *Ergonomics*, **34**(3), 265–276.

WÆRSTED, M. and WESTGAARD, R.H., 1996, Attention-related muscle activity in different body regions during VDU work with minimal physical activity, *Ergonomics*, **39**, 661–676.

WÆRSTED, M., BJØRKLUND, R.A. and WESTGAARD, R.H., 1994, The effect of motivation on shoulder-muscle tension in attention-demanding tasks, *Ergonomics*, **37**(2), 363–376.

WÆRSTED, M., EKEN, T. and WESTGAARD, R.H., 1996, Activity of single motor unit in attention-demanding tasks: firing pattern in the human trapezius muscle, *Eur J Appl Physiol*, **72**, 323–329.

WESTGAARD, R.H. and BJØRKLUND, R., 1987, Generation of muscle tension additional to postural muscle load, *Ergonomics*, **30**(6), 911–923.

WOOD, J.E., MEEK, S.G. and JACOBSEN, S.C., 1989a, Quantitation of human shoulder anatomy for prosthetic arm control – I. surface modelling. *J Biomech*, **22**(3), 273–292.

WOOD, J.E., MEEK, S.G. and JACOBSEN, S.C., 1989b, Quantitation of human shoulder anatomy for prosthetic arm control – II. anatomy matrices. *J Biomech*, **22**(4), 309–325.

CHAPTER TWELVE

Whiplash injuries

MANOHAR M. PANJABI, JONATHAN N. GRAUER,
JACEK CHOLEWICKI AND KIMIO NIBU

INTRODUCTION

Whiplash has been loosely defined as an acceleration injury and most commonly involves an unaware victim in a stationary vehicle being struck from behind. Cervical spine injuries are a significant, but poorly understood, resulting problem.

It is important to characterise such whiplash injuries as they continue to be on the increase. For example, reports from several European countries indicate an alarming increase in the annual number of neck injuries in recent years due to increased traffic density (Kampen, 1993). In Japan, 50 per cent of car-to-car traffic accidents are reported to result in neck injuries (Ono and Kanno, 1993). The clinical symptoms attributed to whiplash include neck and shoulder pain, headache, dizziness, and blurring of vision. Nevertheless, the non-specific nature of these symptoms often leads to undefined diagnoses (Barnley et al., 1994; Gargan and Bannister, 1994; Radanov et al., 1995). The recent scientific monograph by the Quebec Task Force on Whiplash Associated Disorders identified very few objective studies that have documented specific spinal lesions associated with whiplash (Spitzer et al., 1995). Such studies have proven to be particularly challenging due to the intermingled litigation issues (Schrader et al., 1996).

In a survey of cervical spine injuries, the symptoms of pain and headache were present in 25 per cent of the cases five years after accidents (Dvorak et al., 1989). Another study found 28 per cent of whiplash victims with persisting mild symptoms and 12 per cent with significant symptoms at a 10.3 year follow-up (Gargan and Bannister, 1990). A subsequent prospective study found only 38 per cent of the whiplash patients to have returned to baseline at two years follow-up (Gargan and Bannister, 1994).

There is consensus that most whiplash patients suffer from soft tissue injuries (Davis et al., 1993; Jonsson et al., 1994; MacNab, 1971; Maimaris et al., 1988). Patients with more severe injuries show signs of clinical instability (Jonsson et al., 1994), determined using accepted instability criteria (White and Panjabi, 1990). Unfortunately, the presently available imaging methods, such as MRI, do not completely identify such sub-failure injuries of soft tissue which may largely explain the decreased function and pain associated with whiplash trauma.

BIOMECHANICAL BACKGROUND

The mechanism of whiplash has remained unclear over the past 70 years since the term was first coined in 1928 by Crowe. Many laboratory investigations have attempted to determine the whiplash injury mechanisms as it is of value for several reasons. Under-standing the injury mechanism would suggest potential sites of injury, and identify anatomic elements at risk of injury. Additionally, prevention strategies must be tailored to the mode of injury if they are to be effective.

MacNab established the most traditionally accepted concepts of whiplash injuries of the cervical spine approximately 30 years ago (MacNab, 1964, 1966). He studied experi-mental traumas of anaesthetised monkeys and found a predominance of lower cervical anterior element injuries. He hypothesised that hyper-extension of the head and cervical spine was responsible for whiplash injuries.

Penning questioned the ideas put forth by MacNab and postulated that the primary mechanism of whiplash injury is hyper-translation of the head as opposed to hyper-extension (Penning, 1992a, 1992b). He studied lateral radiographs of 'chin-in and chin-out' normal subjects as representative of posterior and anterior head translations. He then compared associated intervertebral sagittal plane rotations with those of actively flexed and extended functional radiographs. He found that the rotations of the cranio-vertebral junction (C0–C2) were greater with simple head translations than with head flexion or extension. This was not the case for the lower cervical intervertebral joints. He thus concluded that upper level flexion injuries should predominate in whiplash trauma.

To understand the injury mechanism, experimental studies have consisted of volun-teers in actual or simulated car collisions (Ewing *et al.*, 1969, 1975, 1976; Matsushita *et al.*, 1994; McConnell *et al.*, 1993; Severy *et al.*, 1955). Such experiments have re-vealed important information concerning the movements of the head and trunk during vehicle impacts. However, by the very nature of human investigations, instrumentation is limited, accelerations are predominantly below injury thresholds, and subjects are aware of impending collisions.

Experiments with whole cadavers have generally studied a limited number of traumas and have monitored relatively few kinematic parameters (Geigl *et al.*, 1994, 1995; Mertz and Patrick, 1967). Cadaveric experiments, although allowing realistic accelerations to be imparted to the test 'subjects', are unable to monitor crucial parameters responsible for injury, i.e. intervertebral motions, which are not accessible for dynamic monitoring.

Mechanical properties and response characteristics of current anthropomorphic dum-mies do not as yet compare favourably with the complex viscoelastic nature of human tissues (Geigl *et al.*, 1995; Svensson, 1993; Svensson *et al.*, 1993). Furthermore, such models can only be as advanced as the kinematic data available for their modelling. As noted above, this information remains limited.

Despite difficulties in defining the whiplash event, understanding the mechanism of whiplash injury remains an important goal. Based upon the MacNab theory of head and neck hyper-extension, the current head-restraint was designed to prevent neck injuries in rear-end collisions by blocking such hyper-extension. Although the head-restraint has helped to limit neck injuries, it has not eliminated them. In a study in Sweden, Nygren *et al.* (1985) found only a 20 per cent decrease in neck injuries after the introduction of the head-restraint. This would suggest that the hyper-extension injury mechanism, first proposed by MacNab more than 30 years ago (MacNab, 1964, 1966), and currently a pre-valent view, needs to be quesioned.

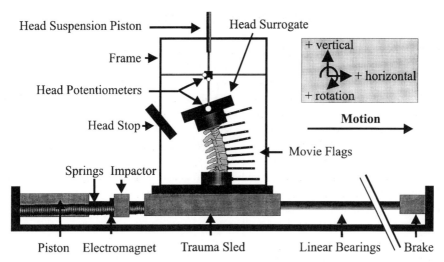

Figure 12.1   Schematic diagram of the bench-top whiplash apparatus. The trauma sled was drawn to the negative horizontal direction with the pneumatic piston and released in the positive horizontal direction. Flexion was defined as positive rotation and extension as negative rotation.

EVOLVING WHIPLASH UNDERSTANDING

A highly instrumented system has been developed in our laboratory to approach the question of the whiplash injury mechanism (Panjabi *et al.*, 1997). This model employs osteo-ligamentous human cadaveric cervical spines, and a specially developed trauma apparatus which simulates rear-end car collisions (Figure 12.1).

Specimens were subjected to incrementally increasing traumas of 2.5g, 4.5g, 6.5g, and 8.5g. Intervertebral rotations were tracked with high speed cinematography at 500 frames per second. Digitised intervertebral data from one specimen traumatised at 6.5g are shown as an example in Figure 12.2. The 30 to 85 msec time period illustrates an initial response phase of the cervical spine with extension at the lower levels and flexion at the upper levels. Beyond 85 msec represents a subsequent response phase of the cervical spine with extension at all levels. This is demonstrated photographically and schematically in Figure 12.3.

Maximal intervertebral flexion and extension rotations were calculated for all cervical levels for each trauma class. Resulting values were compared to physiological limits of rotation of the same specimens as determined by flexibility testing of the intact specimens with loading of up to 1.0 Nm (Grauer *et al.*, 1997). Most notably, the C6–C7 and C7–T1 levels were found to consistently exceed the physiological limits of rotation in extension for all trauma classes studied. Intervertebral rotations for all specimens, when the lowest level was in maximal extension, were averaged. Results are seen in Figure 12.4. As can be seen, the maximal lower level extensions were consistently associated with upper level flexions. In other words, the spine consistently exhibited upper level flexion and lower level extension at the times of maximal lower level extension. In fact, conversion of the spine to complete extension was associated with a relative relaxation of the lower level hyper-extension.

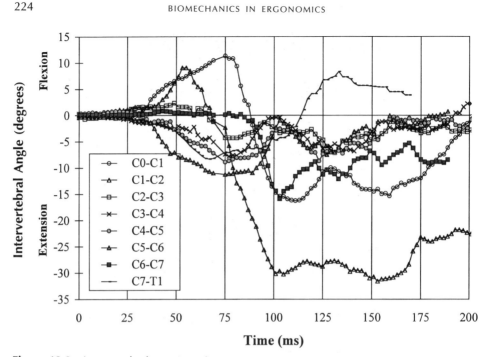

Figure 12.2 Intervertebral rotations from C0–C1 to C7–T1 of a specimen obtained from high speed cinematography during a 6.5g whiplash trauma shown here as a sample data set. Flexion was defined as positive rotation and extension as negative rotation.

Direct information about injuries to the cervical spine was quantified with multi-directional flexibility testing after each incremental trauma (Panjabi *et al.*, 1998). In general, the flexibilities increased after increasing traumas, as one would expect. Physiological values were again compared to cervical-level matched values obtained after each trauma class. Such testing demonstrated that lower level injuries were, in fact, sustained from the whiplash traumas. The lower levels exhibited increases in both extension ranges of motion and neutral zones after 4.5g whiplash trauma. This suggests that the stretching of anterior elements of the lower cervical spine beyond their normal physiological limits resulted in soft tissue injuries.

CURRENT PERSPECTIVE

The above described studies suggest that the mechanism of whiplash injury in rear-end accidents is not as basic as simple neck hyper-extension. Rather, the initially formed S-shaped cervical curvature with extension at the lower levels and concurrent flexion at the upper levels has been identified as the principle injury phase of whiplash with associated lower level extension exceeding physiological limits (Figure 12.5). This has been termed Phase I of the whiplash response.

The subsequent change of the entire cervical spine to extension is consistent with the conversion of the cervical spine to a C-shaped curvature (Figure 12.5). Lower level extension decreases here as compared to Phase I. Consequently, this has been termed Phase II of the whiplash response and has been deemed to have a lesser potential for injury than Phase I.

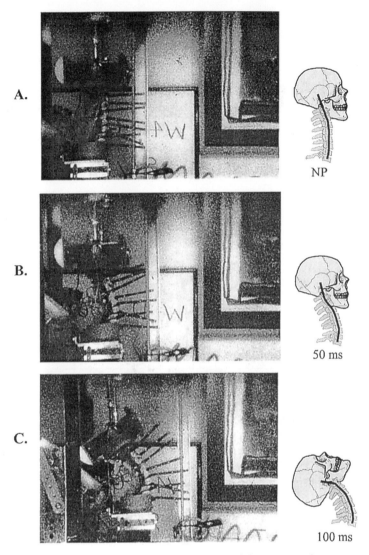

Figure 12.3 Movie still photographs and schematics of the trauma shown in Figure 12.2 illustrating starting neutral position (NP) **(A)**, initial response phase with upper level flexion and lower level extension **(B)**, and the subsequent complete extension of the cervical spine **(C)**.

It was further observed from head potentiometers that the head has increasing posterior translation and decreasing extension with increasing levels of trauma (Cholewicki *et al.*, 1998). This suggests that Phase I of the whiplash becomes more pronounced, and Phase II less so, with increasing levels of trauma.

The previously accepted mechanism of whiplash injury of MacNab was based upon head and neck hyper-extension (MacNab, 1964, 1966). The picture that this mechanism paints is analogous to that of Phase II of the mechanism described above. However, as stated, the Phase II response to whiplash is now believed to be associated with a lesser degree of lower level extension than with Phase I, and thus a lesser potential for causing soft tissue injuries in this region.

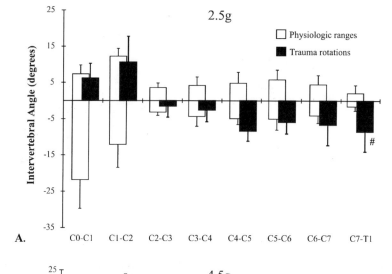

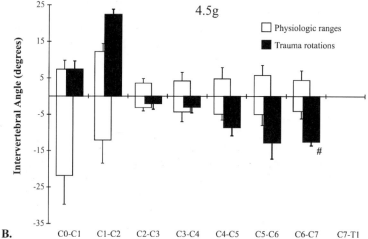

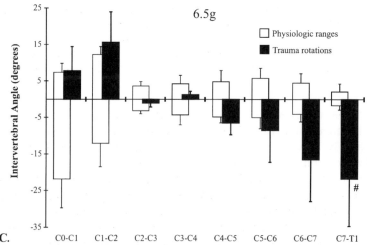

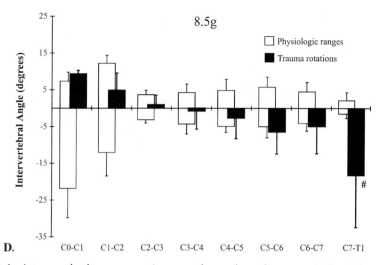

Figure 12.4 Intervertebral trauma motions are shown from the time of whiplash with maximal extensions of the lowest cervical levels C6–C7 or C7–T1 (denoted with #). Physiological ranges are shown on all graphs as a baseline from which to evaluate the trauma induced intervertebral rotations. The figure represents the 2.5g trauma class (n=4) in **(A)**, the 4.5g trauma class (n=2) in **(B)**, the 6.5g trauma class (n=4) in **(C)**, and the 8.5g trauma class (n=2) in **(D)**.

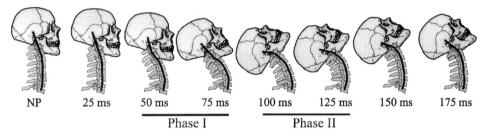

Figure 12.5 Schematic of the trauma shown in Figures 12.2 and 12.3. The spine starts in a neutral position (NP). The 50 to 75 ms time period illustrates the neck forming an S-shaped curvature (Phase I). During this phase, the lower cervical spine intervertebral joints exhibit hyper-extension, exceeding their physiological limits. In the later phase (Phase II), the spine transforms to a C-shape with complete extension. This phase is associated with a lesser degree of the lower level hyper-extension, and thus a lesser potential for injury.

In fact, the above described work did not produce head extensions beyond physiological limits (Grauer *et al.*, 1998). This finding is similar to *in vivo* findings of two recent studies in which whiplash experiments were conducted with volunteers (Matsushita *et al.*, 1994; McConnell *et al.*, 1993) and suggests that injury could not be caused by simple neck extension. The work of MacNab, as well as that of many other early investigators, may have missed the potentially more damaging Phase I response to whiplash because of an inability to monitor individual intervertebral motions continuously.

The S-shaped cervical spine curvature of the Phase I response to whiplash has been previously noted by Svensson *et al.* (1993) in a dummy preparation, but they did not relate this to spinal column injury. Geigl *et al.* (1994) also measured, in one whole cadaveric whiplash trauma, rotations within the cervical spine. They found C0–C4 flexion with simultaneous C4–C7 extension which peaked at 120msec, while the head rotation peaked later at 160msec. These times are somewhat longer than those reported in isolated osteoligamentous work and may reflect the differences in the experimental methodologies. They used a whole cadaver sitting in an automobile seat in a large sled for which there was delay for the trauma pulse to travel from the impact point to the T1 vertebra, via the sled, seat, and thorax.

Finally, the S-shaped curvature was an assumption on which Penning's theory of injury mechanism is based (Penning, 1992a, 1992b). However, Penning worked from this assumption and never established it as fact. He then hypothesised that the cranio-vertebral junction would be the principle site of cervical injury in whiplash. In contrast, experimental findings now show that the lower cervical levels most consistently exceed their physiological motion limits.

ERGONOMIC SIGNIFICANCE

In summary, the kinematic response to whiplash is bi-phasic. Phase I is associated with an initial S-shaped curvature of the neck with upper cervical level flexion and lower cervical level hyper-extension. This hyper-extension of the lower cervical spine has been identified as the mode of whiplash injury. The subsequent Phase II response to whiplash is associated with lesser lower level extension and thus lesser potential for injury.

As the understanding of whiplash continues to be refined, it is hoped that the biomechanical and clinical aspects of this problem can be better addressed. In doing so, the necessary injury prevention, clinical diagnosis, and treatment will be facilitated.

References

BARNLEY, L., LORD, S. and BOGDUK, N., 1994, Clinical review: whiplash injuries, *Pain*, **58**, 283–307.

CHOLEWICKI, J.J., PANJABI, M.M., NIBU, K., GRAUER, J.N. and DVORAK, J., 1998, Head kinematics during *in vitro* whiplash simulation, *Accident Analysis & Prevention*, **30**(4), 469–479.

CROWE, H.E., 1928, Injuries of the cervical spine, Paper presented at the meeting of Western Orthopaedic Association, San Francisco, California.

DAVIS, J.W., PHREANER, D.L., HOYT, D.B. and MACKERSIE, R.C., 1993, The etiology of missed cervical spine injuries, *J Trauma*, **34**, 342–346.

DVORAK, J., VALACH, L. and SCHMID, S.T., 1989, Cervical spine injuries in Switzerland, *J Manual Medicine*, **16**, 7–16.

EWING, C.S., THOMAS, D.J., PATRICK, L.M., BEELER, G.W. and SMITH, M.J., 1969, Living human dynamic response to -Gx impact acceleration. II Accelerations measured on the head and neck, *Proceedings of the 13th Stapp Car Crash Conference*, Society of Automotive Engineers, Warrendale, PA, Paper 690817.

EWING, C.L., THOMAS, D.J., LUSTICK, L., BECKER, E., WILLEMS, G. and MUZZY III, W.H., 1975, The effect of the initial position of the head and neck on the dynamic response of the human head and neck to -Gx impact acceleration, *Proceedings of the 19th Stapp Car Crash Conference*, Society of Automotive Engineers, Warrendale, PA, Paper 751157.

EWING, C.L., THOMAS, D.J., LUSTICK, L., MUZZY, W.H., WILLEMS, G. and MAJEWSKI, P.L., 1976, The effect of duration, rate of onset, and peak sled acceleration on the dynamic response of the human head and neck, *Proceedings of the 20th Stapp Car Crash Conference*, Society of Automotive Engineers, Warrendale, PA, Paper 760800.

GARGAN, M.F. and BANNISTER, G.C., 1990, Long-term prognosis of soft tissue injuries of the neck, *J Bone Joint Surg*, **72B**, 901–903.

GARGAN, M.F. and BANNISTER, G.C., 1994, The rate of recovery following whiplash injury, *European Spine Journal*, **3**(3), 162–164.

GEIGL, B.C., STEFFEN, H., LEINZINGER, P., MUHLBAUER, M. and BAUER, G., 1994, The movement of head and cervical spine during rear-end impact, *Proceedings of the IRCOBI*, Lyon, France, pp. 127–137.

GEIGL, B.C., STEFFAN, H., DIPPEL, C., MUSER, M.H., WALTZ, F. and SVENSSON, M.Y., 1995, Comparison of head-neck kinematics during rear end impacts between standard Hybrid III, RID Neck, volunteers and PMTOs, *Proceedings of the IRCBOI*, Brunnen, Switzerland.

GRAUER, J.N., PANJABI, M.M., CHOLEWICKI, J., NIBU, K. and DVORAK, J., 1997, Whiplash produces an S-shaped curvature of the neck with hyper-extension at lower levels. *Spine*, **22**(21), 2489–2494.

JONSSON, H. JR, CESARINI, K. *et al.*, 1994, Findings and outcome in whiplash-type neck distortions (review), *Spine*, **19**, 2733–2743.

KAMPEN, L.T.B. VAN, 1993, Availability and proper adjustment of head restraints in The Netherlands, *Int. IRCOBI Conf. on the Biomech. of Impacts, Sept. 8–10*, Eindhoven, The Netherlands, pp. 367–378.

MACNAB, I., 1964, Acceleration injuries of the cervical spine, *J Bone Joint Surg*, **46A**, 1797–1799.

MACNAB, I., 1966, Whiplash injuries of the neck, *Manitoba Medical Review*, March, 172–174.

MACNAB, I., 1971, The 'whiplash syndrome', *Orthop Clin North Am*, **2**, 389–403.

MAIMARIS, C., BARNES, M.R. and ALLEN, M.J., 1988, Whiplash injuries of the neck: a retrospective study, *Injury*, **19**, 393–396.

MATSUSHITA, T., SATO, T.B., HIRABAYASHI, K., FUJIMURA, S., ASAZUMA, T. and TAKATORI, T., 1994, X-ray study of the human neck motion due to head inertia loading, *Proceedings of the 38th Stapp Car Crash Conference*, Society of Automotive Engineers, Warrendale, PA, Paper 942208.

MCCONNELL, W.E., HOWARD, R.P., GUZMAN, H.M., *et al.*, 1993, Analysis of human test subject responses to low velocity rear end impacts, *Proceedings of the 37th Stapp Car Crash Conference*, Society of Automotive Engineers, Warrendale, PA, Paper 930889.

MERTZ, H.J. and PATRICK, L.M., 1967, Investigation of the kinematics and kinetics of whiplash, *Proceedings of the 11th Stapp Car Crash Conference*, Society of Automotive Engineers, Warrendale, PA, Paper 670919.

NYGREN, A., GUSTAFSSON, H. and TINGVALL, C., 1985, Effects of different types of headrests in rear-end collisions, *10th International Conference on Experimental Safety Vehicles*, 85–90, NHTSA.

ONO, K. and KANNO, M., 1993, Influences of the physical parameters on the risk to neck injuries in low impact speed rear-end collisions, *Int. Conference on the Biomech. of Impacts, IRCOBI Sept 8–10*, Eindhoven, The Netherlands.

PANJABI, M.M., CHOLEWICKI, J., BABAT, L., NIBU, K. and DVORAK, J., 1997, Simulation of whiplash trauma using whole cervical spine specimens, *Spine*, **23**(1), 286–289.

PANJABI, M.M., NIBU, K. and CHOLEWICKI, J., 1998, Whiplash injuries and the potential for mechanical instability. *Eur Spine J*, **7**(6), (in press).

PENNING, L., 1992a, Acceleration injury of the cervical spine by hypertranslation of the head: Part 1. Effect of normal translation of the head on the cervical spine motion: a radiological study, *Eur Spine J*, **1**, 7–12.

PENNING, L., 1992b, Acceleration injury of the cervical spine by hypertranslation of the head: Part 2. Effect of hypertranslation of the head on the cervical spine motion: discussion of literature data, *Eur Spine J*, **1**, 13–19.

RADANOV, B.P., STURZENEGGER, M. and STEFANO, G.D., 1995, Long-term outcome after whiplash injury: a 2 year follow-up considering features of injury mechanism and somatic, radiologic and psychosocial findings, *Medicine*, **74**, 281–297.

SCHRADER, H., OBELIENIENE, D., BOVIM, G., SURKIENE, D., MICKEVICIENE, D., MISEVICIENE, I. and SAND, T., 1996, Natural evolution of late whiplash syndrome outside the medicolegal context, *Lancet*, **347**, 1207–1211.

SEVERY, D.M., MATHEWSON, J.H. and BECHTOL, C.O., 1955, Controlled automobile rear-end collisions, and investigation of related engineering and medical phenomena. *Can Serv Med J*, **11**, 727–759.

SPITZER, W.O., SKOVRON, M.L., SALMI, L.R., CASSIDY, J.D., DURANCEAU, J., SUISSA, S., and ZEISS, E., 1995, Scientific monograph of the Quebec task force on whiplash-associated disorders: redefining 'whiplash' and its management, *Spine Supplement*, **20**, 10S–73S.

SVENSSON, M., 1993, Neck-injuries in rear-end car collisions – sites and biomechanical causes of the injuries, test methods and preventive measures, Chalmers University of Technology, Dept. of Injury Prevention.

SVENSSON, M.Y., HALAND, Y. and LARSSON, S., 1993, Rear-end collisions – a study of the influence of backrest properties on head-neck motion using a new dummy neck, *Proceedings of the 37th Stapp Car Crash Conference*, Society of Automotive Engineers, Warrendale, PA, Paper 930343.

WHITE, A.A. and PANJABI, M.M., 1990, *Clinical Biomechanics of the Spine*, 2nd Edn, Philadelphia: J.B. Lippincott.

PART FOUR

Low Back

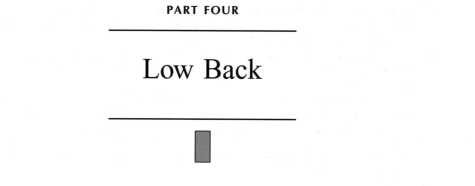

CHAPTER THIRTEEN

Low back pain and whole body vibration

MALCOLM H. POPE, MARIANNE MAGNUSSON
AND DAVID G. WILDER

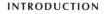

INTRODUCTION

Low back pain (LBP) is the leading major cause of industrial disability in those under the age of 45. The total cost of LBP to the US economy is $90 billion per annum and low back pain accounts for 20 per cent of all work related injuries (Bureau of Labor Statistics, 1982). There is an extensive literature relating exposure to whole body vibration (WBV) to LBP (Backman, 1983; Barbaso, 1958; Cremona, 1972; Fishbein and Salter, 1950; Kelsey and Hardy, 1975; Rosegger and Rosegger, 1960). For example, several studies have related LBP to tractor driving (Dupuis and Christ, 1966; Fishbein and Salter, 1950; Rosegger and Rosegger, 1960). Pathological findings and LBP depend on age and length of exposure (Dupuis and Christ, 1966; Rosegger and Rosegger, 1960). Cremona (1972) reported a 70 per cent LBP prevalence in heavy vehicle equipment users. Hilfert *et al.* (1981) reported greater pathological changes and LBP in drivers of earth moving equipment and the prevalence increased with age. Barbaso (1958) also found an increase in the prevalence of both LBP and pathological changes in bus drivers with time of exposure. Kelsey and Hardy (1975) found the relative risk of herniated nucleus pulposus to be 2.7 in car drivers, and 4.7 for truck drivers.

Many workers have shown transmissibilities greater than 1.0 (i.e. greater output than input) for the first resonant frequency of the seated subject (Bastek *et al.*, 1977; Dieckmann, 1958; Griffin, 1975; Panjabi *et al.*, 1986; Pope *et al.*, 1980; Rosegger and Rosegger, 1960). Resonant frequencies occur between 4 and 6 Hz, due to the upper torso vibrating vertically with respect to the pelvis.

In this chapter we will describe a number of studies, carried out by our group, in order to understand better the relationship between whole body vibration and low back pain.

TWO CENTRE EPIDEMIOLOGICAL STUDY

In this study (Magnusson *et al.*, 1993) vibration exposure was measured according to ISO (1978, 1985), whilst driving on typical roads and met published criteria (Hulshof and Veldhuijzen van Zanten, 1987). The study was carried out in Sweden and the USA. The American workers were significantly shorter and heavier than the Swedish. American bus drivers and sedentary workers were a little older and had been longer on the job than their Swedish colleagues, whereas American truckers were a little younger. The Swedes used tobacco more than the Americans did, and all drivers smoked significantly more than sedentary workers. Bus drivers took more time off work than truckers in both countries. American bus drivers lifted more than truckers and sedentary workers, and Swedish truck drivers lifted more than bus drivers and sedentary workers. Swedish bus drivers were exposed to higher vibration levels, whereas the American truckers were exposed to higher vibration levels than the Swedes. Swedish bus drivers experienced more vibration exposure than did the American bus drivers. This is probably due to the difference in bus types, road conditions, and driving demands. The American truckers were vibrated more than anyone in the study, possibly due to travel on dirt roads and less use of vibration attenuation in seats and cabs.

Swedish and American bus drivers were less satisfied with their working tasks than truck drivers and sedentary workers, and Swedish bus drivers were also less satisfied with their boss. American drivers enjoyed their job more than American sedentary workers. The group with the greatest risk factors were American truck drivers. They had the highest vibration exposure, moderate lifting, and minimal exercise, were overweight and 53 per cent smoked. Although 50 per cent had low back pain recently, only 24 per cent had lost work time for that reason. This group however, reported 100 per cent job enjoyment, the lowest job stress level (21 per cent), 92 per cent boss satisfaction and 97 per cent job satisfaction.

LABORATORY SIMULATIONS

Pope *et al.* (1986) simulated various vibration environments in the laboratory. Under helicopter vibration, volunteers reported a loss of comfort, over a two-hour exposure. There was also a measurable muscle fatigue. Based on these data, recommendations were made to improve the seated posture, and to add vibration dampers to the seats.

Wilder *et al.* (1994) studied the response to whole body vibration in simulated driving. The aim of this study was to compare a truck seat with a gas spring to the standard spring seat. Subject comfort was rated before and directly after exposure to typical vibrations. Muscle fatigue using centre frequency was determined during vibration exposure, and the magnitude and phase of acceleration transfer were calculated from the base plate to the seat pan, and from the seat pan to the bite bar. The mechanical measures showed that the gas spring attenuated the vibration much better.

IN VIVO MEASUREMENTS

Pope *et al.* (1986) studied the response to vibration with transducers rigidly fixed to the lumbar spinous processes compared to those fixed to the skin. Under local anaesthesia, a threaded K-wire was fixed transcutaneously into the spinous process of the third lumbar

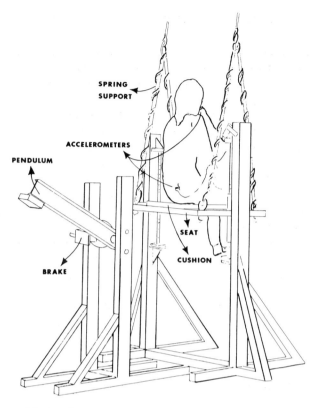

Figure 13.1 Impact test system.

vertebrae. Because of the artifact that was identified in the use of skin mounted transducers, it was elected to use the skeletally mounted transducers in the subsequent studies.
The outcome measure was the transmissibility and phase angle between the pin acceleration and that of the platform.

A new impact system for the human spine was introduced (Pope *et al.*, 1987) (see
Figure 13.1). The apparatus consists of a platform suspended by soft springs and guided
by two linear bearings. The vertical resonance of the system was less than 2 Hz. The
frame resonance was 60 Hz, and the platform rotational resonance was approximately 20
Hz. Rotation was minimised if the subject stood or sat in the centre of the platform. The
impact was applied by a pendulum to the centre of the platform.

In Pope *et al.* (1987) the subject was placed in different controlled sitting postures, and
the transmissibility and phase angle determined in both impact and sinusoidal excitation
conditions. The subjects in the relaxed seated posture experienced a transmissibility peak
at the third lumbar vertebrae at 5 Hz coupled with an attenuation peak between 6 to 8.5
Hz (Figure 13.2). In comparing the relaxed and erect posture, the response curves had the
same general form, except that the peaks were more marked in the relaxed posture. The
Valsalva increased the height of the 5 Hz transmissibility peak, and beyond that point
there was decreasing gain with frequency. Contraction of the glutei resulted in a response
curve which was between that of the relaxed and the Valsalva. Placing a block under the
pelvis to offer rotational support reduced the gain peak and the gain valley. Thus, control
of posture may be a key to obviating the effect of whole body vibration on the spine.
Subjects were also subjected to impacts, whilst seated on various kinds of cushions (Pope

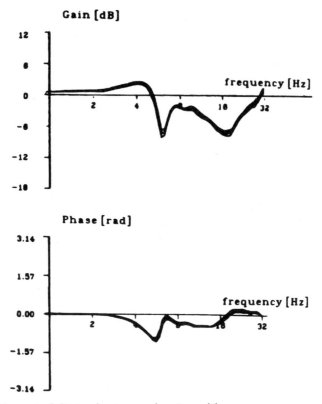

Figure 13.2 Transmissibility and gain as a function of frequency.

et al., 1989a). The least stiff material moved the transmissibility peak below 4 Hz and increased its amplitude. A stiffer material increased the frequency of the transmissibility peak and established a rotational response at higher frequencies. A viscoelastic material had little effect, except at about 8 Hz. The trends between cushion materials were similar in the erect, relaxed and Valsalva postures.

A number of different conditions were explored to establish the effect on the dynamic response of the standing subject (Pope *et al.*, 1989b). In the erect posture, there was a single transmissibility peak at 5.5 Hz. The at-ease posture gave a slightly reduced peak, and a knee-bent posture attenuated the response. A pelvic tilt and Valsalva caused the peak to move to about 7 Hz while a tip toe stance moved the peak to 3 Hz. Standing on foam materials caused the peak to move to lower frequencies, while the wearing of different shoes did not significantly change the response.

PHYSIOLOGICAL MEASURES

Phasic electromyographic activity

The phasic electromyography (EMG) of the erector spinae was measured during whole body vibration (Seroussi *et al.*, 1989). The relationship of the EMG to a given torque demand was found by measuring the electromyographic signal while performing an isometric pull.

The subjects were vibrated at discrete frequencies between 3 and 10 Hz. The electromyographic signals were high-pass filtered, rectified and ensemble averaged. The signals were then converted to torque. From these data, the phase relationship between the input signal, to move the platform, and the resulting torque, was established. The time lag between the input displacement and the peak torque varied from 30 to 100 msec at 3 Hz, and 70 to 100 msec at 10 Hz. WBV added to the net load in the spine due to cyclic muscle forces.

Muscle fatigue

A frequency shift, towards lower frequencies has been shown as an effect of fatiguing contractions (Chaffin, 1973; Komi and Tesch, 1979). The EMG erector spinae was studied under WBV (Hansson et al., 1991; Wilder et al., 1994). To ensure muscular activity, the subjects sat in a forwardly bent position, carrying extra weight on the front of the chest. In this position, the subjects were exposed to: whole body vibration of 5 Hz and 0.2 g root means square acceleration; and static sitting. The mean frequency at both the thoracic and lumbar level, decreased with time. The decrease was accentuated by WBV.

Creep

Spinal height changes were measured on a stadiometer (Magnusson et al., 1992). The stadiometer consists of a column which was tilted slightly backwards. The column was equipped with supports for the head and the pelvis, as well as four pressure sensitive switches, which functioned as posture controls. The posture of the head was controlled by means of glasses equipped with laterally oriented pins attached to the side frame (Figure 13.3). The anterior pin was lined up with one of the posterior pins by means of the image from a mirror in front of the subject. A vertical line on the mirror served as control for head posture in the frontal and transverse planes. A linear variable displacement transducer registered height changes continuously during the exposure. Height changes were measured in 12 female subjects exposed to static sitting and seated whole body vibrations. The procedure enabled discrimination between 'true' height loss and posture change. The vibration input was 5 Hz, the exposure time was five minutes, and the intermissions between the exposure periods were 20 minutes. A larger height loss was demonstrated when the subjects were exposed to vibration, than when not. The height loss was neither time nor order dependent, and did not correlate with either height or weight. In another study it was concluded that an inclined backrest reduces the effects of vibration (Magnusson et al., 1994).

Unexpected load

There are a number of studies which suggest that unexpected load is aetiological for low back pain (Andersson, 1981; Magora, 1973; Manning et al., 1984). When a sudden load is applied the muscles will respond rapidly in order to stabilise the body which leads to overcompensation of the muscles. We hypothesised that subjects who had been exposed to whole body vibration would exhibit a larger latency of response, and a greater response amplitude (Wilder et al., 1995, 1996). The electromyography of the erector spinae

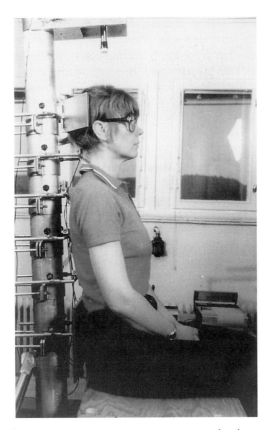

Figure 13.3   The stadiometer – a means to measure accurately changes in stature.

muscle responses was measured in response to a weighted tennis ball falling into an instrumented tray, held in their hands in front of them (Figure 13.4). The weight was dropped onto the tray, and a switch closure indicated the moment of impact. This was compared to the onset of electromyography response. It was established that the response latency was increased, and the response magnitude increased after vertical vibration exposure. Thus, truckers who unload a truck right away could experience soft tissue or muscle injury after whole body vibration. However, we also established that walking for five minutes reversed those effects.

DISCUSSION

Low back pain is multifactorial in origin but there are few risk factors for low back pain which lend themselves to prevention. Risk factors related to the industrial environment are ones over which we have some control. Epidemiological studies have been conducted suggesting that whole body vibration is an important risk factor for low back pain. Vibration also probably combines with other risk factors such as lifting, pushing, and pulling to increase the risk. This is important to the truck driver who loads or unloads the truck. Studies of the occupational environment reveal that many vehicles subject the worker to levels of vibration greater than that recommended by the ISO (1978).

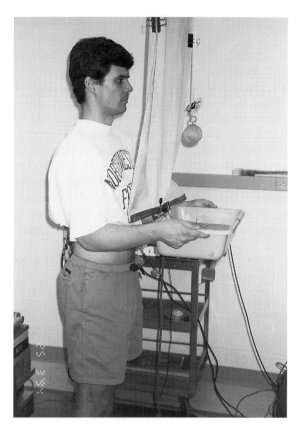

Figure 13.4 Set-up for unexpected load experiment.

It is apparent from whole body vibration data that the human spinal system has a characteristic response to vibrational inputs in a seated posture. The first resonance occurs within a band of 4.5 to 5.5 Hz. Similar, but less tightly defined resonances, are also identified in the 9.4 to 13.1 Hz range. Using direct measures, one can confirm the resonance at 4.5 to 5.5 Hz, but can show how it is markedly affected by the pelvis–buttocks system. The response of the human is due to a combination of a vertical subsystem and a rotational subsystem. The latter is characterised by rocking of the pelvis. Hence, pelvic rocking was shown to be an important factor in the first natural frequency response of the seated individual. Cushions have not been found to be very effective in attenuating the dynamic response and, in fact, increased the response. There are some limitations of these studies. The techniques are highly invasive, and by necessity, limited to a few subjects. The experiments are difficult, and the analyses quite complex.

The muscles are not able to protect the spine from adverse loads. At many frequencies, the muscles' responses are so far out of phase, their forces are added to those of the stimulus. Thus, the muscles have an important role in adding to the effect of vibration. The fatigue that was found in muscles, after whole body vibration, is indicative of the loads in the muscles.

Exposure of the seated subject to whole body vibrations of 5 Hz, in a position that ensured back muscle activity, increased the rate of fatigue in the erector spinae muscles. After whole body vibration, we demonstrated an increased latency in muscle recruitment. This may be due to the fatigue inherent in whole body vibration exposure. This suggests that unloading a vehicle, after exposure to whole body vibration could present a problem for the back.

When the spine is axially loaded it will compress and thus, become shorter. The viscoelastic behaviour of the motion segment of the spine is well described. It was demonstrated that the sitting posture, in itself, always caused height loss in the subjects, provided that the sitting exposure was preceded by a less loading activity. The spinal height change, as measured in the current study of vibration, thus reflected spinal load. An inclined backrest has been shown to reduce the load on the spine and could reduce the effects of vibration in such a position. In summary, after exposure to whole body vibration, the muscles are fatigued and the discs compressed (i.e., less capable of absorbing and distributing load). In this condition, the spine is in a poorer condition to sustain larger loads. Thus, it would seem reasonable to recommend the avoidance of heavy lifting after vibration exposure (i.e., unloading a truck), especially since changes were demonstrated in the ability to respond to a suddenly applied load after whole body vibration.

ACKNOWLEDGEMENT

This work was funded by the NIOSH and AMFO (Swedish Work Environment Fund).

References

ANDERSSON, G.B., 1981, Epidemiologic aspects on low-back pain in industry, *Spine*, **6**(1), 53–60.
BACKMAN, A.L., 1983, Health survey of professional drivers, *Scand J Work Environ Health*, **9**, 36–41.
BARBASO, E., 1958, Sull'incidenza delle alterazioni della colonna vertebrale nel personale viaggiante di una azienda auto-tranviaria, *Med Lavoro*, **49**, 630–634.
BASTEK, R., BUCHHOLZ, C., DENISOV, E.I., *et al.*, 1977, Comparison of the effects of sinusoidal and stochastic octave-band-wide vibrations – a multi-disciplinary study. Part I: Experimental arrangement and physical aspects. Part II: Physiological aspects. Part III: Psychological investigations, *Intl Arch Occup and Environmental Health*, 1977.
BUREAU OF LABOR STATISTICS, 1982, Back injuries associated with lifting (work injury report), *Bulletin 2144*, 1, US Government Printing Office, 1982.
CHAFFIN, D.B., 1973, Localised muscle fatigue – definition and measurement, *J Occup Med*, **15**, 346–354.
CREMONA, E., 1972, Die Wirbelsäule bei den Schwerarbeitern der Eisen-und Stahlindustrie sowie des Bergbaus, *Kommiss Europ Gem Generaldir Soz Angelegenheiten Dok*, Nr 1911/72.
DIECKMANN, D., 1958, A study of the influence of vibration on man, *Ergonomics*, **1**, 347–355, 1958.
DUPUIS, H. and CHRIST, W., 1966, Über das Schwingverhalten des Magens unter dem Einfluss sinusformiger und stochastischer Schwingungen, *Int Z Angew Physiol Arbeitsphysiol*, **22**, 149–166.
FISHBEIN, W.I. and SALTER, L.C., 1950, The relationship between truck and tractor driving and disorders of the spine and supporting structures, *Indust Med Surg*, **19**, 444–445.
GRIFFIN, M.J., 1975, Vertical vibration of seated subjects: effects of posture, vibration level, and frequency, *Aviation, Space, and Environ Med*, **46**(3), 269–276.
HANSSON, T., MAGNUSSON, M. and BROMAN, H., 1991, Back muscle fatigue and seated whole body vibrations. An experimental study in man, *Clin. Biomech*, **6**, 173–178.
HILFERT, R., KÖHNE, G., TOUSSAINT, R. and ZERLETT, G., 1981, Probleme der Ganzkörperschwingungsbelastung von Erdbaumaschinen führrern, *Zentralbl Arb Med*, **31**, 4–5, Part 1: 152–155, Part 2: 199–206.

HULSHOF, C. and VELDHUIJZEN VAN ZANTEN, B., 1987, Whole-body vibration and low-back pain. A review of epidemiologic studies. *Int Arch Occup Environ Health*, **59**, 205–220.

ISO, 1978, *Guide for the Evaluation of Hman Exposure to Whole Body Vibration*, International Standardization Organisation, ISO 2631 (E).

ISO, 1985, *Evaluation of Human Response to Whole Body Vibration*, International Organization for Standardization, Ref. No. 2631 (E).

KELSEY, J.L. and HARDY, R.J., 1975, Driving of motor vehicles as a risk factor for acute herniated lumbar intervertebral disc, *Am J Epidem*, **102**(1), 63–73.

KOMI, P.V. and TESCH, P. 1979, EMG frequency spectrum, muscle structure and fatigue during dynamic contractions in man, *Eur J Appl Physiol Occup Physiol*, **42**, 41–50.

MAGNUSSON, M., ALMQVIST, M., BROMAN, H., POPE, M.H. and HANSSON, T., 1992, Measurement of height loss during whole body vibration, *J Spinal Disorders*, **5**(2), 198–203.

MAGNUSSON, M., WILDER, D.G., POPE, M.H. and HANSSON, T., 1993, Investigation of the long-term exposure to whole body vibration: a 2 country study, *Eur J Phys Med Rehab*, **3**(1), 28–34.

MAGNUSSON, M., POPE, M.H. and HANSSON, T., 1994, The effect of seat back inclination on spine height changes, *Appl Ergonomics*, **25**(4), 294–298.

MAGORA, A., 1973, Investigation of the relation between low back pain and occupation: 4 physical requirements: bending, rotation, reaching and sudden maximal effort. *Scandinavian J Rehab Med*, **5**(4), 186–190.

MANNING, D.P., MITCHELL, R.G. and BLANCHFIELD, L.P., 1984, Body movements and events contributing to accidental and nonaccidental back injuries, *Spine*, **9**(7), 734–739.

PANJABI, M.M., ANDERSSON, G.B.J., JORNEUS, L., HULT, E. and MATTSON, L., 1986, *In vivo* measurement of spinal column vibrations, *J Bone and Joint Surg*, **68A**(5), 695–703.

POPE, M.H., WILDER, D.G. and FRYMOYER, J.W., 1980, Vibration as an etiologic factor in low back pain. *Proc. of Inst. Mech. Engs Conf. on Low Back Pain*, Inst. Mech. Eng., paper C121/80, 1980.

POPE, M.H., WILDER, D.G. and DONNERMEYER, D.D., 1985, Muscle fatigue in static and vibrational seating environments, *Prod. AGARD Conf.*, Italy, 1985.

POPE, M.H., SVENSSON, M., BROMAN, H. and ANDERSSON, G.B.J., 1986, Mounting of the transducer in measurements of sequential motion of the spine, *J Biomech*, **19**(8), 675–677.

POPE, M.H., WILDER, D.G., JORNEUS, L., BROMAN, H., SVENSSON, M. and ANDERSSON, G.B.J., 1987, The response of the seated human to sinusoidal vibration and impact, *J Biomech Eng*, **109**, 279–284.

POPE, M.H., BROMAN, H. and HANSSON, T., 1989a, The dynamic response of a subject seated on various cushions, *Ergonomics*, **32**(10), 1155–1166.

POPE, M.H., BROMAN, H. and HANSSON, T., 1989b, The impact response of the standing subject – a feasibility study, *Clin Biomech*, **4**(4), 195–200.

ROSEGGER, R. and ROSEGGER, S., 1960, Arbeitsmedizinische Erkenntnisse beim Schlepperfahren, *Arch Landtechn*, **2**, 3–65.

SEROUSSI, R.E., WILDER, D.G. and POPE, M.H., 1989, Trunk muscle electromyography and whole body vibration, *J Biomech*, **22**(3), 219–229.

WILDER, D.G., MAGNUSSON, M., FENWICK, J. and POPE, M.H., 1994, The effect of posture and seat suspension design on discomfort and back muscle fatigue during simulated truck driving, *Appl Ergon*, **25**(2), 66–76.

WILDER, D.G., MAGNUSSON, M., POPE, M.H., ROSTEDT, M. and HANSSON, T., 1995, Musculature response to unexpected load in chronic low back pain patients, *Proc. of Intl. Soc. for Study of the Lumbar Spine*, Helsinki, Finland, 1995.

WILDER, D.G., ALEKSIEV, A., MAGNUSSON, M., POPE, M.H., SPRATT, K. and GOEL, V.K., 1996, Muscular response to sudden load: a tool to evaluate fatigue and rehabilitation, *Spine*, **21**(22), 2628–2639.

CHAPTER FOURTEEN

Ergonomic factors in the workplace contribute to disc degeneration

VIJAY K. GOEL, ROBERT E. MONTGOMERY, NICOLE M. GROSLAND, MALCOLM H. POPE AND SHRAWAN KUMAR

INTRODUCTION

Low back pain is the most frequent cause of industrial disability payments and the second most common medical cause of industrial work loss. The total cost of low back pain per year in the USA alone is about $80 billion (Cats-Baril and Frymoyer, 1991). The pain may arise from any of the spinal structures (discs, facets, ligaments, vertebrae, and muscles), but one of the leading causes is the spinal 'instability' resulting from disc degeneration. Epidemiological studies have revealed that ergonomic factors in the workplace, such as chronic vibration exposure during truck driving, can lead to accelerated degenerative changes in the discs and other structures. Understanding the role of mechanical factors in producing disc degeneration is essential for comprehension of low back pain aetiologies and preventative measures.

NORMAL ANATOMY AND PHYSICAL PROPERTIES OF THE INTERVERTEBRAL DISC

In general, the spine may be described as a strong, flexible rod that bends anteriorly, posteriorly, laterally, and rotates while supporting the head, protecting the spinal cord, and acting as an attachment point for the ribs and back muscles. There are five regions of the spine (cranial to caudal): seven cervical (neck), 12 thoracic (posterior to the thoracic cavity), five lumbar (lower back), five sacral (fused into one pelvic bone) and four coccygeal vertebrae. Between all adjacent vertebrae from the second cervical vertebra to the sacrum are intervertebral discs.

The disc is made up of three anatomical structures: the nucleus pulposus, annulus fibrosus, and cartilaginous endplates, shown schematically in Figure 14.1. In a young person, the nucleus pulposus is a viscous gel that is located slightly posterior to the

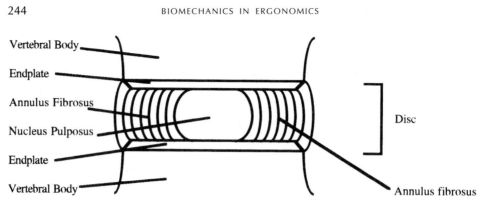

Figure 14.1   Structures of the disc.

middle of the disc and covers about 45 per cent of the disc cross-sectional area. It is surrounded by the annulus fibrosus in the form of eight or more concentric, fibrocartilaginous lamellae embedded in ground substance between the layers. This arrangement allows support for significant loads and enough flexibility to permit spinal mobility.

The structural behaviour of the disc is determined primarily by the nucleus pulposus which attracts and retains water due to its high proteoglycan content (Urban, 1996). The nucleus is 70 to 90 per cent water and is composed of a loose, fibrous strand network suspended in a mucoprotein gel containing mucopolysaccharides (White and Panjabi, 1990).

The annulus fibres are composed of types I and II collagen (Urban, 1996). The inner annulus is primarily type II collagen, while the outer annulus is mostly type I collagen (Eyre and Muir, 1976). The fibres constitute 16 per cent of the annulus volume and are oriented 30° to horizontal in a criss-cross pattern between lamellae. The histochemistry of the annulus changes from the central to peripheral regions. The central portion has a higher glycosaminoglycan content and lower collagen content than the periphery. This gives the central portion a gel-like appearance with more hydrostatic shock-dispersing properties and the peripheral more tensile properties. The fibres in the central portion of the annulus fibrosus connect to the cartilaginous endplates, while the peripheral (Sharpey's) fibres connect to the vertebral bodies. The attachment of Sharpey's fibres to the vertebral bodies is much stronger than where the fibres attach to the endplates in the central annular region (White and Panjabi, 1990). Peripheral annular cells appear spindle shaped, resembling fibrocytes of tendons, while central annular cells appear rounded and are located in the lacunae of chondrocytes (Holm, 1996). These cells maintain the proteoglycan content of the extracellular matrix (Johnstone and Bayliss, 1996). Proteoglycan synthesis occurs most in the mid-annulus region (Bayliss *et al.*, 1988).

The main function of the disc is to resist compression. The nucleus transforms compressive loadings into hydrostatic pressure which is radially directed as tensile stress in the annulus. When the external stresses on the disc are greater than the nucleus swelling pressure, water is lost through the annulus and cartilaginous endplates. Therefore, much water is lost from the disc during the completion of daily activities (Eyre and Muir, 1976).

The cartilaginous endplate is thought to play an important role in the nutrition of the intervertebral disc and hence may be of significance in the aetiology of low back pain (Roberts *et al.*, 1987). According to these authors the endplate is hyaline cartilage with a similar composition to that of articular cartilage. Endplate cartilage becomes bone in adulthood after its growth cartilage has progressed from an active to an irregularly arranged state. The thickness of the endplate is approximately 0.6 mm and is generally thinnest in the central region. The endplate resembles the disc by having a higher proteoglycan and water but lower collagen content in the centre adjacent to the nucleus than at the periphery adjacent to the annulus. There is also a chemical gradient with depth throughout the endplate, with the tissue nearest to the bone having a higher collagen but lower proteoglycan and water content than that nearest the disc. Because of the thinness of the endplate and its similarity in composition to the disc, it has been suggested that the endplate provides little resistance to the diffusion of nutrients such as glucose and oxygen. There are numerous microscopic irregularities throughout the endplate, with either bone or disc tissue protruding into it. Where macroscopic Schmorl's nodes are seen in skeletally mature specimens, there is a significant loss of proteoglycan in both the disc and endplate at that location. Since the disc is the largest avascular tissue, its nutritional status greatly depends on solute transport through the endplate and annulus (Holm, 1996).

There are no nerves present in the substance of the mature human disc (Wyke, 1972). Therefore, nerves do not directly sense degeneration of the disc structure. The altered biomechanics of the surrounding structures and tissues during disc degeneration may cause the perception of pain, though.

In terms of physical properties, the disc is stiffer in compression than tension because of the fluid pressure provided by the nucleus (Markolf and Morris, 1974). A number of studies injecting saline solution to increase nucleus fluid within the disc revealed an associated increase in intradiscal pressure and disc height (Andersson and Schultz, 1982). The vertebral body is about six times stiffer and three times thicker than the disc. Thus, the vertebra deforms about half as much as the disc in compression (Reuber et al., 1982). Reuber et al. also found that a mean disc bulge of up to 2.7 mm may occur (under 800 N of compression and an 11.8 Nm bending moment, maximum) compared to the unloaded state. In this study the posterolateral disc bulge was found to be larger than the posterior bulge. The endplate bulge was also higher in the centre than in the periphery. The bulge in the vertebral endplates under higher loads reduces the straining of the disc fibres and explains why endplates fracture under axial loading. They also found that the disc bulges, tilts, and twists very little during compressive motion. At 800 N of compression the lateral bulge was 1 mm. The disc tilted (on average) 5° for a 10 Nm moment in flexion, extension, or lateral bending. The disc twisted (on average) 2° for a 10 Nm moment. Since the disc is viscoelastic in nature, it also exhibits time-dependent properties such as stress relaxation, creep, and hysteresis.

EPIDEMIOLOGICAL STUDIES RELATING MECHANICAL FACTORS TO DISC DEGENERATION

The outcome of epidemiological studies linking the degenerative changes to mechanical factors has been blurred by the fact that there are a multitude of factors that can lead to low back pain. For example, it is well known that psychological factors often play a role in people complaining of pain or illness. In terms of spinal pain, workers' educational level (low), socioeconomic status (insufficient), intelligence (low), and perception of job performance (unimportant) may all affect the tendency to miss work from low back pain (Bobechko and Hirsch, 1965; Westrin, 1973; White and Panjabi, 1990). Employees who think their work is stressful, anxiety causing, or physically challenging also have increased occurrence of low back pain (Frymoyer et al., 1985; Keegan, 1953; Keim, 1973; Magora, 1970; White and Panjabi, 1990). In addition to these factors another issue that complicates its delineation is the observation that in some people, despite the evidence of severe degenerative changes on radiographs, there is no pain and vice versa.

There are many epidemiological factors which have been correlated with an increased incidence of low back pain. White and Panjabi (1990), based on a survey of epidemiological literature, concluded that driving motor vehicles (especially trucks and heavy equipment), being male, and working as a materials handler are well established risk factors for low back pain. These authors also indicated that jackhammer use, emotionally stressful occupations, and sedentary occupations are probably risk factors for low back pain, but research has been less conclusive on these correlations. Numerous authors have suggested that driving earth moving equipment or tractors poses an increased risk of low back pain. Christ and Dupuis (1966) determined that pathological radiographic changes in tractor drivers occurred 61 per cent of the time when tractor driving over 700 hours per annum and 94 per cent of the time when tractor driving over 1200 hours per annum. The literature also suggests that 70 per cent of heavy-equipment users have low back pain (Cremona, 1972). Backman (1983) found that 40 per cent of bus drivers have low back pain. Based on a survey of 57 000 occupational drivers, Heliovaara (1987) found that they were at high risk for lumbar disc herniation (about 1 per cent were hospitalised for it) when compared to a control group. Whole body vibration has also been implicated as a risk factor by researchers. Seidel and Heide (1986) reviewed 185 articles resulting in 43 000 workers and 24 000 controls and found that there is an increased risk of spinal and peripheral nervous system injuries following intense, long-term whole body vibration that exceeds the ISO Exposure Limit (ISO, 1985). Behrens et al. (1994) reported the highest prevalence of back pain and injury-related back pain from repeated work activities performed while subjected to whole body vibration. Kelsey and Hardy (1975) found that male truck drivers have five times the risk of lumbar disc herniation than non-driving men, probably from the continual sitting and vibrational exposure that is required for truck driving. Another significant finding was that a reduction in the stiffness of the suspension of Grand Prix race cars significantly decreased the incidence and severity of driver low back pain. This may be evidence that shock and vibration are factors contributing to low back pain (Burton and Sandover, 1987).

Other epidemiological studies have also made important contributions towards understanding low back pain aetiology. Many tasks can cause the onset of low back pain in material handling jobs (ordered in decreasing frequency of causing low back pain): lifting, pulling, pushing, carrying, and lowering. Bending, twisting, falling, and slipping are also significant risk factors to low back pain onset (Cady et al., 1979a; Snook et al., 1978, 1980; White and Panjabi, 1990). Nurses have high low back pain incidence because of the heavy physical activity often needed to manipulate the patient and due to the common occurrence of sudden, awkward lifts (Royal College of Nursing, 1980; State of California, 1980; State of Wisconsin, 1973; White and Panjabi, 1990).

It becomes clear from the above review that mechanical factors do contribute to disc degeneration. The next section provides a very brief description of the degenerative changes that occur with time. It is not practical to isolate the contributions of the mechanical factors vis-à-vis the purely age-related changes in the disc. In some people disc degeneration occurs without accompanied instability, pain, and other associated disorders, while in others it does not present any clinical symptoms that necessitate an intervention.

SPINAL DEGENERATION

The process by which disc degeneration occurs is slow and is a cummulative effect of many factors, including mechanical environment, over time. Men start to show signs of degeneration in their 20s, while women begin to have degeneration occur in their 30s. At the age of 50, in both males and females, 97 per cent of the lumbar discs have degenerated. The discs of the lower lumbar region (from the third lumbar vertebra to the sacrum) become the most degenerated with age (Miller *et al.*, 1988). According to Kirkaldy-Willis (1983), the first stage in the spinal degeneration is spinal dysfunction without instability. The second stage still has a mobile nucleus, but the spine has become unstable and has an increased risk of prolapse when subjected to trauma. During the third stage, the spine becomes restabilised due to ligament calcification and osteophytes. The disc degeneration can be assessed as alterations in the appearance and in the chemical composition of the involved structures, and structural behaviour at the macroscopic level (biomechanics).

To characterise the amount of disc degeneration based on morphology, a standard classification was developed by Rolander (1966). The nucleus of a disc with a degeneration grade of 1 is shiny white and macroscopically normal without any structural damage. The nucleus appears gelatinous and separate from the annulus fibrosus. Discs with a degeneration grade of 2 have a normal appearance (including a distinct boundary between the nucleus and annulus) with a more fibrous structure in the nucleus and sometimes a yellowish colour. This type of disc is normal for higher age groups. Discs with a degeneration grade of 3 have clear deterioration of the central structures of the nucleus (which is much drier than normal and usually discoloured), sometimes fissures in the annulus, and a non-distinct boundary between the nucleus and annulus. This disc type is slightly degenerated causing hydrostatic conditions that cannot be maintained. Discs with a degeneration grade of 4 are very degenerated and have marked changes in the nucleus as well as the annulus fibrosus, with ruptures and sequestra in the nucleus or the annulus and/or scarring of the nucleus.

From a chemical perspective, disc degeneration starts with a change in the balance between normal protein polysaccaride and its depolymerisation (Naylor, 1976). As depolymerisation increases, the nucleus increases its fluid uptake, which causes increased intradiscal tension (which Charnley theorised to cause backache). The three different types of disc degeneration noted were normal disc degeneration, subacute or chronic symptomatic degeneration, and acute prolapse of the disc (with different degrees of degeneration). These three types of disc degeneration begin with this disturbed protein polysaccaride equilibrium leading to increased intradiscal pressure as described above. For normal disc degeneration and subacute or chronic symptomatic degeneration, this equilibrium is re-established at a lower level before degenerative processes begin.

Normal disc degeneration happens after repeated cycles of abnormal protein synthesis with increased collagen fibrillation. This may explain the cyclic onset and remission of low back pain. This cycling causes disc scarring, excessive nuclear degeneration, and disc rigidity. Therefore, the disc cannot produce tension or prolapse. This type of degeneration may or may not be accompanied by spinal pain. Subacute or chronic symptomatic degeneration is caused by altered disc biomechanics. Damaging stress produces disruption and/or failure of the annular fibres. Over time, this process may cause prolapse of the nucleus and/or some of the annulus. Intermittent spinal pain occurs before herniation in this process. Acute disc prolapse is when the disc progresses directly from the initial protein polysaccaride imbalance to nuclear or annular prolapse. This type of degeneration may or may not be accompanied by spinal pain.

Some of the biomechanical changes associated with disc degeneration are as follows. Spinal flexibility initially increases but then decreases when degeneration becomes advanced due to decreased disc height (Panjabi, 1996). During compressive loading a degenerated disc is stronger than a normal disc, which indicates that the aetiology of disc herniation is not excessive compression (Virgin, 1951). A degenerated disc bulges more (Roaf, 1960), is less viscoelastic (Kazarian, 1975), and has a lower average failure torque than a normal disc (Farfan *et al.*, 1970). With the progression of disc degeneration, anteroposterior translation increases and axial rotation increases (Panjabi *et al.*, 1982). Unlike young, healthy discs, the lamellae in the central portion of the annulus in degenerated discs bulge medially towards the nucleus (Yasuma, 1990; Yasuma *et al.*, 1986). According to experimentation (McNally and Adams, 1992) and finite element models (Kurowski and Kubo, 1986; Laible *et al.*, 1993; Shirazi-Adl *et al.*, 1984), this annular behaviour changes the load distribution across the disc causing the annulus to undergo non-physiological compression (Hendry, 1958; Hirsch, 1951; Hoof, 1964; Lyons *et al.*, 1981). Disc remodelling occurs in response to these altered stresses (Hoof, 1964; Pritzker, 1977). This remodelling is theorised to cause fibrocartilage to grow rapidly in the inner annulus, as revealed by animal (Lipsom and Muir, 1981) and disc pathology studies (Yasuma, 1990; Yasuma *et al.*, 1986). Degenerated spinal motion segments have a smaller intervertebral foramen than normal specimens due to the decreased disc height (Panjabi *et al.*, 1983). Combined compression and lateral bending produces the largest disc bulge (Reuber *et al.*, 1982).

As the two main load bearing structures in a normal spine, the disc and facets show degenerative changes that may lead to chronic low back pain (Goel and Weinstein, 1990; Herzog, 1991; Modic and Ross, 1991; Saal *et al.*, 1990). The annulus may undergo circumferential tears, rim lesions adjacent to the endplates (delamination), and radial tears over time (Garfin and Ozanne, 1991; Goel *et al.*, 1995). As a person gets older the gel-like nucleus changes into a granular structure, and the number of distinct layers in the annulus fibrosus decreases. Furthermore, the nucleus and annulus interface becomes less evident with age (Andersson, 1992; Kelsey *et al.*, 1984a; Shirazi-Adl, 1989). The chemical composition of the disc also changes as a person gets older. Degeneration may change the ratio of type I and type II collagen in the disc (Brinkley-Parsons and Glimcher, 1984; Eyre and Muir, 1976). Disc metabolism may also change in degenerated discs (Kang and Stefanovic-Racic, 1997). An increase in cellular synthesis of matrix metalloproteinases, which lead to matrix degradation, has also been found in degenerated discs (Kang and Georgescu, 1996; Liu *et al.*, 1991; Sedowofia *et al.*, 1982). Hydration decreases, the annulus collagen network becomes less organised, and proteoglycan content may decrease (Urban, 1992). All of this may lead to a loss of disc height and osteophyte formation later on. In early stages of capsular ligament laxity, changes in the facets involve synovial reaction and cartilage destruction. In later stages, degeneration progresses to subluxation of the facets with osteophyte formation. Other observable changes include: annular bulging, calcification, stenosis, facet joint disease, spondylolisthesis, and ligamentous hypertrophy. The degenerative process is believed to be a cause of low back pain/ sciatica (Hanley, 1991). Disc bulge can cause nerve root impingement and irritation. Low back pain has been theorised to occur from continuous rubbing of the nerve on the bulging disc (Breig, 1978). Investigators have related the symptoms of sciatica to nerve root compression/irritation.

LOADS AND LOAD TYPES ON THE SPINE IN THE WORKPLACE

The lumbar disc is subjected to high compressive loads during normal activities. This is because the centre of gravity of the trunk is anterior to the lumbar region, resulting in

Table 14.1 Compressive load on the L3 disc during normal activities.

Activity	Load (N)
Supine	300
Standing	700
Walking	850
Twisting	900
Bending sideways	950
Straining	1200
Bending forward 20°	1200
Active back hyperextension, prone	1500
Bending forward 20° with 22 lb in each hand	1850
Lifting 44 lb, back straight, knees bent	2100
Lifting 44 lb, back bent, knees straight	3400
Sitting upright, unsupported	1000
Sitting, 100°, seat inclined, 4 cm lumbar support	450
Sitting, 100°, seat inclined and armrest	400
Rising, without arm rest, maximum value	1000
Rising, with arm rest, maximum value	700
Sitting, office chair	500
Sitting, office chair, 20 N arms extended	700
Sitting, forward bent 20°, 100 N each hand	1400

(From Nachemson, 1963, 1965, 1975, 1987).

a moment in the sagittal plane. Large muscle forces are applied to the posterior elements to balance this moment that results in a large compressive reaction force in the disc. Table 14.1 shows the loading on the third lumbar disc (L3) during various activities, which Nachemson (1963, 1965, 1975, 1987) measured by inserting a pressure transducer into the center of the disc *in vivo*. As seen from the table, relatively high compressive loadings occurred in the disc during lifting, sitting, flexion, and hyperextension.

A number of authors have predicted the lumbar disc compression and shear forces during different sagittally symmetric and asymmetric lifting scenarios. Table 14.2 reviews symmetric lifting data, while Table 14.3 reviews asymmetric lifting data (Hooper, 1996). There is obviously a wide variation in disc loading values due to the differences in tasks performed, load lifted, etc.

In Hooper's work (1996) on the consequences of asymmetric lifting on external and internal loads between the third and fifth lumbar vertebra (L3–L5), he found the maximum disc forces occurring at L3–L5 during three different types of asymmetric, 90 N lifts: lifting straight up (0° rotation) and setting the load down, lifting and rotating 45° before setting the load down, and lifting and rotating 90° before setting the load down. His results are shown in Table 14.4.

Another study by Bolte *et al.* (1998) examined the spinal loading while lifting a large recycling barrel which required the barrel to be lifted well above chest height. It was found that the compressive forces on the disc increased as the weight of the barrels increased. The compressive loadings on the disc for the three weights of barrels (90, 135, 180 N) ranged from about 3700 N to 4700 N, while the anteroposterior shear which occurred was about 700 N.

Table 14.2 Review of sagittally symmetric lifting tasks.

Authors (date)	Type of lift	Load (N) lifted	Model	Flexion moment, external (Nm)	Disc comp., internal (N)	Disc level
Eckholm *et al.* (1982)	Leg Back	126	S	160 217	3461 4390	L5–S1
Leskinen *et al.* (1983)	Leg Back	147	D	N/R	5866 6365	L5–S1
Freivalds *et al.* (1984)	Leg	Max.	D	N/R	6000 to 7000	L5–S1
Leskinen (1985)	Leg Back	147	S D S D	N/R	4033 5866 4033 5866	L5–S1
McGill and Norman (1985)	Arms out	177	S Q D	232 345 276	5218 N/R 6391	L4–L5
Buseck *et al.* (1988)	Free Leg	250	D	354 339	N/R	L5–S1
Bush-Joseph *et al.* (1988)	Leg Back Free	150	D	N/R	18% BW 17% BW 17% BW	L5–S1
Schipplein *et al.* (1990)	Free	50–250	D	344	N/R	L5–S1
Gagnon and Smyth (1991)	Lift Lower	32–216	D	N/R	N/R	All major joints
Hanley (1991)	Leg Back	0–180	D	112 161	765 601	L3–L4
Tsuang *et al.* (1992)	Free	150	S Q D	210 250 310	N/R	L5–S1

BW: body weight, N/R: not reported, D: dynamic, S: static, Q: quasistatic.
L3–L4 = between the third and fourth lumbar vertebrae.
L4–L5 = between the fourth and fifth lumbar vertebrae.
L5–S1 = between the fifth lumbar and first sacral vertebrae.
(From Hooper, 1996).

The cascading degenerative process is often the result of cumulative damage to the spinal components induced by chronic loading (Goel and Weinstein, 1990). Many situations may cause chronic loading. For example, during the heavy physical work prevalent among blue collar workers, lifting not only induces large axial compressive forces across the motion segment, but tends to be associated with twisting and bending of the trunk (Andersson, 1981; Brinckmann and Porter, 1994; Chaffin and Andersson, 1984; Chaffin and Park, 1973; Damkot *et al.*, 1984; Frymoyer *et al.*, 1983; Kelsey and White, 1980). The other major class of loading situations associated with low-back pain is static loading influenced by posture (Anderson, 1987; Wood and Badley, 1987). Backache appears to occur with increased frequency in those with sedentary occupations (such as jobs involving

Table 14.3 Review of asymmetric lifting tasks.

Author (date)	Task	Weight (N)	External moments (Nm)	Int. disc lateral shear	Internal disc comp.	Int. disc A/P shear	Level
Kromodihardjo and Mital (1987)	Sym. and asym. lift	292 262	−90–360 F −210–240 LB −60–70 AT	Shear forces lumped	4706 3751	395 529	L5–S1
Jager and Luttmann (1992)	Asym. lift	392	325 F 50 LB 100 AT	200	6000	900	L5–S1
Gagnon and Gagnon (1992)	Asym. lift and lower	114	139 F 54 LB 37 AT	N/R	N/R	N/R	L5–S1
Hooper and Goel (1994)	Sym. and asym. lifts	90	181 F 86 LB 29 AT	74 139	4122 4406	1142 1134	L3–L4 L4–L5

N/R: not reported, F: flexion, LB: lateral bending, AT: axial twist.
L3–L4 = between the third and fourth lumbar vertebrae.
L4–L5 = between the fourth and fifth lumbar vertebrae.
L5–S1 = between the fifth lumbar and first sacral vertebrae.
(From Hooper, 1996).

Table 14.4 Mean maximum disc forces at L3–L4 and L4–L5 while lifting 90 N (quasi-static) in asymmetric postures.

Asymmetry wrt sagittal plane	0° Mean loading (N)	45° Mean loading (N)	90° Mean loading (N)
At disc L3–4			
Lateral shear	35.4	55.5	66.8
Comp.	3764.7	3899.2	3990.4
A/P shear	944.4	1017.8	1031.5
Flex	19.8	21.3	22.0
Twist	0.2	0.5	0.7
Lateral bending	1.7	4.5	6.3
At disc L4–5			
Lateral shear	43.9	91.9	146.7
Comp.	3483.4	4142.3	4290.3
A/P shear	662.2	1000.0	1058.5
Flex	21.5	23.1	23.9
Twist	0.2	0.5	0.7
Lateral bending	0.9	2.4	3.4

(From Hooper, 1996).

prolonged sitting) and in people whose work involves bending over. Vibration from activities like vehicle driving may also compound the problems caused by prolonged sitting (Chaffin and Andersson, 1984).

The above review suggests that in a normal healthy person the major load on the ligamentous spine is axial compression followed by A-P and lateral shear forces and bending moments, especially when the muscle function that protects the ligamentous spine is suboptimal. In addition to this the spine is exposed to chronic vibration and loads that are repetitive in nature. The next section describes the manner in which these types of loads may lead to degeneration from a mechanical perspective.

BIOMECHANICAL BASIS FOR DISC DEGENERATION

Axial forces experienced by a vertebra *in vivo* are of sufficient magnitude to induce fatigue fractures in the bony elements of the motion segment (Saal *et al.*, 1990). Finite element model based studies have revealed that under axial compression the disc may be damaged as well. According to these analyses the intervertebral discs bear most of the load with a small contribution by the facets. At higher compressive loads, however, the inferior facet could also contact the lamina of the vertebra below, suggesting an increased role of the facets in resisting the loads (Shirazi-Adl and Drouin, 1987; Yang and King, 1984). In axial compression failure occurred first in the endplate (and then the annulus) at the junction of the annulus and endplate in the posterolateral region (Natarajan *et al.*, 1994). Farfan (1973) believed that compression failures of the vertebral endplates promoted disc degeneration. The adult disc is avascular, and endplate microfractures can result in vascular ingrowth and subsequent formulation of granular tissue or callus. The callus formed during the healing process may lead to a decrease in the diffusion area for the nutrition of the disc. As a result, the chemistry of the disc and the mechanical behaviour of the constituents may be altered.

Separation of laminae is also an indication of disc degeneration. Interlaminar shear stresses (ILSS) can lead to laminae separation. In response to an axial compressive load of 413 N, a maximum ILSS of 270 kPa was predicted in the posterolateral region of an intact disc, which is consistent with observations that annular tears originate in the posterolateral region of the disc (Goel *et al.*, 1995). A partially or totally denucleated disc (often used to simulate disc degeneration in biomechanical testing) can also lead to laminae separation (Goel and Kim, 1989; Kim, 1988; Kim *et al.*, 1988; Shirazi-Adl, 1992). The effect of a radial incision of the annulus in the posterolateral region was an increase in radial disc bulge and interlaminar stresses compared to the no injury case (Goel *et al.*, 1995). A significant increase in interlaminar stresses did not occur until approximately 70 per cent of the annular depth had been compromised, however. Therefore, in the presence of the chemical and structural changes that occur with aging, ILSS may be an important cause of further degeneration due to laminae separation. This weakens the disc and will hasten the herniation of the nucleus and other degenerative processes.

Cyclic bending of a ligamentous spine, subjected to a 'small' flexion bending moment, led to a tangible increase in motion in the extension mode in comparison to the intact pre-fatigued spinal behaviour (Goel *et al.*, 1988a). This finding suggests that a partial loosening of the disc structure had occurred. The examination of dissected discs revealed fissures in the annulus of a few specimens.

Finite element analysis has also verified that the ligaments are the means of load transfer in flexion (Kim, 1988). Therefore, the ligaments experience large strains in flexion and are vulnerable to rupture. It was found that during flexion the major load bearing elements (up to 7° of flexion) are the disc and the ligaments. Beyond 7° of flexion, however, a large percentage of load is borne by the facets. If, for any reason, the protection provided by the muscles reaches its peak or experiences a decrease (for example, due to disc degeneration, chronic muscular fatigue, or inappropriate posture or load), the ligaments may be called upon to carry higher than normal loads. In such a scenario the capsular ligaments/facets and the disc may be overloaded and thus may become a source of low back pain (Goel *et al.*, 1987).

The testing of hyperflexed specimens in the axial compressive mode (flexion bending plus cyclic axial load) resulted in disc prolapse in younger spinal specimens (Adams and Hutton, 1982a). Wilder *et al.* (1988) observed disc herniation in 75 per cent of calf spinal segments tested under repetitive combined flexion, lateral bending, axial compression, and a constant axial torque, but no older human specimens herniated in this scenario. Shirazi-Adl (1989), Stokes and Greenapple (1985), and Stokes (1987) have also called attention to the vulnerability of the posterolateral portion of the disc. Under simulated loads representing heavy symmetric and asymmetric lifts, maximum annulus fibre strain occurred posterolaterally in the innermost annular layer.

When cyclic axial twist (torsional loads) was applied to *in vitro* specimens, they exhibited discharge of synovial fluid from the apophyseal joint capsules at some stage during testing (Liu *et al.*, 1985). For specimens in which axial rotation exceeded 1.5°, bony failure of the facets and/or tearing of the capsular ligaments was observed. Cyclic torsional loads may lead to weakening and improper functioning of the apophyseal joints and disc. In the absence of synovial fluid the facet joint may exhibit more bony contact and higher friction. These factors are likely to trigger degenerative changes of the facets and/or the disc, in agreement with the work of Farfan *et al.* (1970).

Prolonged sitting postures, alone or in association with vibration exposure, increase the risk of low back pain (Andersson, 1992; Chaffin and Andersson, 1984). From a biomechanical viewpoint the primary load induced on the spine, as a result of a prolonged seated posture, is a 'constant' axial compressive load. As a result of this sustained loading the viscoelastic (creep and relaxation) properties of the disc and to some extent those of the vertebra may be altered (Goel and Weinstein, 1990; Hansson *et al.*, 1987; Shirazi-Adl and Drouin, 1987; Simon *et al.*, 1985). Furlong and Palazotto (1983) formulated viscoelastic axisymmetric finite element models of intact and denucleated discs. Radial stress along the annulus periphery increased with time. It is very likely that, under chronic conditions, the degree of alteration may become so severe that any sudden activity undertaken by a subject after prolonged sitting (like lifting a heavy load) may lead to disc prolapse.

The seated vibration environment is associated with low back pain production (Sandover, 1981). The resonating frequency of the lumbar spine in response to vibration has been found to be about 5 Hz, ranging from about 4 to 6 Hz (Dupuis, 1974; Goel *et al.*, 1988b; Panjabi *et al.*, 1986; Pope *et al.*, 1986; Wilder and Pope, 1996; Wilder *et al.*, 1982a), based on findings from *in vivo* testing of seated and standing subjects, *in vitro* lumbar spinal segment testing, and finite element analyses. Since this is the frequency at which most cars vibrate, driving is a risk factor. Drivers of cars which resonate at a frequency out of this range (Swiss and Japanese) have a lower occurrence of disc herniation than people who drive typical cars that resonate around 5 Hz (Kelsey *et al.*, 1984a). Postures that are very common in the occupational work place (lateral bending and axial rotation) lead to greater transmission of vibrations (Wilder *et al.*, 1982a, 1985). Pope *et al.* (1991) found that greater intervertebral rotations and translations occurred at 5 Hz, confirming the effect of the resonant frequency.

Other aetiologies of low back pain caused by vibration have also been investigated. Sitting, which flattens lumbar lordosis and shifts the line of force of the spine to a point posterior to the effective pivot point of the ischial tuberosities, causes an increased moment arm during vibration that may cause additional pelvic rocking and may amplify vibration (Chaffin and Andersson, 1984). Ligaments have been shown to become softer and weaker from fatigue due to vibrational loading (Hertzberg and Manson, 1980; Riddell *et al.*, 1966; Wiesman *et al.*, 1980). The combination of imposed lateral bend vibration and the flexion–extension response caused by vertical vibration poses the most severe mechanical environment for the lumbar disc because of the greater potential for stretching the posterolateral region, the most common region for disc herniation (Wilder, 1990; Wilder *et al.*, 1982b). Pope *et al.* (1985) showed that measurable fatigue, based on a decrease in median frequency of electromyographic activity, occurred in back muscles during a helicopter vibrational simulation. Due to the vibrational environment fatigued back muscles are not able to protect the spine from adverse loads. At many frequencies the muscles' responses are so completely out of phase that their forces are added to the stimulus.

Goel *et al.* (1988b) found that an increase in load occurs across the disc at the resonant frequency. This may explain the pathophysiology of seated whole-body vibrations. This study found that at resonating frequency, the displacement of the third lumbar vertebral body increased by a factor of three, compared to the static case. The corresponding increase in nucleus pressure was about 150 per cent of the static case (although these increases are dependent on the damping ratio assumed for the model). Since nucleus pressure indicated the load imposed on the spine, the results suggest that the spine is likely to experience excessive loads. The chronic vibration-induced loads may lead to low back pain over time.

A combined finite element and optimisation approach was developed to investigate the effects of muscle dysfunction on the biomechanics of the ligamentous spine under five quasi-static back lifting conditions (Kong *et al.*, 1996). Muscle 'dysfunction' was simulated by decreasing the computed muscle forces. At higher loads and/or at larger flexed postures, muscles were found to play a more crucial role in stabilising the spine, as compared to the passive structures. Muscle 'dysfunction' destabilised the spine, reduced the role of facet joints in transmitting load, and shifted loads to the discs and ligaments. Therefore, muscle 'dysfunction' disturbs the normal functioning of other spinal components and may cause spinal disorders of the disc.

PREVENTATIVE MEASURES

The above review suggests that mechanical factors do play a role in the degenerative process. Thus, it would be beneficial to reduce the effects of loads on the spine by reducing the magnitude of loads on the disc, limiting the extent of chronic exposures, etc.

Physicians and safety professionals recommend squatting posture (straight-back and bent knees) instead of a stooped (flexed spine) posture when lifting a load from the floor (Adams and Hutton, 1982b; Asmussen *et al.*, 1965; Ayoub and El-Bassoussi, 1978; Goel and Weinstein, 1990; Leskinen *et al.*, 1983; White and Panjabi, 1990). Squat lifting is preferred over stoop lifting because the load is transferred to the legs which are stronger than the back, the load is closer to the body (closer to the lumbar spine), if the dimensions of the load are not excessive, resulting in a smaller moment arm (Bendix and Eid, 1983; Goel and Weinstein, 1990; Troup *et al.*, 1983; White and Panjabi, 1990), the ligaments of the low back are subjected to less maximal strain (Anderson, 1983; Poulsen, 1981), the compressive loading on the spine becomes relatively small (Ayoub and El-Bassoussi, 1978; Goel and Weinstein, 1990; Leskinen *et al.*, 1983; White and Panjabi, 1990), and motion is relatively restricted to the sagittal plane so that the spine undergoes very little rotation or lateral bending (Troup and Edwards, 1985). All researchers seem to agree that a load should be lifted or carried as close to the body as possible and that a load should be lifted with a slow, controlled method.

There is significant association between low back pain and lifting improperly with a flexed spine (straighter legs) instead of lifting properly using a squatting technique (White and Panjabi, 1990). When performing lifting with spinal flexion, the load has been shown to be supported by the ligaments (EMG signal dropout), referred to as flexion–relaxation (Floyd and Silver, 1955). Adams and Hutton (1982b) found that the lumbar spine was most at risk in the lordotic posture and when bending forward. Bending forward wedges the lumbar discs, rendering them vulnerable to fatigue injuries during heavy labour. Excessive flexion can cause posterior ligament damage which, followed by a strong contraction of the back muscles, can lead to a prolapsed disc. Axial torsional loads applied to failure caused fractures adjacent to the facets and ultimately failure of the interspinous ligaments. Ligament failure may be another cause of low back pain.

During squat style lifts, nearly all Olympic competitors preserve moderate lordosis (McGill, 1990). The annulus is most resilient against compressive load when in its 'neutral' posture (neither flexed nor extended). This is the only position where all the annular fibres bear equivalent load and stress is equalised (Hickey and Hukins, 1980). When compression is applied to a flexed disc, anterior annulus fibres become disabled and transfer their share of supporting responsibility to the posterior annulus. This may explain the preservation of lordosis during heavy lifts although other mechanisms such as maintenance of muscles at optimal force generating lengths also result from normal lordosis. In addition, facet contact has been suggested to bear significant load when lordosis is maintained (Adams and Hutton, 1980).

Researchers disagree on whether increased intra-abdominal pressure increases or decreases intradiscal pressure. McGill (1990), Krag *et al.* (1986), Nachemson and Morris (1964), and Nachemson *et al.* (1986) found that intradiscal pressure increased and erector spinae activities did not decrease with an increase in intra-abdominal pressure. In order to meet the requirements of the net low back moment during a squat lift, additional extensor activity is necessary to offset the flexor moment produced by the abdominals. This creates a double contribution to spinal joint compression from the abdominals and extensors (McGill, 1990). It seems that the spine prefers to sustain increased compression loads if spinal stability is increased. An unstabilised spine buckles under a very low compressive load, about 20 N according to Lucas and Bresler (1961). Individual muscle components exert lateral and anteroposterior forces on the spine (like guy wires on a mast) to prevent bending and compressive buckling. Activated abdominals also change the trunk into a rigid cylinder to prevent buckling and support shearing through the abdomen. Therefore, intra-abdominal pressure is not a direct reducer of spinal compression but is used to stiffen the trunk and prevent tissue strain and failure due to buckling extensors (McGill, 1990). Abdominal belts worn during material handling or weight lifting increase intra-abdominal pressure, but their utility has not been thoroughly proven. McGill *et al.* (1990) found that from the muscle activity and intra-abdominal pressure data obtained during short duration lifting, they could not justify mandatory abdominal belt use in workers. If abdominal belts really do prevent low back pain, the belt functions as a stiffening device for the trunk, the lower lumbar spine, and lumbosacral joint, thereby preventing overall structural failure of the lumbar spine during lifting. Whether the abdominal belt works through mechanical or psychological factors is also being debated.

Intra-abdominal pressure has been compared in pushing, pulling, and lifting. Researchers found that the largest intra-abdominal pressures occurred when pushing due to rectus abdominis tension, while the smallest pressures occurred when pulling due to back muscle tension (Davis and Troup, 1964). Since the rectus abdominis has a much larger lever arm than the erector spinae muscles, its spinal bending moment and force requirement is smaller. Therefore, the load on the disc is less during pushing than pulling (White and Panjabi, 1990). This is why workers who manoeuvre dollies or gurneys frequently (retail workers, warehouse workers, nurses, etc.) are told to push them instead of pull.

Experimental studies have shown that a reclined, slightly extended posture unloads the spine by lowering intervertebral pressure and paraspinous muscle activity (White and Panjabi, 1990). The optimal seat type and backrest angle, minimising intradiscal pressure and paraspinal muscle activity was found to be having the backrest reclined at 120° and the lumbar support located at 5 cm. The greatest intradiscal pressure was observed when sitting with no lumbar support and the backrest at 90° (Andersson et al., 1977). Another study found that lumbar support affected lumbar lordosis the most, while the angle of the backrest affected disc loads the most (Andersson et al., 1979). This study also found that as backrest angle increased, more body weight was placed on the backrest, which caused a reduction in loading across the disc and less erector spinae force to keep the spine upright. A different study (Kelsey and Hardy, 1975) found that vehicle drivers are at risk for sciatica. Since this study showed that a chair with arm rests and lumbar support decreases intradiscal pressure, drivers who are having low back pain should use vehicle seats with these two features. As described earlier, the fatigue in muscles after vehicular vibration indicates the magnitude of loads in the muscles. Therefore, avoiding lifting soon after vibration exposure is recommended. It is also suggested that people exposed to prolonged vibration (like long distance driving) take frequent rests and walking breaks (Wilder and Pope, 1996).

Some other facts not yet discussed in this chapter may also assist in the prevention of industrial low back pain. Since there is a 50 to 60 per cent chance of low back pain recurring one year after the initial problem (Andersson, 1981), injured employees should be monitored and their condition medically managed because this results in better care, shorter disability, and less expense (Leavitt et al., 1972; Wiesel et al., 1980). The chance of undergoing injury increases by up to three times if the lifting needed for the job is beyond the strength capability of the worker according to isometric strength tests (Chaffin et al., 1978). This is why an employee returning to work involving lifting after having low back pain or injury should participate in an extensive regimen of isometric exercises before resuming work.

People in good physical condition have less risk of low back pain (Cady et al., 1979b). Isometric endurance of the low back muscles may prevent the onset of low back pain (Biering-Sorensen, 1984). Mayer et al. (1987) found that 87 per cent of chronic low back pain patients returned to work after rehabilitation with trunk strengthening exercises. More significantly, all of the patients who returned to work were still there after two years, which indicated a success rate five times the success rate of the control. Frequent aerobic exercises can produce endorphin secretions which help control pain and elevate mood. Some physiological studies have shown that the mechanical pumping which occurs when exercising improves disc nutrition (Holm and Nachemson, 1985; Kraemer et al., 1985; Urban et al., 1982). Improvement of back musculature through exercise may decrease lordosis which has been shown to decrease intradiscal pressure by half (Nachemson, 1963).

White and Panjabi (1990) listed advice for the returning worker after a low back pain episode: do not lift heavy objects, be as close as possible to the object being lifted, avoid bending, avoid axial torsion, change positions frequently, avoid sitting in a low chair, and use chairs with armrests and lumbar support. These recommendations follow the biomechanical basis of the effects of loads on the spine, as described above.

SUMMARY

The disc is made up of three anatomical structures: the nucleus pulposus, annulus fibrosus, and cartilaginous endplates. These components allow the disc to support significant loads, while being flexible enough to allow spinal mobility. The nucleus pulposus is a viscous gel located in the middle of the disc which primarily absorbs spinal compressive loading and transforms it into radially directed tensile forces in the annulus. The annulus fibrosus surrounds the nucleus and consists of concentric, fibrocartilaginous layers (lamellae) embedded in a ground substance found between the layers. The cartilaginous endplates enclose the central portion of the disc, are composed of hyaline cartilage, and allow nutrients and water to flow into and out of the disc.

Epidemiological studies have shown that mechanical factors can increase low back pain which is often caused by an associated increase in disc degeneration. Spinal degeneration occurs with age causing the disc and facets to have altered biomechanics. The degenerative process is believed to be a cause of low back pain/sciatica through disc bulge causing nerve root impingement and irritation. Degeneration begins with spine dysfunction without instability and then progresses to a state of instability and increased injury risk. This flexibility is later restabilised by ligament calcification and osteophyte formation.

Identifying load types and quantifying load magnitudes in the workplace is essential for a better understanding of the aetiology of low back pain. The lumbar disc is subjected to high compressive loads during normal activities. Relatively high compressive loadings were seen in the disc during lifting, sitting, flexion, and hyperextension, implicating these activities as having a higher risk of low back pain. Flexion combined with lateral bending also produced a relatively high compressive loading. Disc compression is high during lifting tasks and has varied from about 4000 to 7000 N in the majority of current studies, depending on the lifting technique and model utilised in each study.

Many biomechanical factors influence disc degeneration. Axial compressive forces on the spine can induce fatigue fractures such as compression failures of the vertebral endplates. The callus formed during healing may lead to a decrease in disc nutrition, which also increases degeneration. Separation of the laminae is also associated with degeneration due to interlaminar shear. A decrease in nucleus hydration and solidification of the gel contents can also lead to laminae separation. Damage to the annulus in the posterolateral region increases radial disc bulge and interlaminar stresses. This may increase the probability for subsequent prolapse. The testing of hyperflexed specimens during flexion bending plus cyclic axial load resulted in disc prolapse. Disc herniation also occurred in 75 per cent of calf spinal segments tested under repetitive combined flexion, lateral bending, axial compression, and a constant axial torque. These findings suggest that combined loadings, especially flexion and lateral bending, may increase the vulnerability of the posterolateral portion of the disc to herniation. Cyclic torsional loads may lead to weakening and improper functioning of the apophyseal joints and disc. Cyclic bending may cause partial loosening of the disc structure and annular fissures. Prolonged sitting postures, alone or in association with vibration exposure, increase the risk of low back pain. As a result of this sustained loading, the viscoelastic (creep and relaxation) properties of the disc may be altered causing the radial stress along the annulus periphery to increase with time. The seated vibration environment is associated with low back pain production. The resonating frequency of the lumbar spine in response to vibration has been found to be about 5 Hz. Due to the vibrational environment fatigued back muscles are not able to protect the spine from adverse loads. An increase in load occurs across the disc at the resonant frequency. The combination of imposed lateral bend vibration and the flexion–extension response caused by vertical vibration poses the most severe mechanical environment for the lumbar disc because of the greater potential for stretching the posterolateral region, the common area for disc herniation. At higher loads and/or at larger flexed postures, muscles were found to play a more crucial role in stabilising the spine, as compared to the passive structures. Muscle 'dysfunction' destabilised the spine, reduced the role of facet joints in transmitting load, and shifted loads to the discs and ligaments.

In order to decrease the loads on the disc to prevent long term degeneration, preventative measures should be taken. A squatting posture (straight-back and bent knees) instead of a stooped (flexed spine) posture should be used when lifting a load from the floor. The load should be lifted with a slow, controlled method and kept as close to the body as possible. Intra-abdominal pressure stiffens the trunk and prevents tissue strain and failure due to buckling by increasing compressive disc loading. Since the rectus abdominis has a much larger lever arm than the erector spinae muscles, its spinal bending moment and force requirement is smaller. Therefore, the load on the disc is less during pushing than pulling, so workers who manoeuvre dollies or gurneys are told to push them instead of pull. Experimental studies have shown that a reclined, slightly extended posture unloads the spine by lowering intervertebral pressure. The optimal seat type and backrest angle, minimising intradiscal pressure, is having the backrest reclined at 120° and the lumbar support located at 5 cm. Since a chair with arm rests and lumbar support decreases intradiscal pressure, drivers who are having low back pain should use vehicle seats with these two features. Since there is a 50 to 60 per cent chance of low back pain recurring one year after the initial problem, injured employees should be monitored and their condition medically managed because this results in better care, shorter disability, and less expense. An employee returning to work involving lifting after having low back pain or injury should participate in an extensive regimen of isometric exercises before resuming work, for this strengthens the muscles and thus may prevent a second recurrence of low back pain. People in good physical condition have less risk of low back pain. When returning to work after a low back pain episode, one should not lift heavy objects, be as close as possible to the object being lifted, avoid bending, avoid axial torsion, change positions frequently, avoid sitting in a low chair, and use chairs with armrests and lumbar support.

ACKNOWLEDGEMENTS

This work was supported in part by the University of Iowa Foundation Spine Research fund.

References

ADAMS, M.A. and HUTTON, W.C., 1980, The effect of posture on the role of the apophyseal joints in resisting intervertebral compressive forces, *J Bone Jt Surg*, **62B**(3), 358.

ADAMS, M.A. and HUTTON, W.C., 1982a, Prolapsed intervertebral disc: a hyperflexion injury, *Spine*, **7**, 184–191.

ADAMS, M.A. and HUTTON, W.C., 1982b, Mechanical factors in the etiology of low back pain, *Orthopedics*, **5**, 1461.

ANDERSON, C.K., 1983, A Biomechanical Model of the Lumbosacral Joint for Lifting Activities, unpublished PhD dissertation, University of Michigan, Ann Arbor.

ANDERSON, J.A.D., 1987, Back pain and occupation, in Jayson, M.I.V. (Ed.), *The Lumbar Spine and Back Pain*, New York: Churchill Livingstone, p. 16.

ANDERSSON, G.B.J., 1981, Epidemiologic aspects on low back pain in industry, *Spine*, **6**, 53.

ANDERSSON, G.B.J., 1992, Intervertebral disk – clinical aspects, presentation at the Workshop on Age-Related Musculoskeletal Soft Tissue Changes, Colorado Springs, CO.

ANDERSSON, G.B.J. and SCHULTZ, A.B., 1982, Effects of fluid injection on mechanical properties of intervertebral discs, *J Biomech*, **12**, 453.

ANDERSSON, G.B.J., ORTENGREN, R. and NACHEMSON, A., 1977, Intradiscal pressure, intra abdominal pressure and myoelectric back muscle activity related to posture and loading, *Clin Orthop*, **129**, 156.

ANDERSSON, G.B.J., MURPHY, R.W., ORTENGREN, R. and NACHEMSON, A., 1979, The influence of back rest inclination and lumbar support on lumbar lordosis, *Spine*, **4**, 52.

ASMUSSEN, E., POULSEN, E. and RASMUSSEN, B., 1965, Quantitative evaluations of the activity of the back muscles in lifting, *Comm Dan Nat Assoc Infant Paral*, **21**.

AYOUB, M.M. and EL-BASSOUSSI, M.M., 1978, Dynamic biomechanical model for sagittal plane lifting activities, in Drury, G.G. (Ed.), *Safety in Manual Materials Handling*, Cincinnati: NIOSH, pp. 78–185.

BACKMAN, A.L., 1983, Health survey of professional drivers, *Scand J Work Environ Health*, **9**, 36–41.

BAYLISS, M.T., JOHNSTONE, B. and O'BRIEN, J.P., 1988, Proteoglycan synthesis in the human intervertebral disc, *Spine*, **12**, 972–981.

BEHRENS, V., SELIGMAN, P., CAMERON, L., *et al.*, 1994, The prevalence of back pain, hand discomfort, and dermatitis in the US working population, *Am J Pub Health*, **84**(11), 1780–1785.

BENDIX, T. and EID, S.E., 1983, The distance between the load and the body with three bi-manual lifting techniques, *Appl Eng*, **14**(3), 185–192.

BIERING-SORENSEN, F., 1984, Physical measurements as risk indicators for low-back trouble over a one year period, *Spine*, **9**, 106.

BOBECHKO, W.P. and HIRSCH, C., 1965, Auto-immune response to nucleus pulposus in the rabbit, *J Bone Joint Surg*, **47B**, 574.

BOLTE, K.M., POPE, M.H., GOEL, V.K. and SPRATT, K., 1998, Spine loading during a lift of a large recycling barrel, accepted to the Orthopedic Research Society.

BREIG, A., 1978, *Adverse Mechanical Tension in the Central Nervous System: An Analysis of Cause and Effect: Relief by Functional Neurosurgery*, Stockholm: Almqvist & Wiksell International.

BRINCKMANN, P. and PORTER, R.W., 1994, A laboratory model of lumbar disc protrusion, *Spine*, **19**, 228–235.

BRINKLEY-PARSONS, D. and GLIMCHER, J., 1984, Is the chemistry of collagen in the intervertebral discs an expression of Wolff's law, *Spine*, **9**, 148–163.

BURTON, A.K. and SANDOVER, J., 1987, Back pain in grand prix drivers: A 'found' experiment, *Appl Ergonom*, **18**(1), 3–8.

BUSECK, M., SCHIPPLEIN, O.D., ANDERSSON, G.B.J. and ANDRIACCHI, T.P., 1988, Influence of dynamic factors and external loads on the moment at the lumbar spine in lifting, *Spine*, **13**(8), 918–921.

BUSH-JOSEPH, C., SCHIPPLEIN, O., ANDERSSON, G.B.J. and ANDRIACCHI, T.P., 1988, Influence of dynamic factors on the lumbar spine moment in lifting, *Ergonomics*, **31**(2), 211–216.

CADY, L.D., BISCHOFF, D.P., O'CONNELL, E.R., THOMAS, P.C. and ALLEN, J.H., 1979a, Letter to the editor: author's response, *J Occup Medicine*, **21**, 720.

CADY, L.D., BISCHOFF, D.P., O'CONNELL, E.R., THOMAS, P.C. and ALLEN, J.H., 1979b, Strength and fitness and subsequent back injuries in firefighters, *J Occup Med*, **21**, 269.

CATS-BARIL, W.L. and FRYMOYER, J.W., 1991, The economics of spinal disorders, in Frymoyer, J.W. *et al.* (Eds), *The Adult Spine*, New York: Raven Press, pp. 58–105.

CHAFFIN, D.B. and ANDERSSON, G.B.J., 1984, *Occupational Biomechanics*, New York: Wiley & Sons.

CHAFFIN, D.B. and PARK, K.S., 1973, A longitudinal study of low back pain as associated with occupational lifting factors, *Am Ind Hyg Ass J*, **34**, 513.

CHAFFIN, D.B., HERRIN, G.D. and KEYSERLING, W.M., 1978, Pre-employment strength testing: an updated position, *J Occup Med*, **20**, 403.

CHRIST, W. and DUPUIS, H., 1966, Urber die Beanspruchung die Wirbelsaule unter dem Einfluss sinusforminger und stochastischer Schwingungen Int. Zeitschrift angewandte Phys., *Arbeitsphys*, **22**, 258–278.

CREMONA, E., 1972, Die Wirbelsaule bei den Schwerarbeiten der Eisen- und Stahlindustrie sowie des Bergbaus, *Kommiss Europ Gem Generaldir Soz Angelegenheitern*, Dok. Nr. 1911/72.

DAMKOT, D.K., POPE, M.H., LORD, J. and FRYMOYER, J.W., 1984, The relationship between work history, work environment and low back pain in men, *Spine*, **9**, 395.

DAVIS, P.R. and TROUP, J.D.G., 1964, Pressures in the trunk cavities when pulling, pushing, and lifting, *Ergonomics*, **7**, 465.

DUPUIS, H., 1974, Belastung durch mechanische Schwingungen und moegliche Gesundheitsschaedigungen im Bereich der Wirbelsaeule, *Fortsch Med*, **92**(14), 618–620.

ECKHOLM, J., ARBORELIUS, U.P. and NEMETH, G., 1982, The load on the lumbo-sacral joint and trunk muscle activity during lifting, *Ergonomics*, **25**, 145–161.

EYRE, D.R. and MUIR, H., 1976, Types I and II collagens in the intervertebral disc: interchanging radial distribution in the annulus fibrosus, *Biochem J*, **157**, 267–270.

FARFAN, H.F., 1973, *Mechanical Disorders of the Low Back*, Philadelphia: Lea & Febiger.

FARFAN, H.F., COSETTE, J.W., ROBERTSON, G.H., WELLS, R.V. and KRAUS, H., 1970, The effects of torsion on the lumbar intervertebral joints: the role of torsion in the production of disc degeneration, *J Bone Joint Surg*, **52A**, 468.

FLOYD, W.F. and SILVER, P.H.S., 1955, The function of the erectores spinae muscles in certain movements and postures in man, *J Physiol*, **129**, 184.

FREIVALDS, A., CHAFFIN, D.B., GARG, A. and LEE, K.S., 1984, A dynamic biomechanical evaluation of lifting maximum acceptable loads, *J Biomech*, **17**(4), 251–262.

FRYMOYER, J.W., POPE, M.H., CLEMENTS, J.H., WILDER, D.G., MacPHERSON, B. and ASHIKAGA, T., 1983, Risk factors in low back pain, *J Bone Joint Surg*, **65A**, 213.

FRYMOYER, J.W., POPE, M.H., COSTANZA, M.C., GOGGIN, J.E. and WILDER, D.G., 1985, Epidemiologic studies of low back pain, *Spine* **5**, 419.

FURLONG, D.R. and PALAZOTTO, A.N., 1983, A finite element analysis of the influence of surgical herniation on the viscoelastic properties of the intervertebral disc, *J Biomech*, **16**, 785–795.

GAGNON, D. and GAGNON, M., 1992, The influence of dynamic lifting factors on triaxial net muscular moments at the L5/S1 joint during asymmetrical lifting and lowering, *J Biomech*, **25**(8), 891–901.

GAGNON, M. and SMYTH, G., 1991, Muscular mechanical energy expenditure as a process for detecting potential risks in manual materials handling, *J Biomech*, **24**(3/4), 191–203.

GARFIN, S.R. and OZANNE, S., 1991, Spinal pedicle fixation, in Weinstein, J.N. (Ed.), *Clinical Efficacy and Outcome in the Diagnosis and Treatment of Low Back Pain*, Raven Press, pp. 137–174.

GOEL, V.K. and KIM, Y.E., 1989, Effects of injury on the spinal motion segment mechanics in the axial compression mode, *Clin Biomech*, **4**, 161–167.

GOEL, V.K. and WEINSTEIN, J.N., 1990, *Biomechanics of the Spine: Clinical and Surgical Perspective*, Boca Raton, FL: CRC Press, Inc.

GOEL, V.K., FROMKNECHT, S., NISHIYAMA, K., WEINSTEIN, J. and LIU, Y.K., 1985, The role of spinal elements in flexion, *Spine*, **10**, 516.

GOEL, V.K., WINTERBOTTOM, J.M., WEINSTEIN, J.N. and KIM, Y.E., 1987, Load sharing among spinal elements of a motion segment in extension and lateral bending, *J Biomech Eng*, **109**, 291.

GOEL, V.K., VOO, L.M., WEINSTEIN, J.N., LIU, Y.K., OKUMA, T. and NJUS, G.O., 1988a, Response of the ligamentous lumbar spine to cyclic bending loads, *Spine*, **13**, 294.

GOEL, V.K., KIM, Y.E. and ZHANG, F., 1988b, Biomechanical effects of vibration on the human spine, *15th Proceedings of the International Society for the Study of the Lumbar Spine*, Miami, April 13–18.

GOEL, V.K., MONROE, B.T., GILBERTSON, L.G. and BRINCKMANN, P., 1995, Interlaminar shear stresses and laminae separation in a disc: finite element analysis of the L3–4 motion segment subjected to axial compressive loads, *Spine*, **20**, 689–698.

HANLEY, E.N., 1991, The cost of surgical intervention for lumbar disc herniation, in Weinstein, J.N. (Ed.), *Clinical Efficacy and Outcome in the Diagnosis and Treatment of Low Back Pain*, Raven Press, pp. 67–90.

HANSSON, T., KELLER, T. and HOLM, S., 1987, The load of the porcine lumbar spine during seated whole body vibration, *XIV Proceedings of the International Society for the Study of the Lumbar Spine*, Rome, Italy, May 24–28, p. 30.

HELIOVAARA, M., 1987, Occupation and risk of herniated lumbar intervertebral disk of sciatica leading to hospitalization, *J Chron Dis*, **40**, 259–264.

HENDRY, N.G.C., 1958, The hydration of the nucleus pulposus and its relation to intervertebral disc degeneration, *J Bone Jt Surg*, **40B**, 132–144.

HERTZBERG, R.W. and MANSON, J.A., 1980, *Fatigue of Engineering Plastics*, New York, NY: Academic Press, p. 64.

HERZOG, R.J., 1991, CT, in Weinstein, J.N. (Ed.), *Clinical Efficacy and Outcome in the Diagnosis and Treatment of Low Back Pain*, Raven Press, pp. 67–90.

HICKEY, D.S. and HUKINS, D.W.L., 1980, Relation between the structure and the annulus fibrosus and the function and failure of the intervertebral disc, *Spine*, **5**(20), 106.

HIRSCH, C., 1951, Studies on the mechanism of low back pain, *Acta Orthop Scand*, **20**(26).

HOLM, S.H., 1996, Nutritional and pathophysiologic aspects of the lumbar intervertebral disc, in Weisel, S.W. and Weinstein, J.N. (Eds), *The Lumbar Spine*, Philadelphia: W.B. Saunders, pp. 244–260.

HOLM, S. and NACHEMSON, A., 1985, Variations in the nutrition of the canine intervertebral disc induced by motion, *Spine*, **8**, 867.

HOOF, A.V.D., 1964, Histological age changes in the annulus fibrosus of the human intervertebral disc: with discussion of the problem of disc herniation, *Gerontolgia*, **9**, 136–149.

HOOPER, D.M., 1996, Consequences of Asymmetric Lifting on External and Internal Loads at the L3–L5 Lumbar Levels, unpublished PhD dissertation, University of Iowa, Iowa City, IA.

HOOPER, D.M. and GOEL, V.K., 1994, Comparisons of three-dimensional kinematics of the legs and lower back during dynamic symmetric and asymmetric lifting, BED, Vol. 28, 1994 Advances in Bioengineering ASME, 333–334.

ISO (International Organization for Standardization), 1985, *Guide for the Evaluation of Human Exposure to Whole Body Vibration*, Ref. No. ISO 2631/1 (E).

JAGER, M. and LUTTMANN, A., 1992, Load on the lumbar spine during asymmetrical bimanual materials handling, *Ergonomics*, **35**(7/8), 783–805.

JOHNSTONE, J.W. and BAYLISS, M.T., 1996, Proteoglycans of the intervertebral disc, in Weinstein, J.W. and Gordon, S.L. (Eds), *Low Back Pain*, Illinois: AAOS, pp. 493–509.

KANG, J.D., GEORGESCU, H.I., *et al.*, 1996, Herniated lumbar discs spontaneously produce matrix metalloproteinases, nitric oxide, interleukin-6 and prostaglandin E_2, *Spine*, **21**, 271–277.

KANG, J.D., STEFANOVIC-RACIC, M., *et al.*, 1997, Toward a biochemical understanding of human disc degeneration and herniation, *Spine*, **22**, 1065–1073.

KAZARIAN, L.E., 1975, Creep characteristics of the human spinal column, *Orthop Clin North Am*, **6**(3).

KEEGAN, J.J., 1953, Alterations of the lumbar curve related to posture and seating, *J Bone Joint Surg*, **35A**, 589.

KEIM, H.A., 1973, Low Back Pain, unpublished Ciba Clinical Symposia, Vol. 25, No. 3.

KELSEY, J.L. and HARDY, R.J., 1975, Driving of motor vehicles as a risk factor for acute herniated lumbar intervertebral disc, *Am J Epidemiol*, **102**, 63.

KELSEY, J.L. and WHITE, A.A., 1980, Epidemiology and impact of low back pain, *Spine*, **5**, 133.

KELSEY, J.L., GITHKENS, P.B., WHITE, A.A., *et al.*, 1984a, An epidemiologic study of lifting and twisting on the job and risk for acute prolapsed lumbar intervertebral disc, *J Ortho Res*, **2**, 61.

KELSEY, J.L., GITHENS, P.B., O'CONNER, T., WEIL, U., CALOGERO, J.A., HOLFORD, T.R., *et al.*, 1984b, Acute prolapsed lumbar intervertebral disc: an epidemiological study with special reference to driving automobiles and cigarette smoking, *Spine*, **9**, 608.

KIM, Y.E., 1988, An Analytical Investigation of Ligamentous Lumbar Spine Mechanics, unpublished PhD dissertation, University of Iowa, Iowa City, IA.

KIM, Y.E., GOEL, V.K. and WEINSTEIN, J., 1988, The role of facets in denucleated discs – an analytical biomechanical study, *34th Orthopedic Research Society*, Atlanta, Georgia, Feb. 1–4.

KIRKALDY-WILLIS, W.H., 1983, *Managing Low Back Pain*, New York: Churchill Livingstone.

KONG, W.Z., GOEL, V.K., GILBERTSON, L.G. and WEINSTEIN, J.N., 1996, Effects of muscle dysfunction on lumbar spine mechanics – a finite element study based on a two motion segments model, *Spine*, **21**, 2197–2207.

KRAEMER, J., KOLDITZ, D. and GOWIN, R., 1985, Water and electrolyte content of human intervertebral discs under variable load, *Spine*, **10**, 69.

KRAG, M.H., BRYNE, K.B., GILBERTSON, L.G. and HAUGH, L.D., 1986, Failure of intraabdominal pressurization to reduce erector spinae loads during lifting tasks, in *Proc North Am Congr Biomech*, August 25–27, Montreal.

KROMODIHARDJO, S. and MITAL, A., 1987, Biomechanical analysis of manual lifting tasks, *J Biomech Eng*, **109**, 132–138.

KUROWSKI, P. and KUBO, A., 1986, The relationship of degeneration of the disc to mechanical loading conditions on lumbar vertebrae, *Spine*, **11**, 726–731.

LAIBLE, J.D., PFLASTER, D.S. *et al.*, 1993, A poroelastic-swelling finite element model with application to the intervertebral disc, *Spine*, **18**, 659–670.

LEAVITT, S.S., BEYER, R.D. and JOHNSTON, T.L., 1972, Monitoring the recovery process: pilot results of a systematic approach to case management, *Ind Med Surg*, **41**(4), 25.

LESKINEN, T.J., 1985, Comparison of static and dynamic biomechanical models, *Ergonomics*, **28**(1), 285–291.

LESKINEN, T.P.J, STAHLHAMMER, H.R. and KUORINKA, I.A.A., 1983, A dynamic analysis of spinal compression with different lifting techniques, *Ergonomics*, **26**(6), 595–604.

LIPSOM, S.J. and MUIR, H., 1981, Proteoglycans in experimental intervertebral disc degeneration, *Spine*, **6**, 194–210.

LIU, Y.K., GOEL, V.K., DEJONG, A., NJUS, G., NISHIYAMA, K. and BUCKWALTER, J., 1985, Torsional fatigue of the lumbar intervertebral joints, *Spine*, **10**, 894.

LIU, J., ROUGHLEY, P.J. and MORT, J.S., 1991, Identification of human intervertebral disc stromelysin and its involvement in matrix degradation, *J Orthop Res*, **9**, 568–575.

LUCAS, D.B. and BRESLER, B., 1961, Stability of the Ligamentous Spine, unpublished Tech. Rep. No. 40, Biomechanics Laboratory, University of California, San Francisco.

LYONS, G., EISENSTEIN, S.M. *et al.*, 1981, Biochemical changes in intervertebral disc degeneration, *Biochemica Biophysica*, **673**, 443–453.

MAGORA, A., 1970, Investigation of the relation between low back pain and occupation, *Ind Med Surg*, **39**, 504.

MARKOLF, K.L. and MORRIS, J.M., 1974, The structural components of the intervertebral disc. A study of their contributions to the ability of the disc to resist compressive forces, *J Bone Jt Surg*, **56A**, 675.

MAYER, T.G., GATCHEL, R.J., MAYER, H., KISHINO, N.D., KEELEY, J. and MOONEY, V., 1987, A prospective two-year study of functional restoration in industrial low back injury. An objective assessment procedure, *JAMA*, **258**, 1763.

MCGILL, S.M., 1990, Loads on the lumbar spine and associated tissues, in Goel, V.K. and Weinstein, J.N. (Eds), *Biomechanics of the Spine: Clinical and Surgical Perspective*, Boca Raton, FL: CRC Press, Inc.

MCGILL, S.M. and NORMAN, R.W., 1985, Dynamically and statically determined low back moments during lifting, *J Biomech*, **18**(12), 877–885.

MCGILL, S.M., NORMAN, R.W. and SHARRATT, M.T., 1990, The effect of an abdominal belt on trunk muscle activity and intra-abdominal pressure during squat lifts, *Ergonomics*, **33**(2), 147–160.

MCNALLY, D.S. and ADAMS, M.A., 1992, Internal intervertebral disc mechanics as revealed by stress profilometry, *Spine*, **17**, 66–73.

MILLER, J.A.A., SCHMATZ, C. and SCHULTZ, A.B., 1988, Lumbar disc degeneration: correlation with age, sex, and spine level in 600 autopsy specimens, *Spine*, **13**(2), 173.

MODIC, M.T. and ROSS, J.S., 1991, MRI, in Weinstein, J.N. (Ed.), *Clinical Efficacy and Outcome in the Diagnosis and Treatment of Low Back Pain*, Chapter 10, Raven Press, pp. 57–66.

NACHEMSON, A.L., 1963, The influence of spinal movement on the lumbar intra discal pressure and on the tensile stresses in the annulus fibrosus, *Acta Orthop Scand*, **33**, 183.

NACHEMSON, A.L., 1965, *In vivo* discometry in lumbar discs with irregular radiograms, *Acta Orthop Scand*, **36**, 418.

NACHEMSON, A.L., 1975, *A Critical Look at the Treatment for Low Back Pain. The Research Status of Spinal Manipulative Therapy*, DHEW Publication No. (NIH) 76–998:21B, Bethesda, MD.

NACHEMSON, A., 1987, in Jayson, M.I.V. (Ed.), *The Lumbar Spine and Back Pain*, London: Churchill Livingstone, p. 191.

NACHEMSON, A.L. and MORRIS, J.M., 1964, *In vivo* measurements of intradiskal pressure, *J Bone Jt Surg*, **46A**, 1077.

NACHEMSON, A.L., ANDERSSON, G.B.J. and SCHULTZ, A.B., 1986, Valsalva maneuver biomechanics: effects on lumbar trunk loads of elevated intraabdominal pressure, *Spine*, **11**(5), 476.

NATARAJAN, R.N., KE, J.H. and ANDERSSON, G.B.J., 1994, A model to study disc degeneration process, *Spine*, **19**, 259–265.

NAYLOR, A., 1976, Intervertebral disc prolapse and degeneration; the biochemical and biophysical approach, *Spine*, **1**, 108.

PANJABI, M.M., 1996, Low back pain and spinal instability, in Weinstein, J.N. and Gordon, S.L. (Eds), *Low Back Pain*, Illinois: AAOS, pp. 367–384.

PANJABI, M.M., GOEL, V. and SUMMERS, D., 1982, Relationship between chronic instability and disc degeneration, Trans. Int. Soc. for Study of Lumbar Spine, Toronto.

PANJABI, M.M., TAKATA, K. and GOEL, V.K., 1983, Kinematics of lumbar intervertebral foramen, *Spine*, **8**(4), 348.

PANJABI, M.M., ANDERSSON, G.B.J., JORNEUS, L., HULT, E. and MATTSSON, L., 1986, *In vivo* measurements of spinal column vibrations, *J Bone Jt Surg*, **68A**, 695.

POPE, M.H., WILDER, D.G. and DONNERMEYER, D.D., 1985, Muscle fatigue in static and vibrational seating environments, *Proc. AGARD Conf.*, Italy.

POPE, M.H., SVENSSON, M., BROMAN, H. and ANDERSSON, G.B.J., 1986, Mounting of the transducer in measurements of segmental motion of the spine, *J Biomech*, **19**(8), 675–677.

POPE, M.H., KAIGLE, A.M., MAGNUSSEN, M., *et al.*, 1991, Intervertebral motion during vibration, *Proc Instn Mech Eng J Eng Med*, **205**, 39–44.

POULSEN, E., 1981, Back muscle strength and weight limits in lifting burdens, *Spine*, **6**, 73–75.

PRITZKER, K., 1977, Aging and degeneration in the lumbar intervertebral disc, *Orthop Clin North Am*, **8**, 65–77.

REUBER, M., SCHULTZ, A., DENIS, F. and SPENCER, D., 1982, Bulging of lumbar intervertebral disks, *J Biomech Eng*, **104**(3), 187.

RIDDELL, M.N., KOO, G.P. and O'TOOLE, J.L., 1966, Fatigue mechanisms of thermoplastics, SPE 22nd Annual Technical Conference, 12, 2–6, *Polymer Eng. Sci.*, **6**, 363.

ROAF, R., 1960, A study of the mechanics of spinal injuries, *J Bone Joint Surg*, **42B**, 810.

ROBERTS, S., MENAGE, J. and URBAN, J.P.G., 1987, Biochemical and structural properties of the cartilage endplate and its relationship to the intervertebral disc, *Spine*, **12**, 658.

ROLANDER, S.D., 1966, Motion of lumbar spine with special reference to stabilizing effect of posterior fusion, *Acta Orthop Scand Suppl*, **90**.

ROYAL COLLEGE OF NURSING, 1980, Back injuries in nurses, *Lancet*, **1**(8163), 325.

SAAL, J.A., SAAL, J.S. and HERZOG, R.J., 1990, The natural history of lumbar intervertebral disc extrusions treated nonoperatively, *Spine*, **15**, 683–686.

SANDOVER, J., 1981, Vibration, posture and low-back disorders of professional drivers, Rep No. DHS 02, May, Dept. of Human Sciences, Univ. of Technology, Loughborough, England.

SCHIPPLEIN, O.D., TRAFIMOW, J.H., ANDERSSON, G.B.J. and ANDRIACCHI, T.P., 1990, Relationship between moments at the L5/S1 level, hip and knee joint when lifting, *J Biomech*, **23**(9), 907–912.

SEDOWOFIA, K.A., TOMLINSON, I.W., *et al.*, 1982, Collagenolytic enzyme systems in human intervertebral disc, *Spine*, **7**, 213–222.

SEIDEL, H. and HEIDE, R., 1986, Long-term effects of whole-body vibration: a critical survey of the literature, *Int Arch Occup Environ Health*, **58**, 1–26.

SHIRAZI-ADL, A., 1989, Strain in fibers of a lumbar disc – analysis of the role of lifting in producing disc prolapse, *Spine*, **14**, 96–103.

SHIRAZI-ADL, A., 1992, Finite element simulation of changes in the fluid content of human lumbar discs, *Spine*, **17**, 206–212.

SHIRAZI-ADL, A. and DROUIN, G., 1987, Load-bearing role of facets in a lumbar segment under sagittal plane loadings, *J Biomechanics*, **20**, 601–613.

SHIRAZI-ADL, A.A.M., SHRIVASTAVA, S.C. and AHMED, A.M., 1984, Stress analysis of the lumbar disc-body unit in axial compression: a three dimensional finite element study, *Spine*, **9**, 120–134.

SIMON, B.R., WU, J.S.S., CARLTON, M.W., KAZARIAN, L.E., FRANCE, I.P., EVANS, J.H. and ZIENKIEWICZ, O.C., 1985, Poroelastic dynamic structural models for rhesus spinal motion segments, *Spine*, **10**, 494–507.

SNOOK, S.H., CAMPANELLI, R.A. and HART, J.W., 1978, A study of three preventative approaches to low back injury, *J Occup Med*, **20**, 478.

SNOOK, S.H., CAMPANELLI, R.A. and FORD, R.J., 1980, A Study of Back Injuries at Pratt and Whitney Aircraft, unpublished data, Liberty Mutual Insurance Co., Research Center, Hopkinton, MA.

STATE OF CALIFORNIA, 1980, Disability work injuries under worker's compensation including back strains per 1000 workers by industry, Department of Industrial Relations, Division of Labor Statistics and Research, San Francisco, California.

STATE OF WISCONSIN, 1973, Workman's compensation data: back injuries, statistical release 3878, Department of Industry, Labor, and Human Relations, Workman's Compensation Division, Bureau of Research and Statistics, Madison, WI.

STOKES, I.A.F., 1987, Surface strains on human intervertebral discs, *J Orthop Res*, **5**, 348.

STOKES, I. and GREENAPPLE, D.M., 1985, Measurement of surface deformation of soft tissue, *J Biomech*, **18**, 1.

TROUP, J.D.G. and EDWARDS, F.C., 1985, Manual Handling and Lifting, unpublished data, Her Majesty's Stationery Office, London.

TROUP, J.D.G., LESKINEN, T., STALHAMMER, H., *et al.*, 1983, A comparison of intra-abdominal pressure increases, hip torque and lumbar vertebral compression in different lifting techniques, *Hum Factors*, **25**, 517–525.

TSUANG, Y.H., SCHIPPLEIN, O.D., TRAFIMOW, J.H. and ANDERSSON, G.B.J., 1992, Influence of body segment dynamics on the loads at the lumbar spine during lifting, *Ergonomics*, **35**(4), 437–444.

URBAN, J.P.G., 1992, The Effect of Physical Factors on Disc Cell Metabolism, presented at the Workshop on Age-Related Musculoskeletal Soft Tissue Changes, Colorado Springs, CO.

URBAN, J., 1996, Disc biochemistry in relation to function, in Weisel, S.W. and Weinstein, J.N. (Eds), *The Lumbar Spine*, Philadelphia: W.B. Saunders, pp. 231–244.

URBAN, J.P., HOLM, S., MAROUDAS, A. and NACHEMSON, A., 1982, Nutrition of the intervertebral disc: effect of fluid flow on solute transport, *Clin Orthop*, **170**, 296.

VIRGIN, W., 1951, Experimental investigations into physical properties of intervertebral disc, *J Bone Joint Surg*, **33B**, 607.

WESTRIN, C.G., 1973, Low back pain sick listing. A nosological and medical insurance investigation, *Scand J Soc Med*, Suppl. **7**(1).

WHITE, A.A. and PANJABI, M.M., 1990, *Clinical Biomechanics of the Spine*, Philadelphia: J.B. Lippincott Co.

WIESEL, S.W., CUCKLER, J.M., DeLUCA, F., JONES, F., ZEIDE, M.S. and ROTHMANN, R.H., 1980, Acute low-back pain: an objective analysis of conservative therapy, *Spine*, **5**, 324.

WIESMAN, G., POPE, M. and JOHNSON, 1980, Cyclic loading in knee ligament injuries, *Am J Sports Med*, **8**, 24–30.

WILDER, D.G., 1990, The Effect of Combined Lateral and Flexion Vibration on the Lumbar Intervertebral Motion Segment, unpublished personal research notes.

WILDER, D.G. and POPE, M.H., 1996, Epidemiological and aetiological aspects of low back pain in vibration environments – an update, *Clin Biomech*, **11**(2), 61–73.

WILDER, D.G., WOODWORTH, B.B., FRYMOYER, J.W. and POPE, M.H., 1982a, Vibration and the human spine, *Spine*, **7**, 243.

WILDER, D.G., POPE, M.H. and FRYMOYER, J.W., 1982b, Cyclic loading of the intervertebral motion segment, Northwest Bioengineering Conf., Mar. 15–16, Dartmouth, IEEE Cat 82CH1747–5, NY, pp. 9–11.

WILDER, D.G., FRYMOYER, J.W. and POPE, M.H., 1985, The effect of vibration on the spine of the seated individual, *Automedica*, **6**, 5–35.

WILDER, D.G., POPE, M.H. and FRYMOYER, J.W., 1988, The biomechanics of lumbar disc herniation and the effect of overload and instability, *J Spinal Dis*, **1**, 6–12.

WOOD, P.H.N. and BADLEY, E.M., 1987, Epidemiology of back pain, in Jayson, M.I.V. (Ed.), *The Lumbar Spine and Back Pain*, New York: Churchill Livingstone, p. 1.

WYKE, B.D., 1972, Articular neurology: a review, *Physiotherapy*, **58**, 94.

YANG, K.H. and KING, A.I., 1984, Mechanism of facet load transmission as a hypothesis for low-back pain, *Spine*, **9**, 557–565.

YASUMA, T., 1990, Histological changes in aging lumbar discs. Their role in protrusions and prolapses, *J Bone Jt Surg*, **72A**, 220–229.

YASUMA, T.E., MAKINO, et al., 1986, Histological development of intervertebral disc herniation, *J Bone Jt Surg*, **68A**, 1066–1072.

CHAPTER FIFTEEN

Models in manual materials handling

M.M. AYOUB AND JEFFREY C. WOLDSTAD

INTRODUCTION

The ergonomics approach to manual materials handling (MMH) tasks defines a Man–Task–Environment System. A generally accepted means of minimising MMH related injuries is to design MMH tasks so that the demands of the tasks are less than the capacities of the individuals performing these tasks. Task design is dependent, in part, on the availability of comparable data for task demands and worker capacities. The generation of the appropriate data is dependent, in part, on being able to identify the pertinent capacity parameters of manual materials handling activities.

In the past, a substantial effort has been directed at determining 'safe' lifting capacities for individuals and groups of individuals. The assumption used for these studies was that there is a relationship between an individual's capacity and his or her injury potential. In other words, a person with a small capacity with respect to a given task demand is more likely to be injured than another person with larger capacities. For the measurement of a safe and permissible lifting capacity three approaches are commonly used. The first approach is the biomechanical approach, the second approach is the physiological approach, and the third is the psychophysical approach. These three approaches and the models developed using the selected criterion under each approach are discussed below.

THE BIOMECHANICAL APPROACH

Using the biomechanical approach, researchers attempt to model directly the mechanical stresses placed upon the internal structures of the body during lifting. The goal of this approach is to accurately estimate how work activities stress the bones, muscles and connective tissues of the body and to predict when these stresses will lead to damage of these structures. This approach is very popular in ergonomics because it closely corresponds with most expert views of the aetiology of injury during manual materials handling (NIOSH, 1981).

Biomechanical models typically model the human body as a series of mechanical links and joints corresponding to the human skeleton. Both external forces, needed to perform the work activity, and internal forces, as a result of muscle contraction, are modelled to estimate the mechanical stresses. Most models focus on estimating only a few mechanical stress parameters related to the injury of interest in the analysis. For manual materials handling the parameter most often selected is the compressive force on the low back, usually the L5/S1 spine segment.

The criterion selected

The criterion selected in most biomechanical analyses of manual materials handling has been greatly influenced by the National Institute for Occupational Safety and Health's (NIOSH) guidelines for Manual Lifting (NIOSH, 1981, 1994). In developing a biomechanical criterion, NIOSH arrived at the following three conclusions based upon a review of the literature (NIOSH, 1994):

(1) The joint between L5 (fifth lumbar) and S1 (first sacral) is the joint of greatest lumbar stress during lifting.

(2) Compressive force (at this joint) is the critical stress vector.

(3) The compressive force criterion that defines increased risk is 3.4 kN.

Support for these assumptions can be found in both NIOSH documents (NIOSH, 1981, 1994) and in epidemiological studies by Herrin et al. (1986), Bringham and Garg (1983), Anderson (1983), and Chaffin and Park (1973). However recent work by Leamon (1994) suggests that more research is needed in this area.

Several other criteria have been used to a lesser extent in biomechanical modelling, including the external hip moment, the external moment at L5/S1 joint, anterior–posterior (A–P) shear force, and lateral shear force. In addition, Marras et al. (1993) have recently proposed using kinematic parameters of the torso as criterion to predict injury (Marras et al., 1993, 1995). Because most models attempt to predict compressive force, A–P shear force, and lateral shear force at the lower back (either L5/S1 or L3/L4), the rest of this section will focus on these criteria.

Estimating the external load moment

All biomechanical models employed to evaluate lifting begin by knowing the external load placed on the body by the task under study. The procedure used for this calculation in different models is essentially the same, with slight differences in the kinematic representations of the body and the anthropometric and body segment data that are used in the calculation. The skeleton of the body is modelled as a series of rigid links or levers connected at frictionless pin joints. With several other assumptions, engineering mechanics is used to calculate the moment created by the force acting at the hands at each joint, beginning with joints closest to the hands and ending at the joint of interest (usually the L5/S1 or L4/L5 intervertebral joints). Implicit in the construction of these models are simplifying assumptions regarding the number and geometric complexity of the joints and bones of the human body.

Biomechanical models are either two-dimensional or three-dimensional and either static or dynamic. For static models, the calculations require information on the orientation of the links in the model (subject's posture), the length of each segment, the mass of each segment, and the location of the centre-of-mass of each segment. Dynamic models require this same information plus the angular joint accelerations, linear acceleration of each segment at the centre-of-mass, and the moment-of-inertia of each link through the centre of mass. A general equation to calculate the static moment at successive joints in a linkage is:

$$\underline{M}_{joint} = \underline{M}_{joint-1} + (\underline{L}_{link} \times \underline{F}_{joint-1}) + (\underline{CM}_{link} \times m_{link}\underline{G}) \tag{15.1}$$

where:

$\underline{M}_{joint}$ is the reactive load moment vector for the joint of interest,
$\underline{M}_{joint-1}$ is the reactive load moment vector for the joint previous to the joint of interest in the linkage,
$\underline{L}_{link}$ is the vector from the position of the joint of interest to the previous joint,
$\underline{F}_{joint-1}$ is the reactive force for the joint previous to the joint of interest,
$\underline{CM}_{link}$ is the vector from the position of the joint of interest to the centre-of-mass position for that link,
m_{link} is the mass of the link, and
$\underline{G}$ is the vector representing acceleration due to gravity.

For dynamic models, an equivalent equation is:

$$\underline{M}_{joint} = \underline{M}_{joint-1} + (\underline{L}_{link} \times \underline{F}_{joint-1}) + (\underline{CM}_{link} \times m_{link}\underline{G}) + (\underline{CM}_{link} \times m_{link}\underline{A}_{link})$$
$$+ (\underline{\ddot{\theta}}_{joint} \times \underline{I}_{link}) \tag{15.2}$$

where:

$\underline{M}_{joint}$ is the reactive load moment vector for the joint of interest,
$\underline{M}_{joint-1}$ is the reactive load moment vector for the joint previous to the joint of interest in the linkage,
$\underline{L}_{link}$ is the vector from the position of the joint of interest to the previous joint,
$\underline{F}_{joint-1}$ is the reactive force for the joint previous to the joint of interest,
$\underline{CM}_{link}$ is the vector from the position of the joint of interest to the centre-of-mass position for that link,
m_{link} is the mass of the link,
$\underline{G}$ is the vector representing acceleration due to gravity,
$\underline{A}_{link}$ is the instantaneous linear acceleration vector of the link centre-of-mass,
$\underline{\ddot{\theta}}_{joint}$ is the angular acceleration of the link about the joint of interest, and
$\underline{I}_{link}$ is the moment-of-inertia of the link through the centre-of-mass.

Anthropometric data needed for these equations can be found in a number of sources including Dempster (1955), Clauser *et al.* (1969) and NASA (1978). Additional details on how to calculate external load moments can be found in Chaffin and Andersson (1991), Winter (1990), Özkaya and Nordin (1991) and Williams and Lissner (1977).

Estimating internal muscle forces

The forces acting on the intervertebral discs are a combination of the external forces at the joints and the internal forces created by muscles and connective tissues. For two-dimensional models, muscle forces are usually estimated by assuming that the erector spinae muscle acts to generate force if the external load moment at the torso is acting to increase torso flexion (i.e., lifting activities) and the rectus abdominus muscle is active if the external load moment at the torso is acting to decrease torso flexion (i.e. pushing down). For static models, the muscle forces can be derived using the conditions of static equilibrium. For dynamic activities, Newton's second law can be used. The most popular two-dimensional static biomechanical model currently in use is the University of Michigan's *2D Static Strength Prediction Program*. In addition to using the erector spinae muscles and the rectus abdominus muscles, this model also adds internal forces due to the interabdominal pressure (IAP) created by the muscles of the torso during lifting activities. The use of interabdominal pressure in biomechanical models has been questioned by several researchers (Mairiaux and Malchaire, 1988; McGill and Norman, 1986) and is not generally included in most three-dimensional models. In addition to disc compressive forces, the University of Michigan's *2D Static Strength Prediction Program* also predicts muscle strength at each joint included in the model.

Estimating internal muscle forces has proven to be difficult for three-dimensional models due to the complexity of the human torso. Because the number of muscles in the torso region is generally greater than the number of force and moment equations, the problem is indeterminate. Optimisation procedures were first employed to solve for the static three-dimensional muscle forces in the torso by Schultz *et al.* (1983). This model was later refined into the minimum-intensity-compression (MIC) model (Bean *et al.*, 1988). The model employs a two-step linear programming approach to estimating the internal muscle forces. The first step in the procedure:

$$\text{Minimise} \quad I \tag{15.3}$$

subject to:

$$\sum_{i=1}^{m} \|f_i\| (r_i \times \underline{\tau}_i) + \underline{M}_{joint},$$

$$\frac{f_i}{A_i} \le I,$$

$$f_i \ge 0,$$

where:

  f_i is the tension in each muscle,
  r_i is the moment arm vector,
  $\underline{\tau}_i$ is the muscle line-of-action vector,
  $\underline{M}_{joint}$ is the reactive load moment for the joint of interest,

finds the minimum–maximum muscle intensity for the muscles being considered in the model. Intensity is defined as the force exerted by the muscle divided by the cross-sectional area of the muscle. The second step in the procedure:

$$\text{Minimise} \quad \|f_i\| \underline{\tau}_i^z \tag{15.4}$$

subject to:

$$\sum_{i=1}^{m} \|f_i\| (\underline{r}_i \times \underline{\tau}_i) + \underline{M}_{joint},$$

$$\frac{f_i}{A_i} \le I^*,$$

$$f_i \ge 0,$$

where:

f_i is the tension in each muscle,
$\underline{r}_i$ is the moment arm vector,
$\underline{\tau}_i$ is the muscle line-of-action vector,
$\underline{M}_{joint}$ is the reactive load moment for the joint of interest,
I^* is the minimum intensity value from the first step in the procedure,

selects muscle forces which satisfy the minimum intensity criteria generated in the first step and also minimises the compressive force on the intervertebral disc. The second step is only needed if multiple optima are found in the first step which seldom occurs in practical application of the model. This model is included in the University of Michigan's *3D Static Strength Prediction Program*. The main output screens of this computer program for a typical lifting task are shown in Figure 15.1.

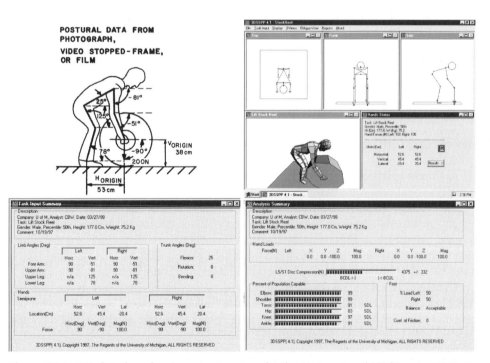

Figure 15.1 Work task and main output screens for the University of Michigan's *3D Static Strength Prediction Program* (reprinted with permission from the University of Michigan, 1998).

A second optimisation model often used to estimate static muscle force in the torso is the sum of cubed intensities (SCI) model first proposed for use in modelling the extremities by Crowminshield and Brand (1981). While similar to the MIC model, this algorithm employs non-linear programming which makes the solution procedure, in general, more difficult. The SCI optimisation model is formulated as:

$$\text{Minimise} \quad \sum_{i=1}^{m} \left(\frac{f_i}{A_i} \right)^3 \qquad\qquad (15.5)$$

subject to:

$$\sum_{i=1}^{m} \|f_i\| \left(\underline{r}_i \times \underline{\tau}_i \right) + \underline{M}_{joint},$$

$$f_i \geq 0,$$

where:

f_i is the tension in each muscle,
$\underline{r}_i$ is the moment arm vector,
$\underline{\tau}_i$ is the muscle line-of-action vector,
$\underline{M}_{joint}$ is the reactive load moment for the joint of interest.

Both the MIC and the SCI optimisation procedures do not restrict the number of muscle forces predicted, but they require information on the cross-sectional area of the muscles, the muscle line of action, and the muscle moment arm vector. This information must be in three dimensions and applicable to the joint of interest in the model. Models are usually formulated using from 10 to 22 different muscles about the torso. Relevant anthropometric values for these parameters can be found a variety of sources (Chaffin et al., 1990; Dumas et al., 1988; Han et al., 1992; Macintosh and Bogduk, 1986; McGill et al., 1988; Schultz et al., 1983; Tracy et al., 1989). A review of different torso anthropometries and their potential effects on optimisation models can be found in McMulkin (1996). Experimental support using electromyographs (EMGs) was provided for the MIC model by Ladin et al. (1989); however, in a direct comparison of the SCI model and the MIC model, both Hughes (1991) and McMulkin (1996) found that the SCI model more closely reflected muscle activation patterns of torso muscles.

A second approach to estimating the internal muscle forces has been to use EMG activity to predict how the muscles respond in different situations. Marras and Sommerich (1991a) present a three-dimensional dynamic model that uses this method. Inputs to the model include the external load moment at the trunk, the trunk flexion angle, trunk angular velocity, and EMG signals from five left/right pairs of muscles: the latissimus dorsi, erector spinae, rectus abdominus, internal oblique, and external oblique. EMGs must be collected for the activity of interest and for maximum exertions of the trunk. A similar EMG based model has been developed by McGill and his colleagues (McGill, 1992; McGill and Norman, 1986). A difference between the model proposed by McGill and that proposed by Marras and Sommerich (1991a) is that the McGill model incorporates the effects of passive tissues into the calculations and it considers muscle activities at several different levels of the torso. Kee and Chung (1996) recently compared the predictions of the Marras and Sommerich (1991a) biomechanical model to those of the MIC model. The MIC model was applied to a dynamic lifting situation by sequentially applying the model at consecutive time intervals throughout the lift. The results of this comparison demonstrated substantial differences between the predictions of the two models, especially for asymmetric tasks.

A third class of biomechanical model has recently been proposed which incorporates both optimisation and EMG components to estimate internal muscle forces. Nussbaum and Chaffin (1996) recently proposed an artificial neural network model that uses EMG signals as a learning tool. The model takes as input the external load moment at the torso and produces as output muscle activities for four left/right pairs of muscles: the latissimus dorsi, erector spinae, rectus abdominus, and external oblique. A quantitative evaluation of the model performed by Nussbaum and Chaffin (1996) indicates remarkable agreement with measured EMG signals. Cholewicki and McGill (1996) have also developed a model that employs both EMG and optimisation techniques. This model estimates muscle forces using EMG signals as inputs and then adjusts to force using an optimisation routine.

The effect of task variables on model predictions

Biomechanical models have been used to evaluate the effects of many different task variables on workers performing manual materials handling tasks. Most biomechanical models are very sensitive to the magnitude of the load and position of the load in relation to the position of the torso. Increasing the load, moving the load away from the body, and moving the load down from waist level to the floor substantially increases the L5/S1 compressive force as shown in Figure 15.2. These estimates were produced using a two-dimensional static model similar to the University of Michigan's *2D Static Strength Prediction Program*.

Static biomechanical models have been reported to under-estimate the forces associated with dynamic activities (Freivalds *et al.*, 1984; Garg *et al.*, 1982; Kim, 1990; Leskinen *et al.*, 1983; Marras and Sommerich, 1991b; McGill and Norman, 1986). The peak compressive force during a dynamic lift activity usually occurs as the load is being accelerated during the motion. For activities with relatively large accelerations, the static estimate of the compressive force at this point is 30–40 per cent lower than the dynamic estimate (Granata and Marras, 1996). Three-dimensional biomechanical models have also shown that asymmetric lift activities result in higher compressive force than symmetric lifts. This occurs for two handed lifts with a twisted body posture (Chen, 1988; Marras and Sommerich, 1991b; Mital and Kromodihardjo, 1986), one handed lifts (Davis *et al.*, 1997), and for team lifts with asymmetric body postures (Marras *et al.*, 1997).

PHYSIOLOGICAL DESIGN APPROACH

Unlike the biomechanical design approach that primarily applies to infrequent lifting, the physiological approach is applicable to repetitive lifting where the load is within the physical strength of the worker. During repetitive handling tasks, a person's endurance is primarily limited by the capacity of the oxygen transport system. As muscles contract and relax, their increased metabolic energy demand requires an increase in the delivery of oxygen and nutrients to the tissues. If this demand for increased oxygen and nutrients cannot be met, the activity cannot be sustained for long.

When a person is engaged in physical work, such as MMH activities, several physiological responses are affected. These include metabolic energy cost, heart rate, blood

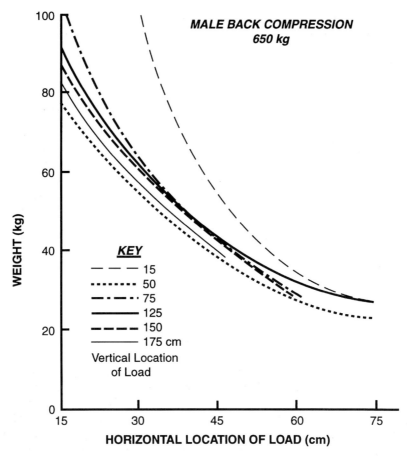

Figure 15.2   Relationship between the load weight, the horizontal distance away from the spine, and the vertical distance of the load from the floor for a constant 650 kg L5/S1 compressive force (from NIOSH, 1981).

pressure, blood lactate and ventilation volume. Of all these responses, metabolic energy expenditure has been the widely accepted physiological response to repetitive handling as it is directly proportional to the workload at steady-state conditions (Aquilano, 1968; Astrand and Rodahl, 1986; Ayoub et al., 1981; Durnin and Passmore, 1967; Hamilton and Chase, 1969; Mital, 1984). For this reason, this discussion will exclusively focus on metabolic energy expenditure rate as the physiological approach design criterion.

Several work- and workplace-related factors affect metabolic energy expenditure rate. Table 15.1 summarises these factors and their net effect on oxygen consumption. For a detailed discussion on the effect of these and personal factors on oxygen consumption the reader is referred to *Manual Materials Handling* by Ayoub and Mital (1989).

There is a need for models that can predict the physiological cost (e.g., oxygen consumption and heart rate) of individuals engaged in repetitive manual materials handling (MMH) tasks. Physiological cost models are used in industry to: determine whether or not the task is within the expected capability of the population; and determine the work/rest schedule for a given task (Asfour, 1980). The literature on physiological cost prediction models for MMH tasks grew in the 1980s. This section will review the existing energy and cardiac cost prediction models for several manual materials handling activities. This by no means is an exhaustive review.

Table 15.1   Net effect of work and workplace factors on metabolic energy.

Factor		
Frequency of handling ($\uparrow$)	All	Increase
Task duration ($\uparrow$)	All	Increase[a]/decrease[b]
Object size ($\uparrow$)	All	Increase
Couplings (good)	All	Decrease
Object shape (various)	All	Unknown
Object weight/force ($\uparrow$)	All	Increase
Load stability/distribution	Lifting, carrying	Unknown
Vertical height ($\uparrow$)	Lifting, lowering	Increase
Distance travelled ($\uparrow$)	Pushing, pulling, carrying	Increase
Speed/grade ($\uparrow$)	Pushing, pulling, carrying	Increase
Asymmetrical handling	Lifting	None

(From Mital *et al.*, 1997).
$\uparrow$ increase; [a] if the weight/force does not change; [b] if the weight/force decreases (e.g., when using the psychophysical methodology).

Energy and cardiac cost for lifting/lowering models

Several researchers have developed prediction models for the energy and cardiac cost responses of individuals engaged in repetitive manual materials handling tasks. Research in this area has been carried out by Aberg *et al.* (1968), Asfour (1980), Chaffin (1967), Frederick (1959), Garg (1976), Karwowski and Ayoub (1984a), Liou and Morrissey (1985), Mital (1983b, 1985), Mital *et al.* (1984) and Morrissey and Liou (1984a, 1984b, 1984c). A list of several energy cost and cardiac cost models is given in Tables 15.2 and 15.3. The cardiac cost models are summarised in Table 15.4.

Frederick (1959) developed a model to predict the consumption of energy for various weights in four different ranges. Chaffin's model (1967) was developed for static weight-holding activities in the sagittal plane. Aberg *et al.* (1968) developed a model based on the principle that mechanical work is related to a change of the positional energy of mass and frictional losses. Garg (1976) and Garg *et al.* (1978) used step-wise regression analysis to develop models for lifting, lowering, and carrying activities. Ayoub *et al.* (1980) provided a review of the energy cost models for manual lifting tasks developed by Aberg *et al.* (1968), Chaffin (1967), Frederick (1959) and Garg (1976).

Asfour (1980) developed and tested energy cost prediction models for manual lifting and lowering using stepwise regression models, and attempted to overcome some of the limitations cited by Ayoub *et al.* (1980) by studying the effect of task variables and their interactions on lifting and lowering tasks. The estimated energy expenditure for 512 tasks was based on frequency of lift or lower (3, 6, 9 times/min), load lifted or lower (6.8, 13.6, 20.4 kg), range of height (floor–76 cm, 76–127 cm, floor–127 cm), box width (38, 66 cm), box length (38, 66 cm), and angle of twist of the body (0, 90 degrees). The models developed were reported later by Asfour *et al.* (1985).

Karwowski and Ayoub (1984a) developed a model to estimate the oxygen consumption associated with the maximum weight (MAW) of lift, determined psychophysically, for frequencies of 0.1, 3, 9, and 12 lifts/min when lifting from floor to table height (76 cm). The inputs to the model are the frequency of lift, maximum acceptable load weight, body weight, and age. This model is presented in Table 15.2.

Table 15.2 Energy cost prediction models for lifting tasks.

Source	Dependent variable	Type of task	Model
Frederick (1959)	Total energy expenditure per hour	Lifting from floor to 20 in, 20 in to 40 in, 40 in to 60 in and 60 in to 80 in	TEE = (Number of lifts/hour)*(lifting height in feet)*(weight of load in pounds)*(energy consumption in gm cal/foot pound)/1000
Garg et al. (1978)	Net metabolic rate (kcal/lift)	Stoop lift (h1 < h2 ≤ 0.81)	NMR = 0.00325*W*(0.81 − h1) + (0.0141*L + 0.0076*G*L)*(h2 − h1)
Garg et al. (1978)	Net metabolic rate (kcal/lift)	Squat lift (h1 < h2 ≤ 0.81)	NMR = 0.00514*W*(0.81 − h1) + (0.0219*L + 0.0062*G*L)*(h2 − h1)
Garg et al. (1978)	Net metabolic rate (kcal/lift)	Arm lift (0.81 < h1 ≤ h2)	NMR = 0.00352*W*(0.81 − h1) + 0.0303*L*(h2 − h1)
Asfour (1980)	Oxygen consumption (ml/min)	Lifting that starts at floor and lowering that ends at floor	VO2 = 545.7538 − 106.4477*TA + 10**−6*F*L**2*(35002.65 − 35058*L) + 17.47*10**−6*F*L*H*WID*LEN*ANG + 16435.22*10**−6*W*F**2
Asfour (1980)	Oxygen consumption (ml/min)	Lifting that starts at table height and lowering that ends at table height	VO2 = 371.5055 − 51.9573*TA + 10**−6*W*F**2*(31856.54 − 2332.8*F) + 12684.91*10**−6*F*L**2 + 12.31*10**−6*F*H*L*W*LEN*ANG
Mital (1983b) and Mital et al. (1984)	Change of oxygen consumption with time (%)	Lifting (males)	CVO2 = 103.763 − 13.497*T + 2.142*T**2 − 0.117**3 + 0.00013*EXP(T)
Mital (1983b) and Mital et al. (1984)	Change of oxygen consumption with time (%)	Lifting (females)	CVO2 = 101.726 − 2.305*T + 0.00003*EXP(T)
Mital et al. (1984)	Oxygen consumption (l/min)	Lifting from floor to knuckle	VO2 = 1.527 − 0.207*G − 0.005*Stature + 0.0013*Back Strength − 0.0002*Chest Width**2 + 0.203*LOG (Shoulder Strength) − 0.408*LOG (Back Strength) − 0.02*Shift Duration + 0.161*LOG(F) + 0.002*F*Lifting Capability − 0.0007*F*Box Size
Mital et al. (1984)	Oxygen consumption (l/min)	Lifting from knuckle to shoulder	VO2 = 0.047 − 0.117*G − 0.003*Age + 0.0005* Chest Depth**2 − 0.00001*Composite Strength**2 − 0.00005*

Table 15.2 (Cont'd)

Source	Dependent variable	Type of task	Model
			Back Strength**2 − 0.175*LOG (Arm Strength) − 0.0084*Shift Duration + 0.004*F*Lifting Capability + 0.00002*Box Size*Lifting Capability
Mital *et al.* (1984)	Oxygen consumption (l/min)	Lifting from shoulder to reach	VO2 = −0.521 − 0.123*G + 0.004*W + 0.25* LOG(Arm Strength) − 0.008*Shift Duration + 0.004*F*Lifting Capability + 0.0003*Box Size*Lifting Capability
Mital *et al.* (1984) and Mital (1985)	Oxygen consumption (l/min)	Lifting for all heights	VO2 = 0.86 − 0.168*G + 0.00002*W**2 − 0.00012*Arm Strength**2 + 0.279* LOG(Arm Strength) − 0.231*LOG(Back Strength) − 0.013*Shift Duration + 0.004*F*Lifting Capability − 0.00012*Box Size*Lifting Capability
Karwowski and Ayoub (1984a)	Oxygen consumption (l/min)	Lifting from floor to 76 cm above floor	VO2 = 0.1659 + 0.004026*F* Lifting Capability + 0.0026887*Lifting Capability + 0.002873*W − 0.005854*Age + 0.032699*F

(From Genaidy and Asfour, 1987; reprinted with permission. Copyright 1987 by the Human Factors and Ergonomics Society. All rights reserved.)

TEE – energy expenditure/hour
NMR – net metabolic rate for the activity performed
VO2 – oxygen consumption (l/min for all studies, except Asfour in ml/min)
CVO2 – change of oxygen consumption with time (%)
W – body weight (kg in Garg *et al.* and Mital *et al.*; pounds in Asfour)
L – amount of load handled (kg in Garg *et al.* and Mital *et al.*; pounds in Asfour)
G – gender (Garg, *et al.*: male = 1, female = 0; Mital *et al.*: male = 1, female = 2)
h1 – vertical height from floor (m); starting point for lift
h2 – vertical height from floor (m); end point for lift
TA – type of task (lifting = 1, lowering = 2)
F – frequency of handling (times/min)
H – height of lift or lower (inches)
WID – box width (inches)
LEN – box length (inches)
ANG – angle of twist (0° twist = 1; 90° twist = 2)
T – shift duration (minutes)

All anthropometric measurements in cm; isometric strengths in kg; lifting capability in kg; box size in inches; age in years; all models are valid for a duration of less than one hour, except those of Mital, which are valid up to 12 hours.

Table 15.3 Energy cost prediction models for lowering tasks.

Source	Dependent variable	Type of task	Model
Garg et al. (1978)	Net metabolic rate (kcal/lower)	Stoop lower (h1 < h2 ≤ 0.81)	NMR = 0.00268*W*(0.81 − h1) + 0.00675*L*(h2 − h1) + 0.0522*G*(0.81 − h1)
Garg et al. (1978)	Net metabolic rate (kcal/lower)	Squat lower (h1 < h2 ≤ 0.81)	NMR = 0.00511*W*(0.81 − h1) + 0.00701*L*(h2 − h1)
Garg et al. (1978)	Net metabolic rate (kcal/lower)	Arm lower (0.81 < h1 < h2)	NMR − 0.00093*W*(h2 − 0.81) + (0.0102*L + 0.0037*G*L)*(h2 − h1)
Asfour (1980)	Oxygen consumption (ml/min)	Lifting that starts at table height and lowering that ends at table height	See Table 15.2
Asfour (1980)	Oxygen consumption (ml/min)	Lifting that starts at floor level and lowering that ends at floor lever	See Table 15.2

(From Genaidy and Asfour, 1987; reprinted with permission. Copyright 1987 by the Human Factors and Ergonomics Society. All rights reserved.)
  NMR – net metabolic rate for activity performed
  W – body weight (kg)
  L – amount of load lowered (kg)
  G – gender (male = 1, female = 0)
  h1 – vertical height from floor (m); end point for lower
  h2 – vertical height from floor (m); starting point for lower
All models are valid for a duration of less than one hour.

Table 15.4 Cardiac cost prediction models for lifting tasks.

Source	Type of Task	Model
Mital (1983b) and Mital et al. (1984)	Lifting for males	CHR = 104.846 − 16.85*Shift Duration + 3.215*Shift Duration**2 − 0.184*Shift Duration**3 + 0.0002*EXP (Shift Duration)
Mital (1983b) and Mital et al. (1984)	Lifting for females	CHR = 100.36 − 16.85*Shift Duration + 0.00004 EXP (Shift Duration)
Mital et al. (1984)	Lifting from floor to knuckle height	HR = −112.342 + 14.677*G − 0.713*Iliac Crest Height − 1.793*Chest Depth + 3.494*Abdominal Depth + 12.078* RPI − 0.0045*(Back Strength) **2 + 18.35*LOG(Arm Strength) + 3.367*Frequency − 0.772*Shift Duration + 1.885*Lifting Capability − 0.01*Box Size*Lifting Capability − 0.48*Age
Mital et al. (1984)	Lifting from knuckle to shoulder height	HR = 1225.276 + 17.693*G + 1.656*Abdominal Depth + 7.37*RPI + 0.62*Back Strength + 0.02*(Knee Height)**2 + 0.0024*(Composite Strength)**2 − 0.0095*(Back Strength)**2 − 279.375*LOG(Stature) + 37.582*LOG(Forearm

Table 15.4 (Cont'd)

Source	Type of Task	Model
		Grip Distance) − 16.853*LOG(Chest Width) − 0.986*Shift Duration + 0.231*Lifting Capability*Frequency + 0.01*Box Size*Lifting Capability
Mital *et al.* (1984)	Lifting from shoulder to reach height	HR = 39.176 + 17.015*G − 0.56*Iliac Crest Height + 0.613*Arm Strength − 0.378*Composite Strength + 25.743*LOG(Back Strength) + 0.003*(Composite Strength)**2 − 0.009*(Back Strength)**2 − 1.32*Shift Duration + 6.43*LOG (Frequency) + 0.067*Frequency*Lifting Capability + 0.005*Box Size*Lifting Capability
Mital *et al.* (1984) and Mital (1985)	Lifting for all heights	HR = 136.943 + 18.565*G + 0.09*(Abdominal Depth)**2 − 0.004*(Back Strength)**2 − 47.227*LOG(Body Weight) + 40.215*LOG(Forearm Grip Distance) − 40.698*LOG (Abdominal Depth) + 11.476* LOG(Arm Strength) + 11.366*LOG(Composite Strength) − 0.96*Shift Duration + 0.246* Frequency*Lifting Capability − 0.009 Box Size*Lifting Capability − 0.425*EXP(H)

(From Genaidy and Asfour, 1987; reprinted with permission. Copyright 1987 by the Human Factors and Ergonomics Society. All rights reserved.)
  Anthropometric measurements in cm
  Isometric strengths in kg
  Frequency in lifts/minute
  Lifting capability in kg
  Box size in inches
  Body weight in kg
  H (height of lift): floor to knuckle = 1, knuckle to shoulder = 2, shoulder to reach = 3
  G (gender): male = 1, female = 2
  Shift duration in hours
  RPI = Height/3*((Body Weight)**0.333)
  Age in years
  HR (heart rate) in beats/min
  CHR (change in heart rate with time) in %
All models are valid for a duration of up to 12 hours.

    Mital (1983a) and Mital *et al.* (1984) developed oxygen consumption and heart-rate prediction models as a function of working time. The maximum weight of lift (MAWL) for these models was determined psychophysically. The oxygen consumption and heart rate associated with the maximum acceptable weight were recorded every two hours for 12 hours. The models are listed in Table 15.2.

    In other studies, Mital (1985) and Mital *et al.* (1984) developed metabolic and cardiac prediction models for lifting tasks. The models were based on task variables as well as anthropometric and strength measurements using experienced subjects. Four lifting frequencies (1, 4, 8, 12 times/min), three height levels (floor to knuckle, knuckle to shoulder, shoulder to reach), and three box sizes (30.5, 45.7, 70.0 cm long in the sagittal plane) were used as the levels of the independent variables. The models developed showed low multiple R-square values (between 0.59 and 0.60). The models are listed in Table 15.2.

Energy and cardiac cost models for carrying

Morrissey and Liou (1984a, 1984b) conducted experiments to develop models to predict the energy cost of two handed carrying of loads in front of the body. Twenty-seven different carrying tasks were used on a level treadmill. The different variables involved in the carrying tasks were treadmill speed (0.89, 1.12, 1.34, 1.56, 1.79 m/sec), container weight (0, 4.5, 11.3, 18.1, 22.7 kg), and container width in the sagittal plane (15.2, 22.8, 30.5 cm). Also included as variables were stature (as percentage of normal stature) and walking speeds. Regression models were developed to predict the steady state heart and metabolic rates; the regression models developed for oxygen consumption and heart rate are given in Tables 15.5 and 15.6.

Morrissey and Liou (1984c) also examined the physiological costs of carrying loads in erect and non-erect postures. Four trained male subjects carried loads on a level treadmill with a range of walking postures, container widths, container weights and walking speeds. The steady state oxygen uptake and heart rate required for task performance were measured and used to develop predictive equations.

Liou and Morrissey (1985) measured female physiological responses to load carrying with a variety of container widths, container weights and walking speeds on a level treadmill. The data obtained were then compared to data from males performing carrying tasks (Morrissey and Liou, 1984b). Regression models were developed to predict oxygen consumption and heart rate from the knowledge of gender, body weight, load carried, walking speed, and container width. The prediction equations for oxygen consumption and heart rate are provided in Tables 15.5 and 15.6.

Evaluation of the models and their limitations

Tables 15.2–15.7 summarise the metabolic and cardiac cost prediction models of various MMH tasks. Asfour (1980) and Ayoub et al. (1980) pointed out the following limitations of the energy cost prediction models developed by Aberg et al. (1968), Chaffin (1967), Frederick (1959), and Garg (1976):

(1) All models are only valid for manual materials handling tasks in the sagittal plane.

(2) They do not take into account the effect of task variables (e.g., frequency, height of handling, box width, and box length) and their interactions.

(3) Subjects were not trained before data collection.

(4) The model developed by Aberg et al. (1968) requires the determination of the body's centre of gravity, which is difficult to perform.

(5) There is a need to measure the individual's standing metabolic rate in order to apply the models developed by Garg et al. (1978).

Asfour (1980) and Ayoub et al. (1980) reported that Garg's model for lifting tasks (1976) is the most flexible of all the metabolic rate prediction models developed prior to 1980. However, this model was based on the assumption that the net total metabolic cost of a

Table 15.5 Energy cost prediction models for carrying tasks.

Source	Dependent variable	Type of task	Model
Garg et al. (1978)	Net metabolic rate (kcal/min)	Carrying loads held at arm's length at sides (in one or both hands)	$NMR = 0.8 + 0.0243*W*V**2 + 0.0463*L*V**2 + 0.0462*L + 0.00379* (W + L)*TG*V$
Garg et al. (1978)	Net metabolic rate (kcal/min)	Carrying loads held against thighs or against waist	$NMR = 0.68 + 0.0254*W*V**2 + 0.048*L*V**2 + 0.114*L + 0.00379*(W + L)*TG*V$
Morrissey and Liou (1984a)	Metabolic rate (watts)	Carrying loads in front of body with both hands	$MR = -181.66 + 7.18*W + 189.45*V**2 + 3.63*L*V**2 + 0.06*L*Z - 3.79*V*(W + L) + 17.76 *(W + L)*(L/W)**2$
Morrissey and Liou (1984b)	Metabolic rate (watts)	Carrying loads in front of body with both hands	$MR = -75.14 + 3.11*W + V**2*(2.72*L + 87.75) + 13.36*(W + L)*((L/W)**2)$
Morrissey and Liou (1984c)	Oxygen consumption (l/min)	Carrying loads in front of body with both hands	$VO2 = 2.74 - 0.03*P + (L/W)*[0.0016*V**2*Z - 6.13*(L/W) + 2.49] + (2.4*10** - 3)*V*(W + L)$
Liou and Morrissey (1985)	Metabolic rate (watts)	Carrying loads in front of body with both hands	$MR = 25.4 + 24.1*G + 0.43*Z*V**2 + (W + L)*(3.16 + 2.54*V**2 + 16*((L/W)**2) - 3.25*V)$

(From Genaidy and Asfour, 1987; reprinted with permission. Copyright 1987 by the Human
Factors and Ergonomics Society. All rights reserved.)
 NMR – net metabolic rate for activity performed
 MR – metabolic rate
 VO2 – oxygen consumption
 L – load carried (kg)
 W – body weight (kg)
 TG – treadmill grade level (%)
 Z – container width with location of hands in front of body (cm)
 P – percent of normal stature
 G – gender (male = 1, female = 0)
 V – walking speed (km/h)
All models are valid for a duration of less than one hour.

series of activities can be estimated by summing their net steady state individual metabolic costs as obtained from their performance separately. This assumption was reported
to be invalid (Asfour, 1980; Genaidy et al., 1985a).

The models developed by Asfour (1980) for lifting and lowering tasks attempted to
overcome the limitations of previous models developed prior to 1980. He employed

Table 15.6   Cardiac cost prediction models for carrying tasks.

Source	Dependent variable	Model
Morrissey and Liou (1984a)	Heart rate (beats/min)	HR = 205.5 + (W + L)*(2.34*(L/W) + 0.38*V**2 − 0.64*V − 1.53)
Morrissey and Liou (1984b)	Heart rate (beats/min)	HR = 192 + 27.39*V*[(V − 1.53) + 1.42(W + L)*(1 − 1.46*(L/W))]
Morrissey and Liou (1984c)	Heart rate (beats/min)	HR = 227.6 − 16.8*W + 15.53*V**2 + 13.2*(L + W) + 0.03*Z*L − 8.9*(L/W)*P
Liou and Morrissey (1985)	Heart rate (beats/min)	HR = 113.28 − 10.62*G + 21.45*V**2 + 2.01*(W + L)*((L/W)**2) + 0.67*L*V**2 − 0.56*(W + L)*V

(From Genaidy and Asfour, 1987; reprinted with permission. Copyright 1987 by the Human Factors and Ergonomics Society. All rights reserved.)
   HR – heart rate
   L – load carried (kg)
   V – treadmill speed (m/sec)
   W – body weight (kg)
   Z – container width with location of hands in front of body (cm)
   P – percentage of normal posture
   G – gender (male = 1, female = 0)
All models are valid for a duration of less than one hour.

Table 15.7   Energy cost prediction models for combined activities.

Source	Type of task	Model
Aberg et al. (1968)	Lifting, lowering, carrying, and dragging	VO2 = k1*W naked + k2*W with clothing*(k3*GCBh + k4*GCBv) + (WWP + WT)*(k5*Lha + k6*Mu*Lhc + k7*Lvu + k8*Ivd)

(From Genaidy and Asfour, 1987; reprinted with permission. Copyright 1987 by the Human Factors and Ergonomics Society. All rights reserved.)
   VO2 – oxygen consumption (l/min)
   W – body weight (kg)
   GCBh – horizontal displacement per time unit of the body's centre of gravity (m/min)
   GCBv – vertical displacement per time unit of the body's centre of gravity up plus down (m/min)
   WWP – weight of work piece (kg)
   WT – weight of the tool (kg)
   Lha – horizontal displacement per time unit of tool and work piece, arm work (m/min)
   Lhc – horizontal displacement per time unit of tool and work piece, carrying or dragging (m/min)
   Lvu – upward vertical displacement per time unit of tool and work piece, lifting (m/min)
   Lvd – downward vertical displacement per time unit of tool and work piece, lowering (m/min)
   Mu – coefficient of friction in horizontal movement
   k1–k7 – constants
All models are valid for a duration of less than one hour.

trained subjects for eight weeks on flexibility, cardiovascular endurance, muscular strength, and muscular endurance (Asfour et al., 1984b). Task variables such as frequency, height, box length, box width, and angle of body twist were incorporated in the models. Based on the database provided by Asfour (1980), Asfour et al. (1986a, 1986b), it is apparent that the frequency, load, height, and box size have a significant effect on the energy expenditure of individuals engaged in lifting and lowering tasks.

Morrissey and Liou's models (Liou and Morrissey, 1985; Morrissey and Liou, 1984a, 1984b, 1984c) were developed for carrying boxes with both hands. Their models did not take into account the effect of task variables and their interaction, except for box width. Mital and Asfour (1983) reported that carrying frequency, distance, and height are important parameters in the design of carrying tasks.

The major limitation of most of the models reported in the literature is that they are applicable only to manual tasks of less than 60 minutes duration. Thus, according to Genaidy and Asfour (1987), future models should address the effect of working time on the physiological responses of individuals engaged in MMH tasks.

The models generated by Mital (1983b, 1985) and Mital et al. (1984) are the only available models for manual lifting over prolonged periods. These models, however, have some limitations. A low correlation was obtained between task variables and oxygen consumption and heart rate. Mital and coworkers attributed the low correlation to the use of the psychophysical methodology to determine the amount of load that can be handled by individuals. Deivanayagam and Ayoub (1979) indicated that oxygen consumption tends to rise gradually over time while the external work output remained the same. This can be attributed to one of the following factors: a progressive accumulative effect of the products of metabolism; changes in blood flow distribution to various parts of the body other that the working muscles; deterioration in mechanical efficiency; or changes in the constitution of metabolic substrate involved in the energy-release processes.

Many investigators have considered manual materials handling tasks as a continuous type of activity. In fact, an MMH task can be regarded as a pulse function of two to three seconds duration. The gross assumption of a continuous MMH activity does not reflect the metabolic and cardiorespiratory peaks obtained at precisely the moment when the physical pulse loading is applied to the human body. Genaidy et al. (1985b) developed the following equations for the working and recovery curves for lowering an 18 kg load at a frequency of 3 times/min from 76 cm above the floor to the floor:

(1)   Working curve: heart rate (beats/min) = $93.35 - 20.85 * \exp(-(\text{time in sec})/1.312)$.

(2)   Recovery curve: heart rate (beats/min) = $92.65 * \exp(-(\text{time in sec})/67.637)$.

PSYCHOPHYSICAL APPROACH

Psychophysics deals with the relationship between human sensations and their physical stimuli. Borg (1962) and Eisler (1962) found that the perception of both muscular effort and force obey the psychophysical function where the sensation magnitude S grows as a power function of the stimulus I. Stevens (1975) indicated that the strength of a sensation (S) is directly related to the intensity of its physical stimulus (I) by means of a power function:

$$S = k * I^n \tag{15.6}$$

where:

Table 15.8 Net effect of work-related factors on acceptable weight/force.

Factor	MMH activity	Net effect
Frequency (↑)	All	Decrease
Task duration (↑)	All	Decrease
Object size (↑)	All	Decrease
Object shape (various)		
Collapsible (e.g. bags)	Lifting, carrying	Increase
Non-collapsible (e.g. metallic)		Increase
(volume increases)		
Non-collapsible (volume does not change)		Unknown
Couplings (good)	All	Increase
Load stability/distribution	Lifting, carrying	Decrease
Vertical lift height (↑)	Lifting, lowering	Decrease
Height of force (↑)	Pulling, pushing	Increase
Application/starting point	Lifting, lowering, carrying	Decrease
Distance travelled (↑)	Pushing, pulling, carrying	Decrease
Speed/grade (↑)	Pushing, pulling, carrying	Decrease
Asymmetrical handling	Lifting, lowering	Decrease

(From Mital *et al.*, 1997).

S = strength of a sensation,

I = intensity of physical stimulus,

k = a constant which is a function of the particular units of measurement that are used,

n = the slope of the line that represents the power function when plotted in log–log coordinates. For example, it is equal to 3.5 for electric shock, and 1.6 for the perception of muscular effort and force. Stevens (1975) suggested an 'n' value of 1.45 for lifting weights.

Snook (1978) stated that psychophysics has been applied to practical problems in many areas, such as the scales of effective temperature, loudness and lightness, and ratings of perceived exertion (RPE). To apply the principle of psychophysics to men at work is to utilise the human capability to judge the subjectively perceived strain at work in order to determine voluntarily accepted work stresses. In terms of MMH activities, it can be used to determine what the subject can handle (capacity) without strain or discomfort. As stated by Legg and Myles (1981), with good subject cooperation and firm experimental control, the psychophysical method can identify loads that subjects can lift repetitively for an eight-hour workday without metabolic, cardiovascular or subjective evidence of fatigue. The measure of capacity used in this approach is 'maximum acceptable weight of lift'. Maximum acceptable weight of lift is generally defined as the maximum weight, determined experimentally that a given person could lift repeatedly for long periods of time without undue stress or fatigue.

A number of personal, work, and environmental factors affect the psychophysical design criterion. The details can be found in Ayoub and Mital (1989). Table 15.8 summarises the net effect of some of the important work factors.

The psychophysical criterion

The use of psychophysics in the study of lifting tasks requires a subject to adjust the weight of load according to his or her own perception of effort such that the repetitive lifting task does not result in overexertion or excessive fatigue. The final weight selected by the subject is considered to be the maximum acceptable weight (MAW) of lift for the given job conditions (frequency of lift, range of lift, container size, etc.). The MAW is the criterion used for design purposes. Because of the popularity of this approach, it has led to the development of capacity models which can predict lifting capacities (or MAW) for several lifting ranges with a reasonable degree of accuracy and confidence (Asfour, 1980; Asfour *et al.*, 1984a, 1985; Ayoub *et al.*, 1978a, 1983; Karwowski and Ayoub, 1984b; Mital, 1983a, 1983b, 1985).

Psychophysical models

McConville and Hertzberg (1966) investigated the optimum size of a container to be lifted with one hand. Boxes of various sizes (height remained constant) were used. The range of lift was from floor to 76 cm height. They indicated that the weight which 95 per cent of the population would be able to lift could be expressed as a function of object width.

Snook (1976) used data from previous studies by Snook *et al.* (1970) and Snook and Ciriello (1974) to develop a simple model to estimate the object weight to be lifted, based on frequency using a container size of $34 \times 48 \times 14$ cm for floor to knuckle lift. These models are in the form:

$$Y = 14.23 + 5.53 \ X \quad \text{for males} \tag{15.7}$$

$$Y = 13.64 + 1.6 \ X \quad \text{for females} \tag{15.8}$$

where:

Y = MAW of lift (kg),
X = frequency of lift in log seconds.

McDaniel (1972) developed a regression model to predict the acceptable weight of lift. The lifting task was defined as the maximum weight the subject was able to lift four times/min for a period of 45 min without strain or unusual fatigue. The range of lift was from the floor to the standing knuckle height of the subject.

Dryden (1973) conducted a similar study to that of McDaniel. The subjects were asked to lift a tote box from their standing knuckle height through a range of 51 cm. The frequency of lift was six lifts/min. Subjects were allowed to adjust their workloads by adding or removing weights from the tote box. A model to predict load of lift was developed using chest circumstance and dynamic endurance as independent variables.

Knipfer (1974) used female and male subjects to develop regression models for prediction of the load of lift. Subjects were asked to lift the box from standing shoulder height through a 51-cm range. The frequency of lift was six lifts/min. The independent variables of the model were back strength, shoulder strength, and age.

Aghazadeh (1974) conducted experiments and also used data by McDaniel (1972), Dryden (1973) and Knipfer (1974) to develop new predictive models. His approach was to establish the relationships between the lifting capacity for lifting from floor to knuckle height and the other two levels of lift, namely, lifting from knuckle height to shoulder height and from shoulder height to reach height. In addition, he included two other task variables – frequency of lift and box size. He simplified the prediction model using the relationship between the levels of lift and considering fewer operator variables and some task and container variables. The simplified model does not have as good an average error ratio as the individual models reported by McDaniel (1972), Dryden (1973) and Knipfer (1974). However, the simplified model has the following advantages (Ayoub and El-Bassoussi, 1976):

(1) One model is used for all three levels of lift.

(2) One model is used for both males and females and such does not have gender as a variable.

(3) The model requires only two measurements of maximum isometric strengths: back strength and leg strength.

Table 15.9 shows these above-mentioned models, as summarised by Genaidy *et al.* (1988). Tables 15.10 and 15.11 give values for C_1, C_2, and C_3 for the models developed by Aghazadeh.

Ayoub *et al.* (1978b) conducted a study using industrial subjects to generate capacity data. Based on those data predictive models for the working population as well as individuals for different height levels as a function of operator and task variables were developed. Six different levels of lift were utilised (floor to knuckle, floor to shoulder, knuckle to shoulder, knuckle to reach, and shoulder to reach height) at rates of two, four, six and eight lifts/min. Three different box sizes were: $12 \times 7 \times 12$, $12 \times 7 \times 18$, and $12 \times 7 \times 24$ (width × depth × length, in). Various strength and anthropometric measurements were recorded for each subject. A stepwise linear regression analysis was employed to select the best prediction model. These models estimated an individual's lifting capacity.

Mital and Ayoub (1980) improved on the predictive models for lifting from data developed by Ayoub *et al.* (1978a). These models, in the form of regression equations, predicted an individual's MAW by using isometric strengths and personal characteristics (age, sex, and anthropometric variables). These revised models are shown in Table 15.12. Table 15.13 shows the multipliers to correct the predicted lift from the models for frequencies ranging from one to eight lifts/min.

Asfour (1980) proposed psychophysical lifting/lowering capacity models for two height ranges (start at floor or at 30 in above the floor). The variables incorporated in the models were the subject's body weight, frequency of lift, box size (width and length), and angle of body twist.

Garg and Ayoub (1980) conducted a psychophysical study to develop lifting capacity models by using a single strength (static or dynamic) variable. These models are attractive because of their simple form. They showed that the static vertical lift strength measured at the origin of lift significantly underestimated the dynamic lifting capacity as determined by psychophysical methodology. When the static vertical lift strength was performed closer to the body, such a bias was eliminated. They concluded that specific static strength tests must be carefully constructed to predict accurately a person's dynamic lifting capacity.

The arguments against lifting capacity models based on static strength tests are that actual lifting is dynamic in nature although temporary static components are involved (Aghazadeh and Ayoub, 1985; Kamon *et al.*, 1982). Consequently, dynamic strength

Table 15.9 Summary of psychophysical models.

Researchers	Dependent variables	Height level	Male	Female	Both	Model
McConville and Hertzberg (1966)	Maximum weight of lift*	Floor to knuckle	X			Predicted lift = 60 – (width of box in inches
Poulsen (1970)	Maximum weight of lift	Floor to table			X	Predicted lift = 1.40 (max. isometric back st.) – 0.50 (body wt)
		Table to head			X	Predicted lift = 0.50 (sum of right and left max. isometric arm push)
McDaniel (1972); Ayoub and El-Bassoussi (1976)	Load of lift**	Floor to knuckle	X			Predicted lift = 172.36 + 0.02 $(ht)^2$ – 2.73 (static end.)^2 + 0.02 (RPI)(arm st.) + 0.05 (RPI)(back st.) – 2.51 (F1/dynamic end.)
	Load of lift	Floor to knuckle		X		Predicted lift = – 24.03 + 0.19 $(RPI)^2$ + 0.006 (arm st.)(leg st.)
	Load of lift	Floor to knuckle			X	Predicted lift = 11.93 – 1.12 (back st.) + 0.16 $(RPI)^2$ + 0.005 (back st.)^2 – 8.81 (static end.)^2 – 0.1 (sex)(F1) + 0.06 (ht) (RPI) + 0.03 (RPI)(leg st.) – 0.002 (back st.)(leg st.) – 0.03 (leg st.)(stat. end.) + 0.11 (static end.)(F1)
Dryden (1973)	Load of lift	Knuckle to shoulder	X			Predicted lift = 0.0 + 0.83 (chest circumference) + 0.56 (dynamic end.)
Ayoub and El-Bassoussi (1976)	Load of lift	Knuckle to shoulder		X		Predicted lift = 0.0 + 3.81 (RPI) – 1.47 (ht)(F1/1000) – 0.31 (RPI)(static end.) + 1.23 (percent fat)(F1/1000)
	Load of lift	Knuckle to shoulder			X	Predicted lift = 25.12 + 0.38 (sex) (dynamic end.)
Knipfer (1974)	Load of lift	Shoulder to reach	X			Predicted lift = 4.91 + 0.2 (back st.) – 0.02 (shoulder st.) + 0.43 (age)
Aghazadeh (1974)	Load of lift	Floor to knuckle, knuckle to shoulder, shoulder to reach	X			Predicted lift = $(C_1 S + C_2)C_3$ (C_1, C_2 = factor of freq. and height of lift; S = (back st. × leg st.)/1000
Ayoub and El-Bassoussi (1976)	Load of lift	Shoulder to reach		X		Predicted lift = 0.34 (wt) + 0.84 (dynamic end.) + 0.34 (forearm circumference)
	Load of lift	Shoulder to reach			X	Predicted lift = 5.23 (sex) + 0.005 (shoulder st.) + 0.19 (horizontal push st.)
	Load of lift	Floor to knuckle, knuckle to shoulder, shoulder to reach			X	Predicted lift = 13.19 + 13.85 (sex) + 0.26 (dynamic end.)

Table 15.9 (Cont'd)

Researchers	Dependent	Height level variables	Male	Female	Both	Model
Ayoub et al. (1978a)	Load of lift + body weight	Floor to knuckle			X	Predicted lift = −72.17 −28.33 (sex) + 24.24 (wt code) + 0.14 (arm st.) − 0.55 (age) + 1.23 (shoulder ht) + 0.06 (back st.) + 4.91 (abdominal depth) + 1.76 (dynamic end.)
	Load of lift + body weight	Floor to shoulder			X	Predicted lift = 145.41 − 16.17 (sex) + 11.93 (wt code) + 0.19 (arm st.) − 0.6 (age) + 1.44 (shoulder ht) + 0.08 (back st.) + 6.47 (abdominal depth) + 2.61 (dynamic end.)
	Load of lift + body weight	Floor to reach			X	Predicted lift = −41.27 − 19.45 (sex) + 16.18 (wt code) + 0.21 (arm st.) − 0.84 (age) + 0.76 (shoulder ht) + 0.07 (back st.) + 6.22 (abdominal depth) + 1.43 (dynamic end.)
	Load of lift + body weight	Knuckle to shoulder			X	Predicted lift = −55.16 − 18.45 (sex) + 11.70 (wt code) + 0.27 (arm st.) − 0.61 (age) + 0.77 (shoulder ht) + 0.11 (back st.) + 6.29 (abdominal depth) + 1.42 (dynamic end.)
	Load of lift + body weight	Knuckle to reach			X	Predicted lift = −79.19 − 18.92 (sex) + 17.27 (wt code) + 0.3 (arm st.) − 0.5 (age) + 1.09 (shoulder ht) + 0.02 (back st.) + 5.15 (abdominal depth) + 2.12 (dynamic end.)
	Load of lift + body weight	Shoulder to reach			X	Predicted lift = −37.44 − 19.58 (sex) + 20.35 (wt code) + 0.1 (arm st.) − 0.6 (age) + 0.89 (shoulder ht) + 0.1 (back st.) + 4.73 (abdominal depth) + 1.09 (dynamic end.)

(From Ayoub et al., 1980; reprinted with permission. Copyright 1980 by the Human Factors and Ergonomics Society. All rights reserved.)

$RPI = \text{body ht}/\sqrt[3]{\text{body wt}}$

F1 = 100 × duration of the step exercise (s)/2 × pulse recovery sum
* Maximum weight subjects could lift for non-repetitive lifting
** Maximum weight subjects were willing to lift for repetitive lifting
Lift ht* = 127 cm for floor to shoulder and 76 for shoulder to shoulder
See Table 15.10 for C_1 and C_2; see Table 15.11 for C_3.

Table 15.10 Factors for predicting acceptable amount of lift for different heights at different frequencies.

Frequency		C_1	C_2
		Knuckle height	
Frequency of	1	1.87	20.1
	2	1.77	19.1
	3	1.66	17.9
	4	1.57	16.9
	5	1.48	15.9
	6	1.37	14.7
		Shoulder height	
Frequency of	1	2.49	43.6
	2	2.37	33.9
	3	2.22	29.5
	4	2.09	26.7
	5	1.97	24.6
	6	1.82	22.4
		Reach height	
Frequency of	1	1.87	25.1
	2	1.79	26.8
	3	1.68	23.0
	4	1.57	20.6
	5	1.48	18.9
	6	1.37	17.2

(From Ayoub *et al.*, 1978b).

Table 15.11 Factors for box size.

Box length (dimension in sagittal plane)	Box size factor, C_3
10	1.00
12	0.98
14	0.95
16	0.93
18	0.90
20	0.88
22	0.86
24	0.83
26	0.81
28	0.78
30	0.76

(From Ayoub *et al.*, 1978a).

should play a more important role in lifting than static strength. In recent years, several researchers have developed psychophysical lifting capacity models based on dynamic strength tests.

Pytel and Kamon (1981) adapted a portable commercially available device ('Mini-Gym', model 101) to measure isokinetic dynamic strength. A lifting experiment was

Table 15.12 Coefficients for models for predicting maximum acceptable weight of lift (MAW) plus body weight (pounds).

Height of lift	Constant term	Sex code*	Arm st.	Age	Shoulder ht.	Back st.	Abdominal depth	Dynamic end.	(Arm st.)²	(Age)²
FK	-19.444	-15.630	1.051	-0.661	—	—	—	10.250	-0.004	—
FS	-108.770	-7.109	1.372	-1.894	—	0.448	7.685	14.809	-0.007	0.016
FR	-850.993	—	1.449	-2.253	10.687	0.078	8.026	18.193	-0.007	0.018
KS	-148.125	-6.688	1.521	-2.161	1.015	—	7.658	14.881	-0.008	0.020
KR	-194.177	-6.679	1.394	-2.011	1.391	—	7.129	18.460	-0.006	0.017
SR	-904.215	—	0.964	-0.759	10.131	0.110	15.026	18.078	-0.004	—

Height of lift	Shoulder height²	Back strength²	Abdominal depth²	Dynamic end.²	Mean W (males)	Mean W (females)	Mean error (W) (pre.–actual)	SD of error in W	Std. error of mean for W	R²
FK	0.004	-0.001	0.146	-1.213	61.170	37.120	-8.620	20.630	2.360	0.850
FS	0.005	0.0003	—	-1.682	51.210	21.080	-0.120	19.800	2.490	0.903
FR	-0.034	—	—	-1.945	29.120	28.140	2.610	23.280	2.880	0.877
KS	—	0.0004	—	-1.598	54.470	31.970	-4.910	22.100	2.530	0.893
KR	—	-0.0004	—	-1.988	53.540	26.220	-7.460	19.590	2.260	0.902
SR	-0.031	—	-0.174	-1.915	42.620	25.780	12.080	20.680	2.350	0.873

(From Mital and Ayoub, 1980; reprinted with permission. Copyright 1980 by the Human Factors and Ergonomics Society. All rights reserved.)
Note: Age is in years; strengths (arm and back) are in pounds; body dimensions are in centimetres; dynamic endurance is in minutes.
* Sex code: 0 for males; 1 for females
FK: floor to knuckle; FS: floor to shoulder; FR: floor to reach; KS: knuckle to shoulder; KR: knuckle to reach; SR: shoulder to reach.

Table 15.13 Multipliers to adjust the maximum acceptable weight of lift for frequency.

Height of lift	Sex	Frequency (lifts/min)					
		1	2	4	5	6	8
Floor to knuckle	Male	1.093	1.067	1.015	1.0	0.985	0.934
	Female	1.214	1.134	1.053	1.0	0.946	0.785
Floor to shoulder	Male	1.081	1.056	1.008	1.0	0.992	0.934
	Female	1.165	1.113	1.007	1.0	0.992	0.975
Floor to reach	Male	1.126	1.089	1.016	1.0	0.984	0.827
	Female	1.144	1.106	1.030	1.0	0.970	0.956
Knuckle to shoulder	Male	1.110	1.074	1.002	1.0	0.984	0.930
	Female	1.280	1.210	1.070	1.0	0.930	0.790
Knuckle to reach	Male	1.244	1.172	1.028	1.0	0.971	0.895
	Female	1.017	1.009	1.008	1.0	0.991	0.935
Shoulder to reach	Male	1.071	1.059	1.036	1.0	0.964	0.874
	Female	1.196	1.147	1.049	1.0	0.950	0.901

(From Mital and Ayoub, 1980; reprinted with permission. Copyright 1980 by the Human Factors and Ergonomics Society. All rights reserved.)

Table 15.14 Prediction models developed by Kamon *et al.* (1982).

LC = 1.04*EF + 330;	r = 0.49
LC = 1.65*ES + 251;	r = 0.47
LC = 0.46*BE + 380;	r = 0.51
LC = 0.54*LS + 304;	r = 0.47
IL = 0.96*BE + 254;	r = 0.65

where:

  LC = lifting capacity (Newtons)
  EF = elbow flexion, maximal contraction one arm
  ES = elbow strength, dynamic flexion of two arms (isokinetic strength)
  BE = back extension, maximum voluntary contraction
  IL = isometric lift, static simulated lift
  LS = lifting strength, simulated dynamic lift motion

designed to lift a tote box (44 cm × 30 cm × 12 cm) with handles from the floor to 113 cm height. A simple psychophysical model was developed using a simple strength test procedure, a concise form of the prediction models. However, R^2 values were relatively low in this study. Only one lifting range (floor to 113 cm height) and one lifting frequency were studied.

Kamon *et al.* (1982) employed the same test procedure as Pytel and Kamon (1981) to test 228 male steelmill workers. Two psychophysical lifting models were developed by using a single static strength measure (back extension maximum voluntary contraction) or a single dynamic strength measure (lifting strength). The generated models are in the form of linear regression equations as shown in Table 15.14.

Aghazadeh (1983) studied the relationship between box/bag lifting capacity and the subject's strength test. Three task-related variables and five operator-related variables

Table 15.15   Prediction models for the maximum acceptable weight of lift using dynamic strength.

Model code	Constant term	CONTAINR coefficient	LIFTTYPE coefficient	FRQNCY coefficient	DYNSTKS coefficient	R^2
BXBDG	54.72	−9.68	−0.11	−2.21	0.27	0.726
BGD	43.18	−	−0.18	−1.91	0.21	0.594
BXD	37.21	−	−0.03	−2.52	0.34	0.775
BXBGDKS	41.37	−7.52	−	−2.21	−0.36	0.778
BXBGDFS	51.02	−9.68	−	−2.21	0.27	0.706
BGDKS	29.94	−	−	−1.87	0.30	0.725
BGDFS	43.96	−	−	−1.94	0.11	0.452
BXDKS	30.24	−	−	−2.55	0.41	0.795
BXDFS	41.82	−	−	−2.49	0.27	0.798

(From Aghazadeh, 1983).
Container code: CONTAINR = 1 for box and 2 for bag
Lift type code: LIFTTYPE = 20 for knuckle to shoulder height lift and 50 for floor to shoulder height lift
Frequency code: FRQNCY = 2 for 2 lifts/min and 6 for 6 lifts/min
Knuckle to shoulder dynamic strength code: DYNSTKS, units are in foot pounds
General models for box and bag lifting (code BXBGD)
Models for bag lifting only (code BGD)
Models for box lifting only (code BXD)
Models for box and bag lifting from knuckle to shoulder height (code BXBGDKS)
Models for box and bag lifting from floor to shoulder height (code BXBGDFS)
Models for bag lifting from knuckle to shoulder height (code BGDKS)
Models for bag lifting from floor to shoulder height (code BGDFS)
Models for box lifting from knuckle to shoulder height (code BXDKS)
Models for box lifting from floor to shoulder height (code BXDFS).

were studied. Task variables were container type (bag or box), frequency of lift (two or six lifts/min) and lifting ranges floor to shoulder and knuckle to shoulder (FS and KS). Operator-related variables were static strength (arm, stooped back, standing back, composite, shoulder and leg), dynamic strength measured using Cybex isokinetic strength equipment (FS and KS), endurance (static and dynamic), PWC, subject's height and weight. Nine dynamic models and nine static models were developed (see Table 15.15). Both static models and dynamic models could predict the maximum acceptable lifting capacity with a reasonable degree of accuracy (R^2 with the range of 0.452 to 0.862). Aghazadeh and Ayoub (1985) developed models for prediction of weight lifting capacity of individuals incorporating static strengths and dynamic strengths of the individual in a simulated lifting position and task variables: height and frequency of lift. It was concluded that both the dynamic and static models could predict the maximum acceptable amount of lift with a reasonable degree of accuracy. The use of the dynamic model resulted in less absolute error between the actual and predicted load than the static model (reduction of 44 per cent).

Jiang (1984) developed prediction models for both individual and combined MMH activities and examined the relationship between individual and combined MMH activities. MMH capacity was defined as the maximum weight the subject was willing to handle plus his or her body weight for a period of one hour under the variable task conditions. Each activity was conducted under three different frequencies: one time maximum, one handling per min, and six handlings per min. The prediction models for the capacities of individual MMH activities were developed based on the isoinertial six feet weight incremental lifting test or the isometric back strength test. The isoinertial 6-ft incremental weight lifting test was proved to be the best predictor for the individual MMH activities. Since this type of strength test involved both static strength to overcome the inertial resistance and dynamic strength to move the weight to a pre-assigned location, it was recommended as the most promising single screening test.

Jiang *et al.* (1986) developed models to predict capacity for combined material handling activities. Four individual MMH activities were studied: lifting from floor to knuckle height (LFK); lifting from knuckle to shoulder height (LKS); lowering from knuckle to floor height (LOW); and carrying for 3.4 m (C). Three combined MMH activities were studied: lifting from floor to knuckle height and carrying 3.4 m (LC); lifting from floor to knuckle height, carrying 3.4 m, and lifting from knuckle to shoulder height (LCL); and lifting from floor to knuckle height, carrying 3.4 m, and lowering from knuckle to floor height (LCLO).

Three different approaches were used for the modelling of combined MMH capacities: modelling based on one limiting individual MMH capacity, modelling based on isoinertial 1.83 m maximum strength, and modelling based on fuzzy-set theory (the fuzzy-set theory model will be omitted from this discussion). Models were developed using simple and multiple regression, and were evaluated according to goodness of fit (in terms of R^2 values) and PRESS statistics. Both advantages and disadvantages were found for both model types. Unfortunately, these models have yet to be fully validated.

The basis for the *first* approach uses the limiting individual MMH capacity as a predictor. The limiting capacity usually occurs at the most stressful individual activity (or at the weakest joint of the body) used in handling the task. The limiting activity was derived from the minimal capacity of all the individual capacity elements that made up the MMH task. The individual models (for each of the three combined MMH activities – at each of the three frequency conditions) and their corresponding limiting activity and R^2 values are shown in Table 15.16.

The key advantage of these limiting activity-based models is found in the incredibly high R^2 values. Thus, these models had the best fit to the experimental data, in terms of R^2 values. As a result, if the limiting individual MMH capacity is known, the combined MMH capacity can be predicted accurately, using the individual MMH capacity. The close relationship between combined activity and limiting individual activity provides a good framework for job design/redesign that involves combined MMH activity. Several disadvantages exist, however. First, the relationship between combined and individual limiting capacities has not been developed. Next, in order to have the best predicted results, these models should only apply within the range of the independent variables used in this study. Furthermore, it should be again noted that this study only encompassed the participation of 12 (male) subjects, a small sample. Finally, the testing procedure for limiting individual activities should follow the testing procedure used in this study.

The basis for the *second* approach uses isoinertial strength of lifting from floor to a height of 1.83 m (this isoinertial strength test will be denoted at T1). The principle involved in the modelling came from an effort to match an individual's physical condition to his MMH capacities. These models were developed and selected according to simplicity, goodness of fit, and representation of variables. Table 15.17 shows the individual

Table 15.16   Combined activity models by Jiang *et al.* (1986).

Combined activity	R^2	Limiting activity
LCM = 0.762 + (0.953*LFKM)	0.952	LFKM
LCLM = 3.015 + (0.973*LKSM)	0.967	LKSM
LCLOM = −17.805 + (1.602*LFKM)	0.966	LFKM
LC1 = 16.903 + (0.809*LFK1)	0.980	LFK1
LCL1 = −4.201 + (1.022*LKS1)	0.963	LKS1
LCLO1 = 27.777 + (0.685*LFK1)	0.915	LFK1
LC6 = −1.449 + (0.969*LFK6)	0.941	LFK6
LCL6 = 7.126 + (0.883*LKS6)	0.932	LKS6
LCLO6 = 6.272 + (0.867*LFK6)	0.920	LFK6

Lifting F-K (LFK):
 LFKM – LFK at the frequency of one time maximum
 LFK1 – LFK at the frequency of 1 handling/min
 LFK6 – LFK at the frequency of 6 handlings/min
Lifting K-S (LKS):
 LKSM – LKS at the frequency of one time maximum
 LKS1 – LKS at the frequency of 1 handling/min
 LKS6 – LKS at the frequency of 6 handlings/min
Lowering K-S (LOW):
 LOWM – LOW at the frequency of one time maximum
 LOW1 – LOW at the frequency of 1 handling/min
 LOW6 – LOW at the frequency of 6 handlings/min
Two hand front carrying for 14 feet (C):
 CM – C at the frequency of one time maximum
 C1 – C at the frequency of 1 handling/min
 C6 – C at the frequency of 6 handlings/min
Lifting F-K + carrying 14 ft (LC):
 LCM – LC at the frequency of one time maximum
 LC1 – LC at the frequency of 1 handling/min
 LC6 – LC at the frequency of 6 handlings/min
Lifting F-K + carrying 14 ft + lifting K-S (LCL):
 LCLM – LCL at the frequency of one time maximum
 LCL1 – LCL at the frequency of 1 handling/min
 LCL6 – LCL at the frequency of 6 handlings/min
Lifting F-K + carrying 14 ft + lowering K-F (LCLO):
 LCLOM – LCLO at the frequency of one time maximum
 LCLO1 – LCLO at the frequency of 1 handling/min
 LCLO6 – LCLO at the frequency of 6 handlings/min

models for each of the three combined MMH activities at each of the three frequency conditions and their corresponding R^2 and PRESS values.

Some of the advantages of isoinertial strength-based models include: (1) combined MMH capacities can be predicted by simple strength testing which can be conducted in less than five minutes; (2) the combined MMH capacity can be predicted from strength testing, directly; (3) no knowledge of individual capacities is required; and (4) the isoinertial strength tests are more representative of actual industrial lifting activities than other tests. The disadvantages of isoinertial strength-based models are very similar to those dis-

Table 15.17   Models to predict combined activities using 6 ft incremental lift test.

The models	R^2
$LCM = 129.749 - (1.642*T1) + (0.029249*T1^2)$	0.913
$LCLM = 165.945 - (2.545*T1) + (0.028413*T1^2)$	0.885
$LCLOM = 126.811 - (1.884*T1) + (0.033231*T1^2)$	0.916
$LC1 = 144.735 - (2.312*T1) + (0.027586*T1^2)$	0.947
$LCL1 = 75.280 - (0.009*T1) + (0.007132*T1^2)$	0.854
$LCLO1 = 139.556 - (2.092*T1) + (0.024567*T1^2)$	0.923
$LC6 = 99.641 - (1.042*T1) + (0.015411*T1^2)$	0.790
$LCL6 = 98.427 - (0.999*T1) + (0.014337*T1^2)$	0.811
$LCLO6 = 120.787 - (1.734*T1) + (0.020301*T1^2)$	0.846

(From Jiang *et al.*, 1986).

advantages presented above, for the limiting-activity-based models. First, a small sample size of 12 subjects was used to develop the above models. Also, the application of these models should be within the range of the T1 values used in this study (47.7–79.5 kg). Finally, the testing procedure using T1 in this study should be followed in order to measure the isoinertial strength of T1.

Most MMH prediction models have focused on lifting activities. Few models however were developed to predict capacity for lowering, pushing, pulling, and carrying tasks. These are briefly presented in Tables 15.18, 15.19, 15.20 and 15.21.

All of the models presented above can be used to predict individual capacities. Models to estimate population capacities have also been developed. Ayoub *et al.* (1983) developed population models to estimate the lifting capacities for the various percentiles of the population. These models were based on the data generated by Ayoub *et al.* (1978a) (see earlier section for more details on the variables in the study). Table 15.22 shows these models for both males and females.

CONFLICTS BETWEEN CRITERIA BASED ON THE VARIOUS APPROACHES

It is not surprising that criteria based on the principles of biomechanics, psychophysics, and physiology often provide MMH limits that are in conflict. These conflicts pose confusion for practitioners, and make selecting a proper limit troublesome. An example of the conflicts between the criteria is shown in Figure 15.3, which illustrates recommended loads as a function of frequency for a floor to shoulder lift. The example is based on Kim's (1990) models using a 650 kg spinal compression limit and a 1 l/min physiological criteria for males. The biomechanical approach results in high-recommended weights for high-frequency tasks and the physiological approach results in high-recommended loads at low frequencies. The figure also illustrates how the psychophysical approach may be in conflict with the physiological approach. The most conservative approach to these conflicts is to consider all criteria simultaneously in order to estimate the recommended weight for lift as was proposed by Kim (1990). The NIOSH equations of 1981 and 1991 use an approach considering all three criteria to estimate the recommended weight limit (RWL).

Table 15.18 Lowering capacity prediction models.

Source	Height of lower	Gender	Model	R^2
Asfour (1980)	HL1	Male	LC = 7.2904 −0.4887*(10** − 6)*BS1*BS2*AT*F*HL1 + 613153.53*(10** − 6)*BW − 145.03*(10** − 6)*BS*(F**3)	0.72
	HL2	Male	LC = 0.9868 − 48.2692*(10** − 6)*F*BS1*BS2*AT + 367670.51*(10** − 6)*BS − 65.25*(10** − 6)*BW*(F**3)	0.70
Mital (1983c)	All	Both	LC = 15.12 − 7.85*(1/BS1) + 131.53*(1/HL3) − 0.092*(1/F) − 2.75*LN(F) + 1.58*G*HL + 0.344*G*F + 0.034*BS1*HL + 0.002*HS3*F + 0.33*HL*F	0.94

(From Genaidy *et al.*, 1988; reprinted with permission. Copyright 1988 by the Human Factors and Ergonomics Society. All rights reserved.)
HL1: height of lower above the floor (cm)
HL2: height of lower above table height (cm)
LC: lowering capacity (kg)
BS1: box length (cm)
BS2: box width (cm)
AT: angle of twist (dge)
F: frequency of lower (times/min)
BW: body weight (kg)
G: gender (G = 0 for male and 1 for female)
HL: height of lower (HL = 1 for floor to knuckle, 2 for knuckle to shoulder, and 3 for shoulder to reach)
HL3: vertical distance of lower (cm).
The model developed by Mital (1983c) was based on the data generated by Snook (1978); all models are applicable only for the free-style lifting technique.

Table 15.19 Pushing capacity prediction models.

Source	Gender	Model	R^2
Mital (1983c)	Male	PC = 17.29 − 0.166*HD − 11.45*F + 0.0013*(HD**2) + 5.60*(F**2) + 0.001*(1/F) + 0.047*HD*F	0.968
	Female	PC = 10.31 − 0.133*HD − 16.15*F − 0.154*LN(F) + 6.17*EXP(F) + 0.056*HD*F	0.960

(From Genaidy *et al.*, 1988; reprinted with permission. Copyright 1988 by the Human Factors and Ergonomics Society. All rights reserved.)
PC: pushing capacity (kg)
HD: horizontal distance of push (m)
F: frequency of push (times/min).
The model developed by Mital (1983c) was based on the data generated by Snook (1978).

Table 15.20   Pulling capacity prediction models.

Source	Gender	Model	R^2
Mital (1983c)	Male	PC = 18.48 − 0.685*F − 0.0003*(VD**2) + 0.003*VD*F − 0.5*LN(F)	0.978
	Female	PC = 15.03 − 0.394*F − 0.0003*(VD**2) − 0.331*LN(F)	0.945

(From Genaidy et al., 1988; reprinted with permission. Copyright 1988 by the Human Factors and Ergonomics Society. All rights reserved.)
PC: pulling capacity (kg)
VD: vertical distance of pull (m)
F: frequency of pull (times/min).
The model developed by Mital (1983c) was based on the data generated by Snook (1978).

Table 15.21   Carrying capacity prediction models.

Source	Gender	Model	R^2
Mital (1983c)	Male	CC = 77.27 − 12.46*LN(VD) − 2.4*LN(HD) − 0.011*(1/F) − 2.01*LN(F)	0.962
	Female	CC = 46.49 − 0.239*HD − 7.12*LN(VD) − 0.0073*(1/F) − 1.44*LN(F) + 0.0003*VD*HD*F	0.955

(From Genaidy et al., 1988; reprinted with permission. Copyright 1988 by the Human Factors and Ergonomics Society. All rights reserved.)
CC: carrying capacity (kg)
VD: height at which load is carried (cm)
F: frequency of carry (times/min)
HD: horizontal distance of carry (m).
The model developed by Mital (1983c) was based on the data generated by Snook (1978).

Table 15.22   Lifting capacity prediction models.

Gender	Height of lift	Frequency (times/min)	Box size	Model
Male	F-K	0.1 < F < 1.0	12 < BS < 18	LC = [57.2*F**(−0.184697)] + [1.65*(18 − BS)] + [Z*16.86*F**(−0.174197)]
	F-K	0.1 < F < 1.0	BX > 18	LC = [57.2*F**(−0.184697)] + [0/8*(18 − BS)] + [Z*16.86*F**(−0.174197)]
	F-K	1.0 < F < 12.0	12 < BS < 18	LC = [57.2 − 2.0*(F − 1)] + [1.65*(18 − BS)] + [Z*(16.86 − 0.5943*(F − 1))]
	F-K	1.0 < F < 12.0	BS > 18	LC = [57.2 − 2.0*(F − 1)] + [0.8*(18 − BS)] + [Z*(16.86 − 0.5964*(F − 1))]
Male	F-S	0.1 < F < 1.0	12 < BS < 18	LC = [51.2*F**(−0.184697)] + [1.65*(18 − BS)] + [Z*15.09*F**(−0.174197)]
	F-S	0.1 < F < 1.0	BS > 18	LC = [51.2*F**(−0.184697)] + [0.8*(18 − BS)] + [Z*15.09*F**(−0.174197)]
	F-S	1.0 < F < 12.0	12 < BS < 18	LC = [51.2 − 2.0*(F − 1)] + [1.65*(18 − BS)] + [Z*(15.09 − 0.5338*(F − 1))]
	F-S	1.0 < F < 12.0	BS > 18	LC = [51.2 − 2.0*(F − 1)] + [0.8*(18 − BS)] + [Z*(15.09 − 0.5338*(F − 1))]

Table 15.22 (Cont'd)

Gender	Height of lift	Frequency (times/min)	Box size	Model
Male	F-R	$0.1 < F < 1.0$	$12 < BS < 18$	$LC = [49.1*F**(-0.184697)] + [1.65*(18 - BS)] + [Z*14.47*F**(-0.174197)]$
	F-R	$0.1 < F < 1.0$	$BS > 18$	$LC = [49.1*F**(-0.184697)] + [0.8*(18 - BS)] + [Z*14.47*F**(-0.174197)]$
	F-R	$1.0 < F < 12.0$	$12 < BS < 18$	$LC = [49.1 - 2.0*(F - 1)] + [1.65*(18 - BS)] + [Z*(14.47 - 0.5119*(F - 1))]$
	F-R	$1.0 < F < 12.0$	$BS > 18$	$LC = [49.1 - 2.0*(F - 1)] + [0.8*(18 - BS)] + [Z*(14.47 - 0.5119*(F - 1))]$
Male	K-S	$0.1 < F < 1.0$	$12 < BS < 18$	$LC = [52.8*F**(-0.138650)] + [1.10*(18 - BS)] + [Z*14.67*F**(-0.156762)]$
	K-S	$0.1 < F < 1.0$	$BS > 18$	$LC = [52.8*F**(-0.138650)] + [0.8*(18 - BS)] + [Z*14.67*F**(-0.156762)]$
	K-S	$1.0 < F < 12.0$	$12 < BS < 18$	$LC = [52.8 - 2.0*(F - 1)] + [1.10*(18 - BS)] + [Z*(14.67 - 0.5534*(F - 1))]$
	K-S	$1.0 < F < 12.0$	$BS > 18$	$LC = [52.8 - 2.0*(F - 1)] + [0.8*(18 - BS)] + [Z*(14.67 - 0.5534*(F - 1))]$
Male	K-R	$0.1 < F < 1.0$	$12 < BS < 18$	$LC = [50.0*F**(-0.138650)] + [1.10*(18 - BS)] + [Z*13.89*F**(-0.156762)]$
	K-R	$0.1 < F < 1.0$	$BS > 18$	$LC = [50.0*F**(-0.138650)] + [0.8*(18 - BS)] + [Z*13.89*F**(-0.156762)]$
	K-R	$1.0 < F < 12.0$	$12 < BS < 18$	$LC = [50.0 - 2.0*(F - 1)] + [1.10*(18 - BS)] + [Z*13.89 - 0.5240*(F - 1))]$
	K-R	$1.0 < F < 12.0$	$BS > 18$	$LC = [50.0 - 2.0*(F - 1)] + [0.8*(18 - BS)] + [Z*13.89 - 0.5240*(F - 1))]$
Male	S-R	$0.1 < F < 1.0$	$12 < BS < 18$	$LC = [48.4*F**(-0.138650)] + [1.10*(18 - BS)] + [Z*13.45*F**(-0.156762)]$
	S-R	$0.1 < F < 1.0$	$BS > 18$	$LC = [48.4*F**(-0.138650)] + [0.8*(18 - BS)] + [Z*13.45*F**(-0.156762)]$
	S-R	$1.0 < F < 12.0$	$12 < BS < 18$	$LC = [48.4 - 2.0*(F - 1)] + [1.10*(18 - BS)] + [Z*(13.45 - 0.5074*(F - 1))]$
	S-R	$1.0 < F < 12.0$	$BS > 18$	$LC = [48.4 - 2.0*(F - 1)] + [0.8*(18 - BS)] + [Z*(13.45 - 0.5074*(F - 1))]$
Female	F-K	$0.1 < F < 1.0$	$12 < BS < 18$	$LC = [37.4*F**(-0.187818)] + [1.10*(18 - BS)]*[Z*6.87*F**(-0.251605)]$
	F-K	$0.1 < F < 1.0$	$BS > 18$	$LC = [37.4*F**(-0.187818)] + [0.4*(18 - BS)] + [Z*6.87*F**(-0.251605)]$
	F-K	$1.0 < F < 12.0$	$12 < BS < 18$	$LC = [37.4 - 1.1*(F - 1)] + [1.10*(18 - BS)] + [Z*(6.87 - 0.1564*(F - 1))]$
	F-K	$1.0 < F < 12.0$	$BS > 18$	$LC = [37.4 - 1.1*(F - 1)] + [0.40*(18 - BS)] + [Z*(6.87 - 0.1564*(F - 1))]$
Female	F-S	$0.1 < F < 1.0$	$12 < BS < 18$	$LC = [31.1*F**(-0.187818)] + [1.10*(18 - BS)] + [Z*5.71*F**(-0.251605)]$
	F-S	$0.1 < F < 1.0$	$BS > 18$	$LC = [31.1*F**(-0.187818)] + [0.4*(18 - BS)] + [Z*5.71*F**(-0.251605)]$
	F-S	$1.0 < F < 12.0$	$12 < BS > 18$	$LC = [31.1 - 1.1*(F - 1)] + [1.10*(18 - BS)] + [Z*(5.71 - 0.1300*(F - 1))]$
	F-S	$1.0 < F < 12.0$	$BS > 18$	$LC = [31.1 - 1.1*(F - 1)] + [0.4*(18 - BS)] + [Z*(5.71 - 0.1300*(F - 1))]$

Table 15.22   (Cont'd)

Gender	Height of lift	Frequency (times/min)	Box size	Model
Female	F-R	0.1 < F < 1.0	12 < BS < 18	LC = [28.1*F**(−0.187818)] + [1.10*(18 − BS)] + [Z*5.16*F**(−0.251605)]
	F-R	0.1 < F < 1.0	BS > 18	LC = [28.1*F**(−0.187818)] + [0.4*(18 − BS)] + [Z*5.16*F**(−0.251605)]
	F-R	1.0 < F < 12.0	BS > 18	LC = [28.1 − 1.1*(F − 1)] + [0.4*(18 − BS)] + [Z*(5.16 − 0.1175*(F − 1))]
Female	K-S	0.1 < F < 1.0	12 < BS < 18	LC = [30.8*F**(−0.156150)] + [0.55*(18 − BS)] + [Z*5.66*F**(−0.258700)]
	K-S	0.1 < F < 1.0	BS > 18	LC = [30.8*F**(−0.156150)] + [0.2*(18 − BS)] + [Z*5.66*F**(−0.258700)]
Female	K-S	1.0 < F < 12.0	12 < BS < 18	LC = [30.8 − 1.1*(F − 1)] + [0.55*(18 − BS)] + [Z*(5.66 − 0.1289*(F − 1))]
	K-S	1.0 < F < 12.0	BS > 18	LC = [30.8 − 1.1*(F − 1)] + [0.2*(18 − BS)] + [Z*(5.66) − 0.1289*(F − 1))]
Female	K-R	0.1 < F < 1.0	12 < BS < 18	LC = [27.3*F**(−0.156150)] + [0.55*(18 − BS)] + [Z*5.01*F**(−0.258700)]
	K-R	0.1 < F < 1.0	BS > 18	LC = [27.3*F**(0.156150)] + [0.2*(18 − BS)] + [Z*5.01*F**(−0.258700)]
	K-R	1.0 < F < 12.0	12 < BS < 18	LC = [27.3 − 1.1*(F − 1)] + [0.55*(18 − BS)] + [Z*(5.01 − 0.1141*(F − 1))]
	K-R	1.0 < F < 12.0	BS > 18	LC = [27.3 − 1.1*(F − 1)] + [0.20*(18 − BS)] + [Z*(5.01 − 0.1141*(F − 1))]
Female	S-R	0.1 < F < 1.0	12 < BS < 18	LC = [26.4*F**(−0.156150)] + [0.55*(18 − BS)] + [Z*4.85*F**(−0.258700)]
	S-R	0.1 < F < 1.0	BS > 18	LC = [26.4*F**(−0.156150)] + [0.2*(18 − BS)] + [Z*4.85*F**(−0.258700)]
	S-R	1.0 < F < 12.0	12 < BS < 18	LC = [26.4 − 1.1*(F − 1)] + [0.55*(18 − BS)] + [Z*(4.85 − 0.1104*(F − 1))]
	S-R	1.0 < F < 12.0	BS > 18	LC = [26.4 − 1.1*(F − 1)] + [0.2*(18 − BS)] + [Z*(4.85 − 0.1104*(F − 1))]

(From Ayoub et al., 1983).
F: frequency of lift
BS: box size (inches)
LC: lifting capacity (pounds)
F-K: floor to knuckle
F-S: floor to shoulder
F-R: floor to reach
K-S: knuckle to shoulder
K-R: knuckle to reach
S-R: shoulder to reach
Z: score of population percentage from normal tables (Z = −1.6449 for 95%, Z = −1.2816 for 90%, Z = −1.0364 for 85%, Z = −0.6745 for 75%, Z = 0.0 for 50%, Z = 0.6745 to 25%, Z = 1.0364 for 15%, Z = 1.2816 for 10%, and Z = 1.6449 for 5%).
Models are based on the data generated by Snook (1978) and Ayoub et al. (1978a) and are applicable only for the free-style lifting technique.

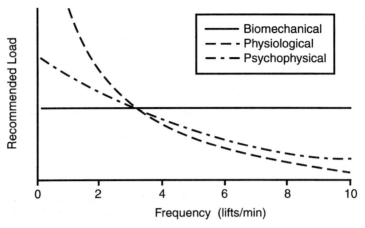

Figure 15.3 Example of conflict among biomechanical, psychophysical, and physiological criteria (based on Kim's (1990) models).

THE FUTURE OF MANUAL MATERIALS HANDLING MODELLING

As documented in this chapter, previous research to model and understand the adverse effects of manual materials handling tasks on workers has come from three distinctly different approaches. Each has provided insight into the hazards of individual task components that are often encountered in many jobs. Unfortunately, each approach is specifically directed at task components and none of these approaches has proven effective at dealing with jobs in their entirety. At the present time typical manual material handling jobs have a variety of different work components that make it difficult to apply any of the three methods in a pure sense. Workers are often required to lift, carry, hold, and lower loads that vary in location and weight throughout the workday. Typical of this are the many warehousing operations currently done manually in the United States. These jobs have so many different tasks components that it is impractical to analyse each task, and even if this could be done, there is currently no agreed method of aggregating task indices of risk into a job index of risk. Workers are also increasingly being asked to rotate between several different jobs with one of the jobs having a large manual materials handling component. In addition, ten and twelve hour work shifts have become common at many work sites.

The variety of different work tasks being done by typical industrial workers presented a problem for the task oriented models presented in this chapter. Ergonomics practitioners are often confused by conflicting recommendations provided by different models and even by the same model for different tasks performed by a worker within a workday. It is the authors' opinion that future modelling efforts should and will concentrate on providing insight into the musculoskeletal risks of jobs and careers, instead of tasks. Whether this is done by combining the task level approaches documented in this chapter into a composite measure, or through an entirely different method is not entirely clear at this time. However, the greatest need in preventing manual materials handling injuries is understanding the cumulative effects of work tasks done over days, years, and even a work career.

References

ABERG, U., ELGSTRAND, K., MAGNUS, P. and LINDHOLM, A., 1968, Analysis of components and prediction of energy expenditure in manual tasks, *The International Journal of Production Research*, **6**, 189–196.

AGHAZADEH, F., 1974, Lifting Capacity as a Function of Operator and Task Variables, Unpublished MS thesis, Texas Tech University, Lubbock, TX.

AGHAZADEH, F., 1983, Simulated Dynamic Lifting Strength Models for Manual Lifting, Unpublished doctoral dissertation, Texas Tech University, Lubbock, TX.

AGHAZADEH, F. and AYOUB, M.M., 1985, A comparison of dynamic- and static-strength models for prediction of lifting capacity, *Ergonomics*, **28**(10), 1409–1417.

ANDERSON, C.K., 1983, A Biomechanical Model of the Lumbosacral Joint for Lifting Activities, Unpublished doctoral dissertation, The University of Michigan, Ann Arbor, Michigan.

AQUILANO, N.J., 1968, A physiological evaluation of time standards for strenuous work as set by stopwatch time study and two predetermined motion time data systems, *Journal of Industrial Engineering*, **19**, 425–432.

ASFOUR, S.S., 1980, Energy Cost Prediction Models for Manual Lifting and Lowering Tasks, Unpublished doctoral dissertation, Texas Tech University, Lubbock, TX.

ASFOUR, S.S., AYOUB, M.M. and GENAIDY, A.M., 1984a, A psychophysical study of the effect of task variables on lifting and lowering tasks, *Journal of Human Ergology*, **13**, 3–14.

ASFOUR, S.S., AYOUB, M.M. and MITAL, A., 1984b, Effects of an endurance and strength training programme on the lifting capability of males, *Ergonomics*, **27**, 435–442.

ASFOUR, S.S., AYOUB, M.M. and GENAIDY, A.M., 1985, Computer models for the prediction of lifting and lowering capacity, in *IEEE 1985 Proceedings of International Conference on Cybernetics and Society*, Tucson, AZ: IEEE Systems, Man, and Cybernetics Society, pp. 1092–1096.

ASFOUR, S.S., AYOUB, M.M. and GENAIDY, A.M., 1986a, A data base of physiological responses to manual lowering, in Karwowski, W. (Ed.), *Trends in Ergonomics/Human Factors III*, Amsterdam: Elsevier, pp. 811–818.

ASFOUR, S.S., AYOUB, M.M., GENAIDY, A.M. and KHALIL, T.M., 1986b, A data base of physiological responses to manual lifting, in Karwowski, W. (Ed.), *Trends in Ergonomics/ Human Factors III*, Amsterdam: Elsevier, pp. 801–809.

ASTRAND, P.O. and RODAHL, K., 1986, *Textbook of Work Physiology*, 3rd edn, New York: McGraw-Hill.

AYOUB, M.M. and EL-BASSOUSSI, M.M., 1976, Dynamic biomechanical model for sagittal lifting activities, *Proceedings of the 6th Congress of International Ergonomics Association*, pp. 355–359.

AYOUB, M.M. and MITAL, A., 1989, *Manual Materials Handling*, London: Taylor & Francis.

AYOUB, M.M., BETHEA, N.J., DEIVANAYAGAM, S., ASFOUR, S.S., BAKKEN, G.M., LILES, D., et al., 1978a, *Determination and Modeling of Lifting Capacity*, Final Report HEW [NIOSH] 5R010H-00545-02, Lubbock, TX: Texas Tech University.

AYOUB, M.M., DRYDEN, R.D., McDANIEL, J.W., KNIPFER, R.E. and AGHAZADEH, F., 1978b, Modeling of lifting capacity as a function of operator and task variables, in *Safety in Manual Materials Handling*, DHEW (NIOSH) Publication No. 78–185, Department of Health Education and Welfare, National Institute for Occupational Safety and Health, Cincinnati, OH.

AYOUB, M.M., MITAL, A., ASFOUR, S.S. and BETHEA, N.J., 1980, Review, evaluation, and comparison of models for predicting lifting capacity, *Human Factors*, **22**, 257–269.

AYOUB, M.M., BETHEA, N.J., BOBO, M., BURFORD, C.L., CADDEL, K., INTARANONT, K., et al., 1981, *Mining in Low Coal, Vol. 1, Biomechanics and Work Physiology*, Final Report, US Bureau of Mines, Contract No. H03087022.

AYOUB, M.M., SELAN, J.L. and JIANG, B.C., 1983, *A Mini-Guide for Lifting*, Lubbock, TX: Department of Industrial Engineering, Texas Tech University.

BEAN, J.C., CHAFFIN, D.B. and SCHULTZ, A.B., 1988, Biomechanical model calculation of muscle forces: a double linear programming method, *Journal of Biomechanics*, **21**, 59–66.

BORG, G.A.V., 1962, *Physical Performance and Perceived Exertion*, Lund: Gleerup.

BRINGHAM, C.J. and GARG, A., 1983, The Role of Biomechanical Job Evaluation in the Reduction of Overexertion Injuries: A Case Study, Paper at the 23rd Annual American Industrial Hygiene Association Conference, Philadelphia, PA.

CHAFFIN, D.B., 1967, The Development of a Prediction Model for the Metabolic Energy Expended During Arm Activity, Unpublished doctoral dissertation, University of Michigan, Ann Arbor, MI.

CHAFFIN, D.B. and ANDERSSON, G.B.J., 1991, *Occupational Biomechanics*, 2nd edn, New York: John Wiley & Sons.

CHAFFIN, D.B. and PARK, K.S., 1973, A longitudinal study of low-back pain as associated with occupational weight lifting factors, *American Industrial Hygiene Association Journal*, **31**, 513–525.

CHAFFIN, D.B., REDFERN, M.S., ERIG, M. and GOLDSTEIN, S.A., 1990, Lumbar muscle size and locations from CT scans of 96 women of age 40 to 63 years, *Clinical Biomechanics*, **5**, 9–16.

CHEN, H.C., 1988, Biomechanical Stresses During Asymmetric Lifting – A Dynamic Three-Dimensional Approach, Unpublished doctoral dissertation, Texas Tech University, Lubbock, TX.

CHOLEWICKI, J. and MCGILL, S.M., 1996, Mechanical stability on the in vivo lumbar spine: implications for injury and chronic low back pain, *Clinical Biomechanics*, **11**(1), 1–15.

CLAUSER, C.W., MCCONVILLE, J.T. and YOUNG, J.W., 1969, *Weight, Volume and Center of Mass of Segments of the Human Body*, AMRL-TR-69-70, Aerospace Medical Research Laboratories, OH.

CROWMINSHIELD, R.D. and BRAND, R.A., 1981, A physiologically based criterion of muscle force prediction in locomotion, *Journal of Biomechanics*, **14**(11), 793–801.

DAVIS, K.G., MARRAS, W.S. and GRANATA, K.P., 1997, The effect of task asymmetry and number of hands on spinal loading, *Proceedings of the Human Factors and Ergonomics Society 41st Annual Meeting*, Albuquerque, NM.

DEIVANAYAGAM, S. and AYOUB, M.M., 1979, Prediction of endurance time for alternating workload tasks, *Ergonomics*, **22**, 279–290.

DEMPSTER, W.T., 1955, *Space Requirements of the Seated Operator*, WADC-TR-55-159, Aerospace Medical Research Laboratories, OH.

DRYDEN, R.D., 1973, A Predictive Model for the Maximum Permissible Weight of Lift from Knuckle to Shoulder Height, Unpublished doctoral dissertation, Texas Tech University, Lubbock, TX.

DUMAS, G.A., POULIN, M.J., ROY, B., GAGNON, M. and JOVANOVIC, M., 1988, A three-dimensional digitization method to measure trunk muscle line of action, *Spine*, **13**(5), 532–541.

DURNIN, J.V.G.A. and PASSMORE, R., 1967, *Energy, Work and Leisure*, London: Heinemann Educational.

EISLER, H., 1962, Subjective scale of force for a large muscle group. *Journal of Experimental Psychology*, **64**(3), 253–257.

FREDERICK, W.S., 1959, Human energy in manual lifting, *Modern Materials Handling*, **14**, 74–76.

FREIVALDS, A., CHAFFIN, D.B., GARG, A. and LEE, K.S., 1984, A dynamic biomechanical evaluation of lifting maximum acceptable loads, *Journal of Biomechanics*, **17**, 251–262.

GARG, A., 1976, *A Metabolic Rate Prediction Model for Manual Materials Handling Jobs*, Unpublished doctoral dissertation, University of Michigan, Ann Arbor, MI.

GARG, A. and AYOUB, M.M., 1980, What criteria exist for determining how much load can be lifted safely? *Human Factors*, **22**, 475–486.

GARG, A., CHAFFIN, D.B. and HERRIN, G.D., 1978, Prediction of metabolic rates for manual materials handling jobs, *American Industrial Hygiene Association Journal*, **39**, 661–674.

GARG, A. CHAFFIN, D.B. and FREIVALDS, A., 1982, Biomechanical stresses from manual load lifting: a static vs dynamic evaluation, *Transactions of the American Institute of Industrial Engineers*, **14**, 272–281.

GENAIDY, A.M. and ASFOUR, S.S., 1987, Review and evaluation of physiological cost prediction models for manual materials handling, *Human Factors*, **29**(4), 465–476.

GENAIDY, A.M., ASFOUR, S.S., KHALIL, T.M. and WALY, S.M., 1985a, Physiologic issues in manual materials handling, in Eberts, R. and Eberts, C.G. (Eds), *Trends in Ergonomics/ Human Factor II*, Amsterdam: Elsevier, pp. 571–576.

GENAIDY, A.M., ASFOUR, S.S. and MUTHUSWAMY, S., 1985b, Modeling of physiologic responses to manual work: a systems approach, in *IEEE Proceedings of the International Conference on Cybernetics and Society*, Tucson, AZ: IEEE Systems, Man, and Cybernetics Society, pp. 1107–1110.

GENAIDY, A.M., ASFOUR, S.S., MITAL, A. and TRITA, M., 1988, Psychophysical capacity modeling in frequent manual materials handling activities, *Human Factors*, **30**(3), 319–337.

GRANATA, K.P. and MARRAS, W.S., 1996, Biomechanical models in ergonomics, in Bhattacharya, A. and McGlothlin, J.D. (Eds), *Occupational Ergonomics – Theory and Application*, New York, NY: Marcel Dekker.

HAMILTON, B.J. and CHASE, R.B., 1969, A work physiology study of the relative effects of pace and weight in a carton handling task, *Transactions of the American Institute of Industrial Engineers*, **1**, 106–111.

HAN, J.S., AHN, J.Y., GOEL, V.K., TAKEUCHI, R. and McGOWAN, D., 1992, CT-based geometric data of human spine musculature. Part 1. Japanese patients with chronic low back pain, *Journal of Spinal Disorders*, **5**(4), 448–458.

HERRIN, G.D., JARIEDI, M. and ANDERSON, C.K., 1986, Prediction of overexertion injuries using biomechanical and psychophysical models, *American Industrial Hygiene Association Journal*, **47**, 322–330.

HUGHES, R.E., 1991, Empirical Evaluation of Optimization-Based Lumbar Muscle Force Prediction Models, Unpublished doctoral dissertation, University of Michigan, Ann Arbor, MI.

JIANG, B., 1984, Psychophysical Capacity Modeling of Individual and Combined Manual Materials Handling Activities, Unpublished doctoral dissertation, Texas Tech University, Lubbock, TX.

JIANG, B., SMITH, J.L. and AYOUB, M.M., 1986, Psychophysical modelling for combined manual materials-handling activities, *Ergonomics*, **29**(10), 1173–1190.

KAMON, E., KISER, D. and PYTEL, J.L., 1982, Dynamic and static lifting capacity and muscular strength of steelmill workers, *American Industrial Hygiene Association Journal*, **43**(11), 853–857.

KARWOWSKI, W. and AYOUB, M.M., 1984a, Effect of frequency on the maximum acceptable weight of lift, in Mital, A. (Ed.), *Trends in Ergonomics/Human Factors I*, Amsterdam: Elsevier, pp. 167–172.

KARWOWSKI, W. and AYOUB, M.M., 1984b, Fuzzy modeling of stresses in manual lifting tasks, *Ergonomics*, **27**, 641–649.

KEE, D. and CHUNG, M.K., 1996, Comparison of prediction models for the compression force on the lumbosacral disc, *Ergonomics*, **39**(12), 1419–1430.

KIM, H., 1990, Model for Combined Ergonomic Approaches in Manual Materials Handling Tasks, Unpublished doctoral dissertation, Texas Tech University, Lubbock, TX.

KNIPFER, R.E., 1974, Predictive Models for the Maximum Acceptable Weight of Lift, Unpublished doctoral dissertation, Texas Tech University, Lubbock, TX.

LADIN, Z., MURTHY, K.R. and DELUCA, C.J., 1989, Mechanical recruitment of low-back muscles: theoretical predictions and experimental validation, *Spine*, **14**(9), 927–938.

LEAMON, T.B., 1994, Research to reality: a critical review of the validity of various criteria for the prevention of occupationally induced low back pain, *Ergonomics*, **37**(12), 1959–1974.

LEGG, S.J. and MYLES, W.S., 1981, Maximum acceptable repetitive lifting workloads for an 8-hour work day using psychophysical and subjective rating methods, *Ergonomics*, **24**(12), 907–916.

LESKINEN, T.P.J., STALHAMMER, H.R., KUORINKA, I.A.A. and TROUP, J.D.G., 1983, The effect of inertial factors on spinal stress when lifting, *Engineering in Medicine*, **12**, 87–89.

LIOU, Y.H. and MORRISSEY, S.J., 1985, Predicting male and female physiological costs of load carriage, in Eberts, R. and Eberts, C.G. (Eds), *Trends in Ergonomics/Human Factors II*, Amsterdam: Elsevier, pp. 633–639.

MACINTOSH, J.E. and BOGDUK, N., 1986, The biomechanics of the lumbar multifidus, *Clinical Biomechanics*, **1**(4), 205–213.

MAIRIAUX, P.H. and MALCHAIRE, J., 1988, Relation between intra-abdominal pressure and lumbar stress: effect of trunk posture, *Ergonomics*, **31**(9), 1331–1342.

MARRAS, W. and SOMMERICH, C., 1991a, A three dimensional motion model of loads on the lumbar spine, I: model structure, *Human Factors*, **33**, 123–137.

MARRAS, W. and SOMMERICH, C., 1991b, A three dimensional motion model of loads on the lumbar spine, II: model validation, *Human Factors*, **33**, 139–149.

MARRAS, W.S., LAVENDER, S.A., LEURGANS, S.E., RAJULU, S.L., ALLREAD, W.G., FATHALLAH, F.A. and FERGUSON, S.A., 1993, The role of dynamic three-dimensional trunk motion in occupationally-related low back disorders: the effects of workplace factors, trunk position and trunk motion characteristics on risk of injury, *Spine*, **18**, 617–628.

MARRAS, W.S., LAVENDER, S.A., LEURGANS, S.E., FATHALLAH, F.A., FERGUSON, S.A., ALLREAD, W.G. and RAJULU, S.L., 1995, Biomechanical risk factors for occupationally-related low back disorders, *Ergonomics*, **28**, 377–410.

MARRAS, W.S., DAVIS, K.G., KIRKING, B.C. and GRANATA, K.P., 1997, Spine loading and trunk kinematic changes during team lifting, *Proceedings of the Human Factors and Ergonomics Society 41st Annual Meeting*, Albuquerque, NM.

McCONVILLE, J.T. and HERTZBERG, H.T., 1966, *A Study of One Hand Lifting*, Wright-Patterson AFB, Ohio, Aerospace Medical Research Laboratory, Technical Report, AMRL-TR-66-17.

McDANIEL, J.W., 1972, Prediction of Acceptable Lift Capability, Unpublished doctoral dissertation, Texas Tech University, Lubbock, TX.

McGILL, S.M., 1992, A myoelectrically based dynamic three dimensional model to predict loads on lumbar spine tissues during lateral bending, *Journal of Biomechanics*, **25**, 395–414.

McGILL, S.M. and NORMAN, R.W., 1986, Partitioning of the L4-L5 dynamic moment into disc, ligamentous, and muscular components during lifting, *Spine*, **11**(7), 666–678.

McGILL, S.M., PATT, N. and NORMAN, R.W., 1988, Measurement of the trunk musculature of active males using CT scan radiography: Implication for force and moment generating capacity about the L4/L5 joint, *Journal of Biomechanics*, **21**(4), 329–341.

McMULKIN, M.L., 1996, Investigation and Empirical Evaluation of Inputs to Optimization-Based Biomechanical Trunk Models, Unpublished doctoral dissertation, Virginia Polytechnic Institute and State University, Blacksburg, VA.

MITAL, A., 1983a, The psychophysical approach in manual lifting – a verification study, *Human Factors*, **25**, 485–491.

MITAL, A., 1983b, Prediction of maximum weights of lift acceptable to male and female industrial workers, *Journal of Occupational Accidents*, **5**, 223–231.

MITAL, A., 1983c, Generalised model structure for evaluating/designing manual materials handling jobs, *International Journal of Production Research*, **21**, 401–412.

MITAL, A., 1984, Comprehensive maximum acceptable weight of lift database for regular 8-hour workshifts, *Ergonomics*, **27**, 1127–1138.

MITAL, A., 1985, Models for predicting maximum acceptable weight of lift and heart rate and oxygen uptake at that weight, *Journal of Occupational Accidents*, **7**, 75–82.

MITAL, A. and ASFOUR, S.S., 1983, Material handling capacity of workers, *Material Flow*, **1**, 89–100.

MITAL, A. and AYOUB, M.M., 1980, Modeling of isometric strength and lifting capacity, *Human Factors*, **22**, 285–290.

MITAL, A. and KROMODIHARDJO, S., 1986, Kinetic analysis of manual lifting activities: Part II – Biomechanical analysis of task variables, *International Journal of Industrial Ergonomics*, **1**, 91–101.

MITAL, A., SHELL, R.L., MITAL, C., SANGHAVI, N. and RAMANANN, S., 1984, *Acceptable Weight of Lift for Extended Workshifts*, Tech. Report Grant No. 1-R01-OH-01429-01 & 2, Cincinnati, OH: NIOSH.

MITAL, A., NICHOLSON, A.S. and AYOUB, M.M., 1997, *A Guide to Manual Materials Handling*, London: Taylor & Francis.

MORRISSEY, S.J. and LIOU, Y.H., 1984a, Development of models for predicting metabolic costs of carrying loads with a range of container sizes, in Mital, A. (Ed.), *Trends in Ergonomics/ Human Factor I*, Amsterdam: Elsevier, pp. 173–178.

MORRISSEY, S.J. and LIOU, Y.H., 1984b, Metabolic costs of load carriage with different container sizes, *Ergonomics*, **27**, 847–853.

MORRISSEY, S.J. and LIOU, Y.H., 1984c, Predicting the metabolic costs of carrying loads in erect and stooped task postures, in Mital, A. (Ed.), *Trends in Ergonomics/Human Factors I*, Amsterdam: Elsevier, pp. 179–184.

NASA, 1978, *Anthropometric Source Book*, NASA Reference Publication No. 1024, National Aeronautics and Space Administration.

NIOSH, 1981, *Work Practices Guide for Manual Lifting*, NIOSH Technical Report No. 81–122, UD Department of Health and Human Services, National Institute for Occupational Safety and Health, Cincinnati, OH.

NIOSH, 1994, *Applications Manual for the Revised NIOSH Lifting Equation*, NIOSH Technical Report No. 94–110, US Department of Health and Human Services, National Institute for Occupational Safety and Health.

NUSSBAUM, M.A. and CHAFFIN, D.B., 1996, Evaluation of artificial neural network modelling to predict torso muscle activity, *Ergonomics*, **39**(12), 1431–1444.

ÖZKAYA, N. and NORDIN, M., 1991, *Fundamentals of Biomechanics: Equilibrium, Motion, and Deformation*, New York: Van Nostrand Reinhold.

POULSEN, E., 1970, Prediction of maximum loads in lifting from measurements of back muscle strength, *Progressive Physical Therapy*, **1**, 146–149.

PYTEL, J.L. and KAMON, E., 1981, Dynamic strength test as a predictor for maximal and acceptable lifting, *Ergonomics*, **24**(9), 663–672.

SCHULTZ, A.B., HADERSPECK, K., WARWICK, D. and PORTILLO, D., 1983, Use of lumbar trunk muscles in isometric performance of mechanically complex standing tasks, *Journal of Orthopaedic Research*, **1**, 77–91.

SNOOK, S.H., 1976, Psychophysiological indices – what people will do. *Report on International Symposium: Safety in Manual Materials Handling*, State University of New York at Buffalo: NIOSH, pp. 63–67.

SNOOK, S.H., 1978, The design of manual handling tasks, *Ergonomics*, **21**, 963–985.

SNOOK, S.H. and CIRIELLO, V.M., 1974, Maximum weights and workloads acceptable to female workers, *Journal of Occupational Medicine*, **16**, 527–534.

SNOOK, S.H., IRVINE, C.H. and BASS, S.F., 1970, Maximum weights and workloads acceptable to male industrial workers, *American Industrial Hygiene Association Journal*, **31**, 579–586.

STEVENS, S.S., 1975, *Psychophysics: Introduction to its Perceptual, Neural, Social Prospects*, Wiley.

TABOUN, S.M., 1986, Models of Individual and Combined Materials Handling Tasks, Unpublished doctoral dissertation, University of Windsor, Windsor, Ontario, Canada.

TRACY, M.F., GIBSON, M.J., SZYPRYT, E.P., RUTHERFORD, A. and CORLETT, E.N., 1989, The geometry of the muscles of the lumbar spine determined by magnetic resonance imaging, *Spine*, **14**(2), 186–193.

WILLIAMS, M. and LISSNER, H.R., 1977, *Biomechanics of Human Motion*, 2nd edn (B. Le Veau, Ed.), Philadelphia: Saunders.

WINTER, D.A., 1990, *Biomechanics and Motor Control of Human Behavior*, 2nd edn, New York: John Wiley & Sons.

PART FIVE

Whole Body Mechanics

CHAPTER SIXTEEN

Posture

STEPHAN KONZ

Posture will be considered 'the configuration of the body's head, trunk and limbs in space'. This chapter will consider the following: non-perfect bodies; measuring/recording posture; static posture; dynamic posture; and external factors.

NON-PERFECT BODIES

Sometimes we forget that everyone does not have a perfect body.

Spine

The spine is concave backwards in two areas (cervical and lumbar) and concave forwards in one area (thoracic). Lordosis is an increase in lumbar curvature – a swayback posture, with the stomach protruding. (Pregnancy gives a temporary increase in lordosis, leading to standing farther from a worksurface, but compensating by bending the torso forward and extending the arms more (Paul and Frings-Dresen, 1994).) Kyphosis is an increase in thoracic curvature – shoulders roll forward, the person slouches, becomes a hunchback. Scoliosis is a bending of the spine to the side (i.e. from a front view).

Legs

Leg length discrepancy (LLD) is the technical name for differences in leg length in the same person. Contreras *et al.* (1993), summarising studies with N = 2377, reported that 40 per cent of people had LLD ≤ 5 mm, 30 per cent had LLD ≤ 9 mm, 20 per cent had LLD ≤ 11 mm and 10 per cent had LLD ≤ 14 mm.

Joints

Other imperfections can affect posture. These problems can be from many causes (injuries, aging, disease, etc.).

For information on the knee and hip, see Nordin *et al.* (1997: Chapter 38, Epidemiology of the lower extremity; Chapter 39, Biomechanics of the hip and knee; Chapter 40, Clinical evaluation of the hip and knee; and Chapter 41, Treatment of common disorders of the hip and knee).

For information on the foot and ankle, see Nordin *et al.* (1997: Chapter 43, Epidemiology of foot and ankle disorders; Chapter 44, Anthropometry of the human foot; Chapter 45, Biomechanics of the ankle joint complex and the shoe; Chapter 46, Clinical and functional evaluation of the foot and ankle; and Chapter 47, Treatment and indications for surgical treatment of foot and ankle injuries).

MEASURING/RECORDING POSTURE

Note that the effects of posture include: body orientation in space; force by muscles to maintain that orientation; and duration the orientation is held. Table 16.1 describes the terminology. There are two general applications: laboratory and field.

Laboratory

A laboratory has the characteristics of precision, repeatability and organisation of data gathering. Thus relatively elaborate equipment can be used.

For photography, consider whether two-dimensional or three-dimensional views are desired. Generally, the view is made with a video camera – probably on a sampling basis. Generally, markers are placed on the person to aid in identifying specific body locations during the analysis. When the marker locations are digitised, they usually will be entered into a computer (manually or automatically) and various angles calculated.

Table 16.1   Terminology for body position descriptions.

Planes
- Sagittal: Divides the body into left and right
  - Medial (Y): Close to the centre
  - Lateral (+Y or −Y): Away from medial on left (+Y) or right (−Y)
- Coronal: Divides the body into front and back
  - Anterior (+X): Front or ventral side
  - Posterior (−X): Back or dorsal side
- Transverse: Divides the body into top and bottom
  - Superior (+Z): Closer to head
  - Inferior (−Z): Closer to feet

Limbs
- Proximal: Closer to the torso
- Distal: Farther from the torso

Wrist/hand motions
- Flexion (bend hand down) vs Extension (bend hand up)
- Radial deviation (bend horizontal hand towards thumb) vs Ulnar deviation (bend horizontal hand towards little finger)
- Pronation (rotation towards palm down) vs Supination (rotation towards palm up)

Goniometers give the angle directly. The simple units have two arms and the experimenter reads the included angle visually. The more complex units operate electronically and give continuous readouts – allowing collection of data over time without distracting the subject (Boocock et al., 1994).

Field

Occasionally a scientist will take apparatus into a field situation and use equipment to record posture. Ergonomists or engineers however, will normally want only approximate information and do not want to 'interfere' with production.

In these cases, the analyst can either take a video of the job (and analyse it in the office) or observe in 'real time' and record the results on a form. A number of forms have been developed which give simple categories (standing straight, standing with back bent less than 45°, standing with back bent 45–90°, etc.). For an example, see the OWAS system (Karhu et al., 1977). When multiple angles need to be recorded and the job is variable (not exactly repeating), real time recording will be inaccurate (DeLoose et al., 1994). The use of a videotape of a number of cycles is recommended, which can be analysed at leisure. An additional advantage of a video is that duration of a posture can be recorded as well as orientation.

STATIC POSTURE

Standing

Table 16.2 gives some dimensions for US adults. A large portion of the variation in human stature is in leg length; the torso is relatively constant in height. Weights of various body segments for adult males (as a percentage of total weight) are: head = 7.3 per cent, torso = 50.7 per cent, one total arm and hand = 4.9 per cent, one total leg and foot = 16.1 per cent.

The mean distance between the inside of the two feet, when standing, is about 100 mm, between foot centrelines is about 200 mm, and between outside edges is about 300 mm (Rys and Konz, 1994). Yet mean height for males is 1750 mm. Thus there is a base of

Table 16.2 Selected dimensions (cm) of nude US adult civilians.

	Mean		Standard deviation	
	Females	Males	Females	Males
Stature	162.9 (100%)	175.6 (100%)	6.4	6.7
Crotch height	74.1 (45%)	83.7 (48%)	4.4	4.6
Knee height	51.5 (32%)	55.9 (32%)	2.6	2.8
Foot length	24.4 (15%)	27.0 (15%)	1.2	1.3
Foot breadth	9.0 (6%)	10.1 (6%)	0.5	0.5

The percentages show the dimension as a percentage of stature height. Shoes add 25 mm height for males and 15 mm for females. Shoes add 0.9 kg to body weight. From Konz (1995), with permission.

Table 16.3 Standing zones vs stress.

Zone	Force moments	Stress	Height of hand	
			Maximum	Minimum
1	2	4.2	Standing on tiptoe	Upper reach
2	1	2.3	Upper reach	Shoulder
3	0	1.0	Shoulder	Trunk bending ≤20°, knees straight
4	1	2.3	Trunk bending ≤20°, knees straight	Knee height
5	3	7.0	Knee height	

Adapted from Swat and Krzychowicz (1996). It is assumed that the 'free comfort boundaries' are trunk forward ≤20°, to the sides ≤10°, backwards ≤5°, and twisting ≤5°. Force moments are calculated from trunk, knee and ankle bending.

only 200–300 mm for a structure of 1750 mm. The base can be increased if the person stands with one foot forward; this also reduces twisting stress if the turn is to the side opposite the forward foot.

This structure has two supports up to the waist and then one support (the spine). Thus there is sway – especially front to back. Sway is increased by lack of vision and by certain noise frequencies (Sakellari and Soames, 1996). When standing, the centre of gravity passes from the ear opening forward of the spine (even L4–L5) so the body normally has a forward bending moment, counteracted by ligament and back muscle forces and soleus muscles of the calf.

'Quiet standing' is actually a highly dynamic event as there is incessant weight shifting from side to side. Satzler *et al.* (1993) recorded foot movements for 120 minutes of standing; people moved a foot approximately every 90 seconds.

Venous pressure in the ankle of sedentary people is approximately equal to hydrostatic pressure from the right auricle. Pollack and Wood (1949) reported 56 mm Hg for sitting and 87 mm Hg for standing; Nodeland *et al.* (1983) reported 48 mm Hg for sitting and 80 mm Hg for standing. However, walking about ten steps drops venous ankle pressure to about 22 mm Hg.

Table 16.3 details stress for work at various standing zones. An empty hand is assumed; the stress is magnified if the hand holds an object such as a handtool. Table 16.4 lists risks for various postures as a function of angle and duration.

Sitting

The concept that people sit with back straight and head up is fictional. For example, Graf *et al.* (1995) divided back postures of seated people into 'forward' (head over centre of thighs), 'middle' (head over buttocks), and 'backwards' (head behind buttocks). The first point is that positions were not constant at middle but varied (changing about ten times per hour). The second point is that the postures varied greatly with task (assembly, office, listening, VDU and cashier). Van Riel *et al.* (1995) also emphasised the differences for head position among tasks.

Table 16.4 Posture checklist for neck, trunk and legs.

Job studied	Percent time posture used in job		
	Never	<1/3	≥1/3
Neck			
1. Mild forward bending (>20°)	0	0	X
2. Severe forward bending (>45°)	0	X	*
3. Backward bending (>20°)	0	X	*
4. Twisting or lateral bending (>20°)	0	X	*
Trunk			
5. Mild forward bending (>20°)	0	X	*
6. Severe forward bending (>45°)	0	*	*
7. Backward bending (>20°)	0	X	*
8. Twisting or lateral bending (>20°)	0	X	*
General body/legs			
9. Standing stationary	0	0	X
(no walking or leaning)			
10. Standing, using footpedal	0	0	*
11. Knees bent or squatting	0	0	*
12. Kneeling	0	X	*
13. Lying on back or side	0	0	*

Total X = _____ Total * = _____

Comments:

From Keyserling *et al.* (1992). A zero indicates insignificant risk; an X indicates a potential risk; a star indicates a significant risk.

Other postures

Table 16.5 gives dimensions for some other working postures.

DYNAMIC POSTURE

Walking/running

When walking, the activity of one leg has a shorter swing phase (when the foot is passed forward) and a longer support (stepping, contact) phase (when the foot is on the ground). The support phase starts at heel strike and ends at toe-off; it has an earlier passive section and a later active (propulsion) section. Since the swing phase is shorter than the support phase, heel strike of the opposite limb occurs during the propulsion section of the support phase. During a slip, instead of stopping, the heel continues to move and the leading foot moves out in front of the body.

The length of stride (L) divided by stature height (h) varies linearly with velocity: $L/h = 0.67$ at $v = 0.8$ m/s and $L/h = 0.9$ at 1.7 m/s.

Table 16.5 Selected body dimensions of males in common working positions
(Annis and McConville, 1996).

Dimension	Mean, mm	Std. dev.	Mean/height
Overhead reach			
Breadth	377	17.3	22
Fist height	2141	82.9	122
Maximum height	2240	85.9	128
Horizontal length			
Knee bent	1484	53.6	85
Knee straight	1778	59.7	101
Supine			
Arm reach	747	32.6	43
Bent knee height	502	22.9	29
Height			
Squatting	1117	49.3	64
Kneeling height	1304	45.0	74
Bent torso	1309	70.1	75
Breadth			
Bent torso	448	22.4	26
Maximum squatting	562	54.1	32
Leg length, kneeling	672	33.5	38

Mean age = 29 years, height = 1752 mm, weight = 73 kg.

Walking changes to running, for normal size adults, at about 2.5 m/s (5.6 miles/h)
since it uses less energy (for the same speed). In running, both feet are off the ground for
part of the stride. Peak force is about $3 \times$ body weight at about 0.1 s after contact.

Stepping

Descending stairs demands a quite different gait than that for ascending. Most stair falls
occur while descending.

For descent, the leading foot swings forward over the nosing edge and stops its
forward motion when it is directly over the tread below; the toe is pointed downward.
Meanwhile the heel of the rear foot begins to rise, starting a controlled fall downward
towards the tread. The heel of the forward foot is then lowered and the weight transferred
to the forward foot. The rear foot then begins to swing forward. Problems are overstep-
ping the nosing with the forward foot, catching the toe of the forward foot, and snagging
the heel of the rear foot on the nosing as it swings past.

For ascent, the leading foot has a toe-off, swing, and first contact with the upper step.
The foot is roughly horizontal. The ball of the foot is well forward on the tread. The rear
foot then rises on tiptoe, pushing down and back. The rear leg then begins the swing
phase. The primary problem is catching the toe, foot or heel of either foot on the stair
nosing. Another problem is slipping by the rear foot when it pushes backward.

Falls

Falls can occur from slips (unexpected horizontal foot movement), trips (restriction of foot movement) and stepping-on-air (unexpected vertical foot movement).

Slips primarily occur during foot pushoff and heel strike. During pushoff, the person falls forward (less common and less dangerous). If a slip occurs during heel strike, the person falls backward. During a slip, there is normally a 'lubricant' (water, oil, grease, dust, ice) either on the surface or on the shoe heel.

Outdoor trips often occur from uneven surfaces which the person expects to be even. Indoor trips tend to be from objects on the floor or stairs. Usually there is a visual problem.

Stepping-on-air can occur on steps with unequal riser distances, when there is a hole in the ground, and when there is 'no ground'. Very often it occurs with 'single steps' (small changes in elevation) such as curbs and one-step changes in floor level. Often stepping-on-air has a visual cause.

Falls which occur when the person is carrying something are especially dangerous. The object carried decreases stability as a function of the torque above the ankle (weight × object height above ankle). Other problems are that the arms cannot be used for balance (to prevent a fall), to grab a railing, or to break the fall impact.

Manual material handling

Cumulative trauma to the back is due primarily to manual material handling. Some statistics (Khahil, 1991) are:

■ On any given day, 6 500 000 people in the USA are in bed with back pain.

■ A total of 75 000 000 Americans have back pain problems.

■ In industrialised countries, 80 per cent of working adults will develop back pain in their career.

■ In the USA, only colds cause more physician visits than back pain. About 50 per cent of all chiropractor visits are due to low-back symptoms.

Note that there is a hierarchy of back problems:

■ low-back *pain*;
■ low-back *impairment* (reduced ability to perform);
■ low-back *disability* (lost time); and
■ low-back *compensation* (reimbursement).

Although personal risk factors are important (Garg and Moore, 1992), the following subsections will concentrate on ergonomic risk factors.

Carrying

Carrying indicates poor job design; replace with pushing or pulling (e.g. carts, conveyors, hoists). Consider a short section of a roller conveyor or belt conveyor (perhaps portable); trucks often are loaded/unloaded using an extendable belt conveyor. Within a workstation, consider balancers, manipulators and robots.

Carrying objects up and especially down stairs and ladders is dangerous as: the hands are not free; and the object may impair vision. Consider hoists and elevators. If the object must be carried on the stair/ladder, keep the hands free (e.g. use a tool belt or a backpack).

Pushing/pulling

Pushing/pulling (at least on a level) does not have to fight gravity and therefore is better than lifting/lowering; three people can push a car but they certainly cannot lift it! In general, pushing is easier than pulling.

Some guidelines for horizontal pushing/pulling perpendicular to the shoulders are:

- Two hands are better than one.
- Force capability goes down as it is exerted more often.
- Females are weaker than males – especially in pushing.
- Push at waist level rather than shoulder or knee level. (Two vertical handles on a cart, rather than one horizontal handle, allows all sizes of people to use optimum posture.)
- Pull at knee level rather than waist or shoulder level. If a two-wheeled cart must be pulled over curbs or steps (as in retail delivery of beverages), larger diameter wheels (larger lever arm) are better.

Arms and shoulders (not the lower back) tend to be limiting when:

- Activity is repetitive (local muscle fatigue).
- Posture is poor:
    - pushing with arms fully extended (arm strength is greatest at 0.5 (reach distance), drops at 0.75 (reach distance) and is lowest at 1.0 (reach distance))(Kumar, 1987);
    - pushing or pulling with one arm;
    - pushing or pulling above the shoulder or below the hip;
    - kneeling (vs standing) reduces capability about 20 per cent;
    - seated (vs standing) reduces capability about 40 per cent.

Lack of a vertical surface to brace against or a slippery foot/floor interface (slippery floor or shoes) reduces capability. For horizontal transfer in and out of a machine, reduce force by replacing frictional contact (e.g. boxes on polished metal tables, pallets on rails) with rolling contact (rollers, wheels, balls).

For horizontal pushing parallel to the shoulders, assume force capability is 50 per cent of perpendicular to the shoulders. For vertical pushing/pulling, sitting decreases capability about 15 per cent vs standing.

Lifting/lowering

Although much remains to be quantified concerning numerical lifting/lowering guidelines, the general concepts are relatively well known.

Table 16.6 gives, in military terms, 'strategy' (big picture) while the various formulas (see below) are 'tactics' (details). There are three 'tactics' approaches which will give numerical values for specific tasks. A note of caution: the three approaches do not give the same answers!

The Center for Ergonomics at the University of Michigan has developed computerised biomechanical models. Several thousand copies have been sold. Prof. Ayoub and Prof. Mital, in contrast, have evaluated many alternatives with a formula; however they have not published the formula but have published the results in tables (Mital et al., 1993).

Table 16.6 Guidelines for lifting (Konz, 1995).

Guideline	Comment
Select individual	
1. Select strong people based on tests.	Anti-discrimination laws have made personnel selection difficult to implement.
Teach technique	
2. Bend the knees.	The squat lift is difficult to implement in practice. The 'free-style' lift (135° angle between upper and lower legs, back angle vs floor is about −10°) requires less energy and is what workers use.
3. Do not slip or jerk.	Minimise peaks of force and torque on the body.
4. Do not twist.	Twisting while erect is bad but the legs and hips can move. Worst is twisting while the torso is at or below the hips. Move the feet.
Design the job	
5. Use machines.	Eliminate stress on the body by using a machine. At a workstation, use balancers, manipulators, turntables, hoists, scissors-lifts and robots. Between workstations, use conveyors, carts and lift-trucks.
6. Move small weights often.	Large loads occasionally put too much stress on the skeletal-muscular system. Reduce the container weight. Weights are smaller when using gravity (e.g. gravity-aided conveyor; lowering instead of lifting).
7. Get a good grip.	Minimise the stress on the wrists and shoulders. The NIOSH lifting guideline reduces permissible load by 5–10% for poor grips.
8. Put a compact load in a convenient container.	The goal is to minimise the torque from the load on the spine. This is done by holding the container close to the body and by having a container with a short dimension vs the shoulders.
9. Keep the load close to the body.	Amplifying guideline 8, reduce reach and disposal distances of the load as well as carrying. This involves reach and disposal distances as well as workstation design.
10. Work at knuckle height.	Knuckle height varies with people; i.e. fixed heights for everyone are poor. Avoid loads below the knees – especially on the floor. Also avoid loads above the shoulders (stress on shoulders and arms as well as back).

The National Institute of Occupational Safety and Health (NIOSH) approach is described in Walters *et al.* (1994). Briefly summarising their approach, the NIOSH group considered: (1) biomechanical criteria (350 kg compressive force on L5–S1); (2) metabolic rate (9.5 kcal/min, multiplied by 70 per cent (due to arm work) and then by 50 per cent (for 1 h), 40 per cent (for 2 h) or 33 per cent (for 8 h); and (3) psychophysiological criteria (75 per cent female, 34 cm wide box, 76 cm vertical displacement and lifting frequency of four lifts/min). The equation is:

$$RWL = LC \times HM \times VM \times DM \times FM \times AM \times CM$$

Table 16.7 Seated work posture vs standing work posture (adapted from Magnusson, 1997).

Advantages of seated	Disadvantages of seated
Provides stability for tasks with high visual and motor control	Increased load on back and neck
Less energy consuming	Risk for decalcification
Less loading on lower extremity joints	Low demands on circulation
Reduces hydrostatic pressure on lower extremity circulation	

where:

RWL = recommended weight limit, kg
LC   = load constant = 23 kg
HM = horizontal multiplier, proportion
VM = vertical multiplier, proportion
DM = distance multiplier, proportion
FM = frequency multiplier, proportion
AM = asymmetry multiplier, proportion
CM = coupling multiplier, proportion.

The maximum load which can be lifted is 23 kg since each of the multipliers is less than 1. Computer programs of the NIOSH approach are available from a number of sources.

From a posture viewpoint, the critical multipliers are HM, VM, DM and AM. Basically, they penalise any material handling not at knuckle height, not close to the body, and with twisting.

Posture variability

Table 16.7 compares sitting vs standing. Note that low back pain is high for both sedentary occupations (due to prolapsed discs) and for heavy work (muscle strain and ligament injury) (Magnusson, 1997). Naturally there is a desire to have 'optimum' posture. This optimum has two dimensions: static and dynamic.

Static

If a joint is not moved, it has a static load. This not only restricts supply of nutrients and oxygen but also restricts removal of metabolic waste products. Thus encourage dynamic

For example, static sitting tends to lead to low back pain, so, when on the job,
occasional standing and walking. Have a sedentary person in the office get the
e copies, get supplies, leave their chair during breaks. A sedentary vehicle
uld adjust seat position and walk occasionally. Off the job, encourage an
e style'.

Dynamic

The minimum stress of a posture is at the 'neutral' position of the joint. Stress increases with departure from neutrality. The stress probably increases non-linearly with departure from neutrality; that is, a departure of 90° is more than twice as stressful as a departure of 45°. The effect of departure direction probably also varies; that is, movement of the wrist of 30° in extension does not have the same penalty as 30° of flexion and the penalty for rotation is not the same as that for flexion/extension. In addition, the stress of departure from neutrality probably varies with the joint.

EXTERNAL FACTORS

Clothing support

Back belts/braces

Somewhat surprisingly, for such a popular product, there has been relatively little experimental study of back belts (Genaidy *et al.*, 1995; Rys and Konz, 1995). Most of the experimental studies have studied lifting/lowering in a laboratory; studies need to be made of industrial lifting (which has much more variety), as well as pushing/pulling, carrying and standing. Belt design should be addressed; there are many designs – intuitively, some should be better than others. In addition, some belts seem to be uncomfortable; Reddell *et al.* (1992) found 58 per cent of the industrial worker participants had discontinued use of a belt before the end of an eight month study. Most studies have concentrated on 'healthy students'; in addition to male/female differences, the effect of belts on people who already have back problems should be addressed. The criteria used have also varied widely.

Until more research is done, my recommendation is to use back belts with caution. They probably will not hurt the worker, assuming the worker does not decide he is Superman, now that he has a belt. In addition, belts should not be considered a substitute for good ergonomics in job design.

Joint braces

There are a variety of braces for the wrist, elbow, knee and ankle. They are to support the joint until it has healed (typically from an injury); they should not be considered a permanent solution.

Shoes

Athletic shoes are divided into running shoes (designed for forward movement) and court shoes (designed for quick side-to-side movement). Boots provide ankle support and protection, typically for outdoor use on uneven ground. Cowboy boots have a large heel to prevent the boot from going through the stirrup. High heels for women are designed so that women arch their back. Shoes without heels (deck shoes) give greater contact with the floor and can reduce slipping.

External support: standing

Standing aids

The key concept is posture variability. As pointed out previously, as few as ten steps of walking will cut ankle venous pressure to 22 mm Hg (from about 83 mm Hg for standing and 51 mm Hg for sitting). Another possibility is to alternate sitting and standing, within the same task or by rotating tasks.

It also is possible to vary posture while standing. Satzler *et al.* (1993) recommended a 100 mm high platform, either flat or angled at 15°. The standing person could shift one foot to the platform as desired (see also Whistance *et al.*, 1995).

Another alternative is a sit/stand stool; the adjustable height seat should have a forward slope of 10–15°. Nijboer and Dul (1987) reported that they were useful in upholstery work even when they could be used for only 15 per cent of the working time.

Mats/carpets

Cushioning the floor can be done everywhere (carpets) or locally (mats). Carpets/mats also act as a frictional surface (reducing slips). Summarising a number of studies on mats:

- Mats improve comfort over hard-surfaced floors. Comfort may increase in the back as well as the legs.
- Mats should compress but not too much. Optimum is about 6 per cent under the shoes of a 70 kg adult.
- Mats should have beveled edges to reduce tripping.
- Mats should have a non-slip surface for the feet and also should not slip on the floor.
- Mats which have to be cleaned periodically (e.g. in food service environments) should be smaller for ease of handling.
- If a person stands on a raised platform, the surface should be resilient (i.e. wood or plastic, not steel). The platform should have a high ratio of surface to holes (i.e. you are not standing on 'knives').

Chairs

A chair supports the body vs gravity. A stool (i.e. no arm or back support) primarily supports the legs (about 32 per cent of body weight). It is difficult to quantify the percentage support from a backrest but common experience indicates the benefits of a back support. Supporting both arms/hands is about 10 per cent of body weight; this percentage decreases as hands are used (e.g. assembly, keyboarding).

Although it is obvious, it will be emphasised that chair selection should consider the task being done while in the chair as well as the individual in the chair.

No hand/arm manipulation

For passive sitting, with no hand/arm manipulation, sitting height is not very critical. The arms can usually be supported by arm rests on the chair. The legs need to be supported, typically by resting on the floor but also perhaps on a footrest. Hamstring length decreases if the knees are flexed, thus decreasing lumbar lordosis; thus all seats should allow for bending the knees at an acute angle (Bridger *et al.*, 1989, 1992); knee angle is especially important for people who are less supple. Thigh clearance is probably not relevant. Although there are some advocates of forward tilted seats, the vast majority of seats tilt to the rear 1–4°. The front of the seat should not exert sharp pressure on the underside of the thighs. The seat should not be contoured as contour seats restrict movement (reducing posture variability). The backrest can be tilted back as desired since hand position is not critical.

Hand/arm manipulation

For active sitting, the position of the hands is important. Hand position determines the vertical location of the seat and also the horizontal location of the backrest. Because the hand position is determined, seat and backrest location will determine head position, both distance from the floor and gaze angle. The eyes typically will focus on the hands (assembly) or an object (infinity for driving). Hand position is more flexible (and body twisting is less) if the seat swivels. If even more flexibility in hand position is needed (greater reach distance), a 'sit/stand' seat can be used; usually this does not support the back.

If the arms are supported, the amount of movement affects the selected alternative. For minimum movement (such as microscope work), typically the arms are supported by arms on the chair; the chair arms may even move in and out or pivot. Another alternative is support by a table: avoid sharp edges and pressure points; also, the table may be slanted (say 10–15°). Driving (support by a wheel) is another variation. For maximum movement while supported, the arms can be supported by slings suspended from a mechanism.

There needs to be room for the lower body. This involves both vertical clearance for the thighs vs the underside of the work surface and no barrier interfering with the horizontal location of the legs.

VDT chairs

The VDT task is a special case of the hand/arm manipulation task. The special case is the static posture of most of the body in combination with intense activity of the fingers.

The static load on the shoulders and forearm can be reduced if an armrest is used (Keller and Strasser, 1996; Paul *et al.*, 1996). Paul *et al.* point out that mouse use requires a pivoting armrest, not just a vertically-adjustable armrest.

Workstation design

The posture used by the operator is influenced by visual requirements and/or reach requirements.

Vision

The viewing angle depends not only on the line of sight of the eyes but also the inclination of the head (often downward). A value for the target of 30–40° below horizontal seems reasonable. Bifocal users tend to tilt their head upward when using VDT screens; minimise this neck strain by using 'work glasses' (single vision lenses with a focal length of about 0.7 m).

Location of a work object typically is a compromise between visual requirements (seeing object comfortably) and hand requirements (work at elbow height). Sometimes the visual requirements can be reduced by: (1) improved lighting; (2) optical aids (magnification mounted on the desk or the head or even using video pictures); or (3) modifying the task (improving size on a VDT screen, such as 12 point rather than 10 point text; better contrast, such as printing on white paper rather than tinted paper; or more viewing time).

Eklund *et al.* (1994) recommended that driver cabins should have narrow window frames and large windows, strategically placed. Mirrors, video monitors, and rotatable seats (with low backrests) can reduce the need for twisting.

Reach

While standing, reach distance is affected by foot position. A space 150 mm × 150 mm × 500 mm wide is sufficient (DeLaura and Konz, 1990).

The object being grasped should be close (to reduce forward bending and thus stress on the back). For example, when reaching for objects on a conveyor, the objects should be on the closer side of the conveyor; accomplish this by a barrier (diverter) on the conveyor. The benefits can be substantial. For example: assume a 70 kg person has a head of 5.1 kg, two arms and hands of 6.9 kg and torso of 35.7 kg. Assume a 0.3 m reach has the centre of gravity of the head 0.15 m forward, arms 0.2 m forward and torso 0.1 m forward. Then the head torque is 0.76 kgm, arm torque is 1.38 kgm and the torso is 3.57 kgm – a total of 5.71 kgm, even with a zero torque from the object! Assume the diverter causes the object to be 0.1 m closer. Then $0.05(5.1) + 0.1(6.9) + 0 = 0.94$ kgm instead of 5.7 kgm!

Although the previous paragraph emphasised horizontal reach distance, if the conveyor is too low (excessive vertical distance), the torque will again be excessive. Modifying the vertical distance implies adjusting operator height or conveyor height. Adjust operator height with a platform; normally it would be a simple wooden structure but it could be motorised to go up and down. Conveyor height is easy to modify for a single operator but is more complex if multiple stations use the conveyor. For example, conveyors can be different heights at different workstations if the conveyor sections are connected by slanting conveyors (powered if uphill). Conveyors for seated operators need to have space for the knees and thighs. (Note: conveyors should be convenient for those working with them, not necessarily easy for engineers to design.)

For the specific situation of keyboarding, vertical extension/flexion movements of the wrist present the greatest risk for carpal tunnel syndrome; minimise extension by having the key top alignment flat (Hedge and Powers, 1995).

References

ANNIS, J. and McCONVILLE, J., 1996, Anthropometry, in *Occupational Ergonomics*, Bhattacharya, A. and McGlothlin, J. (Eds), New York: Dekker.

BOOCOCK, M., JACKSON, J., BURTON, A. and TILLOTSON, K., 1994, Continuous measurement of lumbar posture using flexible electrogoniometers, *Ergonomics*, **37**(1), 175–185.

BRIDGER, R., WILKINSON, D. and VAN HOUWENINGE, T., 1989, Hip joint mobility and spinal angles in standing and in different sitting postures, *Human Factors*, **31**(2), 229–241.

BRIDGER, R., ORKIN, D. and HENNEBERG, M., 1992, A quantitative investigation of lumbar and pelvic postures in standing and sitting: interrelationships with body position and hip muscle length, *International Journal of Industrial Ergonomics*, **9**, 235–244.

CONTRERAS, R., RYS, M. and KONZ, S., 1993, Leg length discrepancy, in *The Ergonomics of Manual Work*, Marras, W., Karwowski, W. and Pacholski, L. (Eds), London: Taylor and Francis, pp. 199–202.

DELAURA, D. and KONZ, S., 1990, Toe space, in *Advances in Industrial Ergonomics and Safety II*, Das, B. (Ed.), London: Taylor and Francis, pp. 297–300.

DELOOSE, M., TOUSSAINT, H., ENSINK, J. and MANGNUS, C., 1994, The validity of visual observation to assess posture in a laboratory-simulated, manual material handling task, *Ergonomics*, **37**(8), 1335–1343.

EKLUND, J., ODENRICK, P., ZETTERGREN, S. and JOHANSSON, H., 1994, Head posture measurements among work vehicle drivers and implications for work and workplace design, *Ergonomics*, **37**(4), 623–639.

GARG, A. and MOORE, S., 1992, Epidemiology of low-back pain in industry, in *Ergonomics: Low Back Pain, Carpal Tunnel Syndrome and Upper Extremity Disorders in the Workplace*, Moore, J. and Garg, A. (Eds), Philadelphia: Henley and Belfus, pp. 593–608.

GENAIDY, A., SIMMONS, R. and CHRISTENSEN, D., 1995, Can back supports relieve the load on the lumbar spine for employees engaged in industrial operations? *Ergonomics*, **38**(5), 996–1010.

GRAF, M., GUGGENBUHL, U. and KRUEGER, H., 1995, An assessment of seated activity and posture at five workplaces, *International Journal of Industrial Ergonomics*, **15**, 81–90.

HEDGE, A. and POWERS, J., 1995, Wrist postures while keyboarding: effects of a negative slope keyboard system and full motion forearm supports, *Ergonomics*, **38**(3), 508–517.

KAHLIL, T., 1991, Ergonomic issues in low back pain: origin and magnitude of the problem, *Proceedings of the Human Factors Society*, pp. 820–824.

KARHU, O., KANSI, P. and KOURINKA, I., 1977, Correcting working postures in industry, a practical guide for analysis, *Applied Ergonomics*, **8**(4), 199–201.

KELLER, E. and STRASSER, H., 1996, Ergonomic evaluation of an armrest for typing via electromyographic and subjective assessment, *Advances in Occupational Ergonomics and Safety I*, Mital, A., Krueger, H., Kumar, S., Menozzi, S. and Fernandez, J. (Eds), Cincinnati, OH: Int. Soc. for Occ. Safety and Health, Vol. 2, pp. 838–845.

KEYSERLING, M., BROUWER, M. and SILVERSTEIN, B., 1992, A checklist for evaluating ergonomic risk factors resulting from awkward postures of the legs, trunk and neck, *International Journal of Industrial Ergonomics*, **9**, 283–301.

KHAHIL, T., 1991, Ergonomic issues in low back pain: origin and magnitude of the problem, *Proceedings of the Human Factors Society*, 820–824.

KONZ, S., 1995, *Work Design: Industrial Ergonomics*, 4th edn, Scottsdale, A2: Publishing Horizons, p. 111.

KUMAR, S., 1987, Arm strength at different reach distances, in *Trends in Ergonomics/Human Factors IV*, Asfour, S. (Ed.), Amsterdam: Elsevier.

MAGNUSSON, M., 1997, Posture, in *Musculoskeletal Disorders in the Workplace*, Nordin, M., Andersson, G. and Pope, M. (Eds), St Louis: Mosby, 77–84.

MITAL, A., NICHOLSON, A. and AYOUB, M., 1993, *A Guide to Manual Material Handling*, London: Taylor and Francis.

NIJBOER, I. and DUL, J., 1987, Introduction of standing aids in the furniture industry, *in Musculoskeletal Disorders at Work*, Buckle, P. (Ed.), London: Taylor and Francis, 227–233.

NODELAND, H., INGEMANSEN, R., REED, R. and AUKLAND, K., 1983, A telemetric technique for studies of venous pressure in the human leg during different positions and activities, *Clinical Physiology*, **3**, 573–576.

NORDIN, M., ANDERSSON, G. and POPE, M. (Eds), 1997, *Musculoskeletal Disorders in the Workplace*, St Louis: Mosby.

PAUL, J. and FRINGS-DRESEN, M., 1994, Standing working posture compared in pregnant and non-pregnant conditions, *Ergonomics*, **37**(9), 1563–1575.

PAUL, R., LUEDER, R., SELNER, A. and LIMAYE, J., 1996, Impact of new input technology on design of chair armrests: investigation on keyboard and mouse, *Proceedings of Human Factors and Ergonomics Society*, pp. 380–384.

POLLACK, A. and WOOD, E., 1949, Venous pressure in the saphenous vein at the ankle in man during exercise and changes in posture, *Journal of Applied Physiology*, **1**, 649–662.

REDDELL, C., CONGLETON, J., HUCHINGSON, R. and MONTGOMERY, J., 1992, An evaluation of a weightlifting belt and back injury prevention class for airline baggage handlers, *Applied Ergonomics*, **23**, 319–329.

RYS, M. and KONZ, S., 1994, Standing, *Ergonomics*, **37**(4), 677–687.

RYS, M. and KONZ, S., 1995, Lifting belts: a review, *International Journal of Occupational Safety and Ergonomics*, **1**(3), 294–303.

SAKELLARI, V. and SOAMES, R., 1996, Auditory and visual interactions in posture stabilization, *Ergonomics*, **39**(4), 634–648.

SATZLER, L., SATZLER, C. and KONZ, S., 1993, Standing aids, *Proceedings of the Ayoub Symposium*, Texas Tech University, Lubbock, TX, pp. 29–31.

SWAT, K. and KRZYCHOWICZ, G., 1996, ERGONON: computer-aided working posture analysis system for workplace designers, *International Journal of Industrial Ergonomics*, **18**, 15–26.

VAN RIEL, M., DERKSEN, J., BURDORF, A. and SNIJDERS, C., 1995, Simultaneous measurements of posture and movements of head and trunk by continuous three-dimensional registration, *Ergonomics*, **38**(12), 2563–2575.

WALTERS, T., PUTZ-ANDERSON, V. and GARG, A., 1994, *Applications Manual for the Revised NIOSH Lifting Guideline*, DHHS (NIOSH) Publication No. PB94-176930.

WHISTANCE, R., ADAMS, L., VAN GEEMS, B. and BRIDGER, R., 1995, Postural adaptations to workbench modifications in standing workers, *Ergonomics*, **38**(12), 2485–2503.

CHAPTER SEVENTEEN

Biomechanical aspects of work seating

JÖRGEN EKLUND

INTRODUCTION

The subject of seating has attracted our attention all through history. Chair design and seating are not only related to ergonomic aspects, such as health and well-being of the sitter and safe and productive conditions. Chairs are also means of expressing status and power. Further, chairs are also pieces of art and craftmanship, and today's furniture industry is well aware of aesthetics as an important property of the chairs. As with many consumer products, chairs are increasingly being used for expressing the personality of the owner or user. These aspects can sometimes support and sometimes counteract the use of ergonomically and biomechanically sound seating.

There is a large number of studies on the subject of ergonomics in seating, and also many reviews in the area, for example, Åkerblom (1948), Asatekin (1975), Corlett (1989), Eklund (1986), Grieco (1986), Kroemer (1991) Lueder and Noro (1994) and Schoberth (1962). These and other publications in ergonomics show that there are many approaches and methods to assess the suitability of a seating arrangement. One crucial aspect of seating is the work and activities performed on the seat. Biomechanical evaluations of such activities are often not reported in the literature. Neither is it fully understood how work and other activities relate to seat design.

Broadly, publications in the field of seating fall into three categories: consequences; evaluation; and design procedures.

CONSEQUENCES

Publications dealing with consequences include epidemiological studies and other studies that assess the risks for discomfort, health impairment or accidents. In the above-mentioned publications, a strong focus has been placed on musculoskeletal problems, in particular back pain, as one of the most important problems related to sitting. There are also studies reporting consequences for performance, including productivity and the quality of work performed.

Table 17.1   Often mentioned sources of impaired safety, health, well-being or performance in seated work.

High or prolonged load on passive structures (back, neck, arm and wrist joints)
Static or high muscle activity (back, neck, shoulders, arms)
Increased venous blood pressure (feet, lower legs)
Increased pressure on internal organs (lungs, digestive system)
Seat surface pressure (buttocks, popliteal area)
Upholstery properties (heat conductivity and moist permeability)

As mentioned above, several studies have established a relationship between sitting and back pain. High risks have been found for long periods of sitting, especially in vehicles (Kelsey, 1975; Magora, 1972). It is considered that in addition to vibrations, the most important risk factors for back pain are the load on the spine (Andersson, 1981) and the spinal posture, especially the degree of kyphosis of the lumbar spine (Keegan, 1953). Increased risk of neck and shoulder pain have also been identified in several studies. Based on these, Kuorinka and Forcier (1995) proposed certain generic risk factors, which can be interpreted for the neck and upper arms as highly frequent movements, postures deviating from the neutral position, and postures held for long periods. Excessive muscle activity is another risk factor, which refers to static, medium or peak levels (Jonsson *et al.*, 1981). Long periods of sitting, especially if the front edge of the seat creates a pressure in the popliteal region, can impair the venous blood flow, increase the blood pressure and cause uncomfortable swelling in the feet and lower legs, and even thrombosis in the lower legs. These effects are also related to inactivity of the calf muscles (Haeger, 1966; Winkel, 1981). The sitting posture decreases the space in the cavities of the trunk, resulting in increased pressure on internal organs such as the lungs and the digestive system. This has been reported to cause impaired oxygen uptake (Burandt, 1970) and stomach trouble, even colon cancer (Gerhardsson *et al.*, 1986). It has been shown that discomfort and pain also impair productivity and affect the quality of the result. The mechanisms identified include compensatory activities, such as rest, lessening of discomfort or pain, avoidance of activities that provoke discomfort and distraction from the main task (Corlett and Bishop, 1976; Eklund, 1995; Lueder, 1985). There are many sources of decreased comfort. Inappropriate pressure from the seat surface and the pressure distribution are discomforting. Build up of heat and moisture in the seat contact area or too high a heat conductivity are other causes of discomfort (Andrén *et al.*, 1975; Elnäs and Holmér, 1981).

EVALUATION

A large number of methods and criteria proposed for evaluation of the appropriateness of seating have been reviewed by Corlett (1989) and Kroemer (1991) among others. In some cases these evaluations refer only to seating arrangements in general, and in other cases to a specific work situation and context. Biomechanical and psychophysical methods have been particularly influential in this respect.

Most methods for evaluation of seating that have been proposed are not standardised and thus are used differently by different investigators. There are few quantified criteria for interpretation of the results, but most criteria are on a qualitative basis. The methods

Table 17.2 Some methods for evaluation of seating.

Loadings
Disk pressure measurements
EMG
Spinal shrinkage
Gravity load
Foot and lower leg volume
Seat surface pressure
Intra-abdominal pressure
Blood pressure and blood flow
Diagnostic measurements

Postures
Spinal curvature
Joint angles (in mid-range of motion)
Head, neck, arm, legs and trunk positions

Comfort
Ratings of discomfort, pain, exertion
Disorders
Well-being
Pleasure
Preferences

Performance
Work speed
Error rate

---

can largely be classified into four groups: loadings of body structures and their effects; posture assessment; perceived comfort; and performance. Some of the most commonly referred methods are listed in Table 17.2.

DESIGN PROCEDURES

The design procedures deal with recommended procedures for the design of seating arrangements. There is an obvious relation between the tasks and the design of the workplace. Sometimes the tasks and workplace design are considered at the same time, and sometimes these factors are given in the beginning of the seating design process.

Procedures for anthropometric design of chairs were proposed early and were one of the first criteria developed for the design of seating (Hooton, 1945). These have been strongly developed over the years (Pheasant, 1996; Roebuck, 1995). Also, more general design recommendations have been proposed as well as specific design procedures for seated workplaces (Corlett and Clark, 1995). These include allowance for access, clearance and maintenance, and even recommended dimensions and measures. More general methods such as Quality Function Deployment and Kansei Engineering have been developed (see Nagamachi, 1994; Norell, 1992), which can be applied to seating design. In addition, specific methods for input to the design process, such as fitting trials, have been developed (Drury and Coury, 1982; Shackel, *et al*., 1969). However, no detailed and structured seat design procedure based on the activities of the work has been published.

BIOMECHANICAL ASPECTS OF SITTING POSTURES

An important reason for musculoskeletal problems is when the sitter is forced into a constrained and awkward posture during work activities, and when there is no possibility to get relief or change posture (van Wely, 1970).

In situations where the person has a free choice of posture, as in leisure sitting or standing, a range of substantially varied postures will be adopted. Branton and Grayson (1967) observed that passengers in trains showed a pattern of gradually slumping in the seat, whereafter they sat up in their seat distinctly. This pattern of movements was cyclically repeated approximately every 20 minutes. Maintaining the head straight means from a biomechanical point of view, that the head is balanced around an equlibrium and a semi-stable position. When the neck is slightly flexed, the extensor muscles in the back of the neck exert a small force in order to counteract the resulting moment. If the person feels a beginning discomfort or tiredness, he or she will make a small posture change to a slightly extended neck, where the flexor muscles start to work and give the antagonistic extensor muscles an opportunity to relax. The same effects can be noticed in standing postures for the lower back and the ankles, and the characteristic body sway in standing contributes to intermittent rest pauses and a more varied pattern of muscle activation (Odenrick, 1985). The possibility to choose free postures provides the opportunity to relax muscles intermittently.

There is another aspect of stability for relaxation. For tasks with hardly any lower arm movements, armrests will decrease shoulder muscle load (Andersson and Örtengren, 1974). To use armrests for tasks that demand hand and arm movements can cause increased shoulder muscle load (Lundervold, 1951). In these situations, mobile armrests have been proposed. The logic behind this is that an increased amount of lower arm support would be possible during these movements, thus decreasing the muscle activity. However, if the sitter needs the armrests for support, for example, when moving in the seat, mobile armrests will not provide sufficient stability. In a similar way, castors can increase the risk for muscular tensions in the legs, but castors with some friction may offer sufficient stability and relaxation, and also provide opportunities to move around in the workplace (Hansson et al., 1984; Lundervold, 1951). A further example is the use of forward sloping seats. A high degree of forward tilt will put load on the feet. When the feet take more than 25 per cent of the body weight, this will result in static leg muscle activity and discomfort (Eklund, 1986). It can be concluded that relaxation requires stability.

If the workplace design in combination with the work demands require for example continuous visual attention downwards, this will result in a flexed neck and long term static muscle load on the extensor muscles of the neck, and no opportunities to relax these muscles other than at intervals. This shows that the demands and restraints from work are the main causes of loadings on the body and also affect postures. In consequence, there will be shorter work periods and longer pause intervals.

The postures adopted at work and in other activities are influenced by the concentration level – compare the postures of someone who takes the first driving lesson with the posture of an experienced taxi driver – the interest and involvement, the social interaction and the emotional state, for example, anger, fear, self-consciousness, discouragement and agression. Many of these aspects are revealed by the body language and consequently by the postures taken (Fast, 1970). The postures have also been shown to affect the mood (Haruki and Suzuki, 1994). Also the climate will influence the posture, i.e., chill causes a tense posture with raised shoulders and the extermities pressed against the body (compare

Sundelin and Hagberg, 1992). Appropriate seating arrangements should not only allow but should also help people to take the postures they prefer. Restrictions due to the task and the workplace design should be avoided.

One of the most commonly discussed aspects of seating is spinal curvature. Since sitting flattens the lumbar spine, the debate has concentrated on how to counteract this. This is a difficult problem especially in forward sitting, as when performing work on a bench or work table. Åkerblom and Staffel (1883) (in Åkerblom, 1948) advocated the use of a lumbar support to counteract kyphosis. Since the force from the backrest tended to push the sitter forwards, a backwards inclination of the seat was proposed, in order to compensate for this force. Another approach was to increase the angle between trunk and thighs, using sit–stand stools (Laurig, 1969), forward inclined seats (Mandal, 1976) and various other shapes of the seat to allow for forwards sloping thighs. It has been shown that increased thigh–trunk angles and also to a certain extent more acute knee angles contribute to preserving the lumbar lordosis (Eklund and Liew, 1991; Keegan, 1953), but other problems of increased surface pressure, shear forces on the skin and sliding forwards on the seat are introduced.

ANALYSIS OF THE WORK SITUATION

From the above, it is obvious that both the physical and mental requirements of work influence the behaviour and thereby the desired properties of the seating arrangement. The choice and design of seats starts with an analysis of the work and the activities to be performed in the seat. The primary aspect is to be able to perform the tasks, i.e., to see the work object or what needs visual control, and to be able to reach and manipulate the objects and to perform the physical activities needed, normally by using hands and sometimes also feet. However, there is a built-in conflict between a comfortable viewing direction and a comfortable position for the hands, since these areas do not coincide. Important aspects in this analysis are presented in Table 17.3.

There may be many different purposes of the analysis. Sometimes only the seat might be in focus while the work, workplace and individuals are given beforehand, and sometimes the purpose is to design a completely new situation for unknown workers. Of course the latter case offers possibilities to create a better total situation since there is an opportunity for mutual adaptation.

ERGONOMIC SEAT DESIGN FEATURES

The design is often related to a user population. The physical properties of this population, including body size and strength are defined. The proportion of the population for which the design should fit is chosen, normally 90 or 95 per cent. The work demands are identified, to form the basis for the design of the seat features (see Corlett and Clark, 1995).

There are a number of recommendations that cannot be listed in a short table. The following text gives an example of how the work demands influence the seat des¹ In tasks which demand twisting of the trunk, it is important that the trunk rot be distributed along the spinal column, not only in the cervical region. Ther backrests should be relatively low or narrow in the upper part in order to let th blades rotate without restriction above the upper edge of the backrest. Tasks th

Table 17.3   A basis for analysis of work demands in seated tasks.

Visual demands
Viewing distances
Viewing directions
Detail size
Colour properties
Texture
Temporal pattern

Physical demands
Work object size, weight, shape and position
Force exertion
Precision
Handgrips
Postures (head, arms, trunk and legs)
Movements
Temporal pattern

Mental and social demands
Decision making
Concentration, prolonged attention
Time pressure
Social interaction, communication

Environmental conditions
Light (level, contrasts, reflexes, glare, light sources)
Noise
Climate
Chemicals
Vibrations

Rest activities
Stability in resting
Ability to relax
Ability to stretch and change posture
Egress and entry

Workplace
Dimensions
Space
Layout
Controls
Technology
Aids

The sitter
Arousal
Education and training
Experience
Stress
Anthropometry
Clothing
Physical, mental and social abilities

Table 17.4 Seat design features and design recommendations.

Seat height	Adjustable, front height corresponds to lower leg length
Seat width	Correspond to largest hip plus clothing
Seat depth	Adjustable, seated thigh length minus 1 dm, or the shortest thigh
Seat angle	Adjustable
Seat shape	Waterfall front edge
Seat padding	Corresponding to at least 2 cm firm padding
Backrest height	Depending on work task
Backrest width	Depending on work task
Backrest inclination	Adjustable, depending on work task
Backrest shape	Lumbar support, shape depending on work task
Backrest padding	Softer than the seat padding
Lateral supports	Stabilising the trunk and body for lateral forces
Arm rests	Adjustable to elbow height, padded
Upholstery	Friction to prevent sliding but not restrict movements, not too high heat conductivity, and moisture permeability

forwards directed forces of the hands should, on the contrary have a high backrest above shoulder level in order to take up the reaction forces. Sometimes, pulling forces can correspondingly be counteracted by a more inclined full-size backrest. Vehicle driving which gives lateral forces on the sitter should increase the stability of the trunk and body by lateral supports, possibly with softer padding. Wooden seats and other seats with low surface friction do not allow for full use of a backrest or a lumbar support, since the buttocks will slide forwards. Armrests are suitable if the work does not require arm movements, and they seem to function well if there are also small rotations in the elbow joint but with the elbow otherwise in a fixed position.

There is a built-in conflict between the advantage of increasing the trunk–thigh angle and the disadvantages that this produces. One disadvantage is that the seat shapes often used in this type of sitting changes the pressure distribution and decreases the weight bearing surface with higher surface pressures as a result, which tends to increase the rate of discomfort from the buttocks. Another disadvantage is that it becomes more difficult to use a backrest since this tends to push the sitter forwards on the seat.

A PROPOSED GENERIC SEAT DESIGN RECOMMENDATION

Based on the consequences that are commonly recognised in the literature, the following mechanical risk factors can be identified:

- static loads
- high load levels
- fixed postures
- lack of rest pauses for the muscles
- load on joints in the outer range of motion
- long-term exposure
- repetitive movements.

There are also several other risk factors, all largely qualitative. This makes the design of work seats complicated. Below, an attempt has been made to summarise the most import-ant criteria for seat design in four generic aspects, namely:

- enhance stability
- keep joints in the mid-range of motion
- minimise gravity induced moments on joints
- enhance variation.

The concept of stability for the sitter has been referred to by many authors. Åkerblom (1948) proposed a backwards inclined seat in combination with a backrest convexity in the lumbar region in order to obtain increased stability for the trunk, Branton and Grayson (1967) observed that train passengers had a tendency to cross their legs or to cross their ankles, which is another means of obtaining better stability for the legs. Seats for vehicles often have a longer seat pan and more pronounced lateral supports compared to other seats, which increases the stability of the legs for sideways movements and thereby decreases other compensations in the form of active muscle forces. The inclined full-size backrest with lateral supports, often used in vehicles, has the same effect for the trunk and improves the stability. Hence, increased stability is one precondition for muscle relaxation.

A commonly recognised risk factor for musculoskeletal problems is work postures where the joints are held in their outer range of motion (van Wely, 1970). Not only are certain structures, such as ligaments, substantially loaded then, but static muscle forces must also counteract the moments caused by these passive structures. However, if pos-tures are held so that the joints are kept in their mid-range of motion, this will minimise the load on the passive structures and also the need for active muscle force. Further, movements around this position enable variation of the loads.

In certain postures, muscle activity is needed to counteract gravity induced moments around the joints. One example of this is upright sitting with a slightly flexed neck, where the extensor muscles resist the moment caused by the gravitational force on the head. A balanced posture is taken when there is no need for active muscle force from neither the extensor, nor the flexor muscles of the neck. In conclusion, postures with no or minim-ised gravity-induced moment on joints decrease the level of static muscle activity.

Static loads and lack of rest pauses have frequently been mentioned as risk factors for musculoskeletal loads. From a physiological point of view, muscles and other stuctures have to be subjected to varied loads and movements (Kuorinka and Forcier, 1995). The term variation cannot of course be defined exactly. The concepts of repetitiveness, dura-tion and level of load have been proposed to describe variation (Winkel and Westgaard, 1992). Also, the pattern of pauses is considered to be of great importance, and methods to describe this have been developed (Linderhed, 1991). In spite of the operational prob-lems, variation is a key factor for the appropriateness of seating.

ERGONOMIC SIGNIFICANCE

on biomechanics and seating often lacks consideration of the tasks per-
sitter. This chapter provides practical recommendations for the analysis of
ands, and recommendations of how to relate these demands to appropriate
f the seat.

References

ÅKERBLOM, B., 1948, *Standing and Sitting Posture*, Stockholm: AB Nordiska Bokhandeln.

ANDERSSON, B., 1981, Epidemiologic aspects on low-back pain in industry, *Spine*, **6**, 53–60.

ANDERSSON, B. and ÖRTENGREN, R., 1974, Lumbar disc pressure and myoelectric back muscle activity during sitting. III. Studies on a wheelchair, *Scandinavian Journal of Rehabilitation Medicine*, **6**, 122–127.

ANDRÉN, E., BRATTGÅRD, S.-O., CARLSÖÖ, S. and SEVERINSSON, K., 1975, Temperatur och fuktighet i sittyta. Analys av skilda sitsmaterial vid olika rumsklimat (Temperature and moisture in the seat surface), Göteborg: Avdelningen för handikappforskning, Göteborgs Universitet.

ASATEKIN, M., 1975, Postural and physiological criteria for seating. A review, *METU Journal of the Faculty of Architecture*, **1**, 55–83.

BRANTON, P. and GRAYSON, G., 1967, An evaluation of train seats by observation of sitting behaviour, *Ergonomics*, **10**, 35–51.

BURANDT, U., 1970, Projekt Arbeitsstuhl, Möbel Interior Design, April, 64–66.

CORLETT, E.N., 1989, Aspects of the evaluation of industrial seating, *Ergonomics*, **32**, 257–269.

CORLETT, E.N. and BISHOP, R.P., 1976, A technique for assessing postural discomfort, *Ergonomics*, **19**, 175–182.

CORLETT, E.N. and CLARK, T.S., 1995, *The Ergonomics of Workspaces and Machines. A Design Manual*, London: Taylor & Francis.

DRURY, C. and COURY, B., 1982, A methodology for chair evaluation, *Applied Ergonomics*, **13**, 195–202.

EKLUND, J., 1986, Industrial Seating and Spinal Loading, unpublished PhD thesis, University of Nottingham.

EKLUND, J., 1995, Relationships between ergonomics and quality in assembly work, *Applied Ergonomics*, **26**, 15–20.

EKLUND, J. and LIEW, M., 1991, Evaluation of seating: the influence of hip and knee angles on spinal posture, *International Journal of Industrial Ergonomics*, **8**, 67–73.

ELNÄS, S. and HOLMÉR, I., 1981, Avkylning i kalla bilsäten. En pilotstudie av värmeledningsegenskaperna hos värmesitsar (Cooling due to cold car seats), Stockholm: Arbetarskyddsstyrelsen.

FAST, J., 1970, *Kroppsspråket (Body Language)*, Bungay, Suffolk: Chancer Press Ltd.

GERHARDSSON, M., NORELL, S., KIVIRANTA, H., PEDERSEN, N. and AHLBOM, A., 1986, Sedentary jobs and colon cancer, *American Journal of Epidemiology*, **123**, 775–780.

GRIECO, A., 1986, Sitting posture: an old problem and a new one, *Ergonomics*, **29**, 345–362.

HAEGER, K., 1966, Passageraretrombos (Passenger thrombosis), *Läkartidningen*, **63**, 2833–2837.

HANSSON, J.-E., ATTERBRANT-ERIKSSON, M., CARLSÖÖ, S. and ROXENHED, S., 1984, Arbetsställningar och möbelutformning vid kontorsarbete (Work postures and furniture design in office work), Arbete och Hälsa 1984:5, Arbetarskyddsstyrelsen, Stockholm.

HARUKI, Y. and SUZUKI, M., 1994, Our posture dictates perception, in Lueder, R. and Noro, K. (Eds), *Hard Facts about Soft Machines*, London: Taylor & Francis, pp. 133–143.

HOOTON, E., 1945, *A Survey in Seating*, Gardner, Massachusetts: Heywood-Wakefield Comp.

JONSSON, B., ERICSON, B.-E. and HAGBERG, M., 1981, Elektromyografiska metoder för analys av belastningen på enskilda muskler och muskulära utröttningseffekter under längre tids arbete (EMG methods for analysis of loads on single muscles and muscular fatigue during long term work), Undersökningsrapport 1981:9, Stockholm: Arbetarskyddsstyrelsen.

KEEGAN, J., 1953, Alterations of the lumbar curve related to posture and seating, *Journal of Bone and Joint Surgery*, **35-A**, 589–603.

KELSEY, J., 1975, An epidemiological study of acute herniated lumbar intervertebral discs, *Rheumatology and Rehabilitation*, **14**, 144–159.

KROEMER, K.H.E., 1991, Sitting at work: recording and assessing body postures, designing furniture for for the computor work station, in Mital, A. and Karwowski, W. (Eds), *Workspace, Equipment and Tool Design*, Amsterdam: Elsevier, pp. 93–112.

KUORINKA, I. and FORCIER, L. (Eds), 1995, *Work Related Musculoskeletal Disorders. A Reference Book for Prevention*, London: Taylor & Francis.

LAURIG, W., 1969, Der Stehsitz als physiologisch günstige Alternative zum reinen Steharbeitsplatz, Arbeitsmedizin, Sozialmedizin, *Arbeitshygiene*, **8**, 219–224.

LINDERHED, H., 1991, A method for analysing the temporal pattern of EMG, in Queinnec, Y. and Daniellou, F. (Eds), *Designing for Everyone. Proceedings of the 11th Congress of the International Ergonomics Association*, London: Taylor & Francis, pp. 45–47.

LUEDER, R., 1985, Adjustable furnishings increase productivity, *Contract*, **27**, 202–205.

LUEDER, R. and NORO, K. (Eds), 1994, *Hard Facts about Soft Machines*, London: Taylor & Francis.

LUNDERVOLD, A., 1951, Electromyographic investigations of position and manner of working in typewriting, *Acta Physiologica Scandinavica* **24** (Suppl. 84), 115–171.

MAGORA, A., 1972, Investigation of the relation between low back pain and occupation. 3 Physical requirements: sitting, standing and weight lifting, *Industrial Medicine and Surgery*, **41**, 5–9.

MANDAL, Å., 1976, Work-chair with tilting seat, *Ergonomics*, **19**, 157–164.

NAGAMACHI, M., 1994, Kansei Engineering: a consumer-oriented technology, in Bradley, G. and Hendrick, H. (Eds), *Human Factors in Organisational Design and Management – IV*, Amsterdam: Elsevier Science, pp. 467–472.

NORELL, M., 1992, Stödmetoder och samverkan i produktutveckling, unpublished PhD thesis, Royal Institute of Technology.

ODENRICK, P., 1985, On Analysis and Clinical Measurements of Gait and Upright Stance, unpublished PhD thesis, Linköping University.

PHEASANT, S., 1996, Bodyspace. *Anthropometry, Ergonomics and Design*, London: Taylor & Francis.

ROEBUCK, J., 1995, *Anthropometric Methods: Designing to Fit the Human Body*, Santa Monica: Human Factors and Ergonomics Society.

SCHOBERTH, H., 1962, *Sitzhaltung – Sitzschaden – Sitzmöbel*, Berlin: Springer Verlag.

SHACKEL, B., CHIDSEY, K. and SHIPLEY, P., 1969, The assessment of chair comfort, *Ergonomics*, **12**, 269–306.

SUNDELIN, G. and HAGBERG, M., 1992, Effects of exposure to excessive draughts on myoelectric activity in shoulder muscles, *Journal of Electromyography and Kinesiology*, **2**, 36–41.

VAN WELY, P., 1970, Design and disease, *Applied Ergonomics*, **1**, 262–269.

WINKEL, J., 1981, Swelling of the lower leg in sedentary work – a pilot study, *Journal of Human Ergology*, **10**, 139–149.

WINKEL, J. and WESTGAARD, R., 1992, Occupational and individual risk factors for shoulder–neck complaints: Part II – The scientific basis (literature review) for the guide, *International Journal of Industrial Ergonomics*, **10**, 85–104.

CHAPTER EIGHTEEN

Climbing biomechanics

DONALD S. BLOSWICK

INTRODUCTION/BACKGROUND

Accidents/injuries

Ladders

Climbing activities are performed as part of many occupational and non-occupational tasks. Injuries from slips and falls or overexertion during climbing activities on ladders frequently result in significant medical expenses and workers compensation costs. According to the US Consumer Product Safety Commission, there were 211 000 injuries associated with ladders in the USA in 1975 (ANSI, 1983). The National Safety Council (1994) indicates that 317 people were killed falling from ladders or scaffolding in 1991. This represents approximately 1 per cent of the total accidental deaths in the United States during that year.

Snyder (1977) noted that between 1966 and 1973 ladders accounted for 31 per cent of all falls in the construction industry in California. In a study by Safety Sciences (1978) it was noted that approximately 8 per cent of a sample of 500 occupational falls surveyed in the United States occurred from ladders. Kari *et al.* (1988) note that ladders account for 1–2 per cent of occupational related accidents. In Oregon, falls from ladders accounted for 457 disabling workers compensation claims or approximately 1.5 per cent of the total claim amount for 1995 (Oregon Department of Consumer and Business Services, 1997).

Injuries resulting from falls from ladders appear to be a serious problem in other countries as well. In both Sweden and Germany ladder accidents account for nearly 2 per cent of all reported occupationally related accidents (Unfallstatistik det gesetzlichen Unfallversicherung in der Bundesrepublik Deutschland, 1984, Annual Report on Occupational Injuries). In Sweden, with a population of approximately 8.5 million, ladder accidents requiring hospital care relating to recreational or leisure use are estimated at approximately five to six thousand per year (Danielsson, 1987), and two thousand relating to professional use (Malmros, 1986).

While the injuries and deaths resulting from ladders have a variety of causes, it is reasonable to assume that the ergonomic or biomechanical 'match' between the task requirements and the user capabilities is an important issue.

Stairs

It has been estimated that in 1975 there were approximately 2×10^{12} stair uses, 2.6×10^8 noticeable missteps, 3.1×10^7 minor accidents, 2.7×10^6 disabling accidents, 5.4×10^5 hospital treatments, and 3.8×10^3 deaths (Archea *et al.*, 1979). The National Safety Council (1994) has estimated that approximately 1200 deaths occurred in 1991 due to falls on stairs or steps. It has been estimated that nearly 1 million people received hospital treatment from injuries resulting from stair accidents, and nearly 50 thousand were hospitalised in the United States in 1990 (Pauls, 1985). Templer (1994) has estimated that between 1.8 and 2.6 million people per year are disabled for at least one day from stair accidents. In Oregon, in 1995, approximately 2400 or 7.9 per cent of total disabling occupational claims were caused by falls down stairs or steps (Oregon Department of Consumer and Business Services, 1997).

General design guidelines

Ladders

Ergonomic/biomechanical issues are certainly a contributing factor to ladder falls. ANSI (1992) suggests that fixed ladders be constructed so that the slant from horizontal is between 75 and 90 degrees. They suggest that there be a 30.5 cm (12 in) distance between rungs, 40.6 cm (16 in) between side rails, a 17.8 cm (7 in) toe clearance behind the rung, and a minimum 1.9 cm (0.75 in) rung diameter. They also suggest that side rails be uniform and allow a power grip along the length of the ladder. ANSI (1990) suggests a 75.5 degree ladder slant for portable ladders, a 30.5 cm (12 in) rung/step separation, and a minimum 30.5 cm (12 in) distance between the side rails. Since portable ladders can be constructed of metal or wood with varying strength characteristics, most other dimensions can vary depending on the type of material used; however, a minimum rung diameter of 2.9 cm (1.125 in) is required for wood ladders (ANSI, 1994). Diffrient *et al.* (1991) recommend that for rung ladders the optimum slant is 75–85 degrees, with rung spacing of 17.8–30.5 cm (7–12 in), and a rung diameter of 1.9–3.8 cm (0.75–1.5 in).

There is considerable variation relating to the slant actually preferred by ladder users. Irvine and Vejvoda (1977) found that the average slant preferred by 20 male subjects was 71.9 degrees. Häkkinen *et al.* (1988) found that climbers preferred a slant of 66 degrees, and Bloswick and Crookston (1992) found that male users preferred a slant of 73.5 degrees for both 13 foot and 18 foot ladders.

Stairs

The three critical issues relating to stair design include the step depth (tread), step height (riser), and handrail size and height. The US Department of Commerce recommends a tread of 27.94–35.56 cm (11–14 in) and a riser of 10.16–17.78 cm (4–7 in). Diffrient *et al.* (1991) recommend a stair slant of 30–35 degrees, resulting in a range of 27.94 cm (11 in) tread $\times$ 17.145 cm (6.75 in) rise to 25.4 cm (10 in) tread $\times$ 17.78 cm (7 in) rise. Templer (1994) suggests that tread depth be at 27.9–35.6 cm (11–14 in) and riser height be 11.7–18.3 cm (4.6–7.2 in). Pauls (1985) notes that US codes and standards are moving towards a requirement that tread depth be no less than 27.9 cm (10.98 in), and riser height be no more than 17.8 cm (7 in).

Diffrient *et al.* (1991) recommend that railings be 76.2–86.4 cm (30–34 in) above the leading edge of the step, with a maximum diameter of 6.7 cm (2.6 in). Templer (1994) notes that while 76.2–86.4 cm (30–34 in) is often required in codes and guidelines, stability requirements would suggest a handrail height of 91–102 cm (36–40 in) and a 3.8 cm (1.5 in) handrail diameter. The US Department of Commerce (Archea *et al.*, 1979) recommends a 0.69–0.79 cm (1.75–2 in) diameter hand rail.

LADDER BIOMECHANICS

Unless otherwise noted all research discussed in this section deals with ladders with 28.0–30.3 cm (11–12 in) rung separation. Ladder slant is defined as degrees from the horizontal.

Body movement

General description

Dewar (1977) defines that one complete climbing cycle or stride begins as one foot is put on a rung and ends when that same foot is again placed on a rung. The stride for the opposite side of the body is displaced in time by 50 per cent of the cycle. During the normal climbing activity the foot is placed on every other rung.

There is a wide variation in hand movements during ladder use. Dewar (1977) defines a 'lateral gait' as when the hands move in synchrony with the foot on the same side, and a 'diagonal gait' as when the hands move in synchrony with the foot on the opposite side. He notes that the diagonal gait is the 'natural' movement pattern. Hammer and Schmalz (1992) however, indicate that the lateral gait is more prevalent, and McIntyre (1983) found that nearly 60 per cent of his subjects applied the lateral gait. Hammer and Schmalz (1992) also note that people frequently change their gait between climbing activities and even within the same ladder ascent or descent.

Dewar (1977) found that for males foot contact ranged from 61 to 63 per cent of total cycle time, independent of the climbing speed and Lee *et al.* (1994) found contact time for males to be 55–58 per cent of total cycle time. Both Dewar (1977) and Häkkinen *et al.* (1988) found that climbers preferred to grip the ladder side or rail as opposed to the ladder rung.

ANSI (1990, 1994) notes that during use of portable ladders, 'When ascending or descending the ladder the user shall face the ladder and maintain a firm hold on the ladder', and when using a fixed ladder, 'When ascending/descending a ladder, the user shall face the ladder and maintain a three point contact at all times. Three point contact consists of two feet and one hand, or two hands and one foot, which is safely supporting a user's weight when ascending/descending ladder'.

McIntyre (1983) notes, however, that there are extended periods in both diagonal and lateral gait patterns when climbers have only two limbs in contact with the ladder. Hammer and Schmalz (1992) note that three point contact as a percentage of total time ranges from approximately 37 per cent of total cycle time at 60 degree ladder slant to approximately 52 per cent of total cycle time when the ladder is vertical.

Body centre of mass/trunk

Dewar (1977) notes that for male subjects the body centre of mass was approximately 7.5 cm (2.95 in) further back (away from the ladder) when using the 75.2 degree ladder as opposed to the 70.4 degree ladder slant. Kinoshita *et al.* (1984) note that during vertical ladder use the body centre of mass was kept further from the ladder during ladder descent than ascent. Lee *et al.* (1994) note that for male subjects the climbing path varied less at a faster speed (106 steps per minute) than at a slower (86 steps per minute) climbing speed. They interpret this as indicating that the individuals displayed less control while climbing at a faster speed. It would appear to this author that the opposite conclusion may be the case and that less variation during the faster speed would indicate more control. McIntyre (1983) notes that the movement of the body centre of mass away from the point of support during use of the steeper ladders indicates a decrease in stability. While this may be true for the 70 to 75 degree ladder slants, the extension of this logic to more extreme ladder slants should be avoided. For example, while climbing a vertical ladder the whole body centre of mass may be some distance outboard from the points of support but the body is in a 'stable' position if the points of support do not slip. On the other hand, a ladder with an extremely shallow slant, say 45 degrees, may be very difficult to use because of the difficulty of balancing on the rungs and reaching the side rails with the hands even though the whole body centre of mass would be nearly over the points of support at the feet.

Extremities

Dewar (1977) found that, when using the opposite leg as a reference, the maximum hip flexion angle for males was approximately 55 degrees and the maximum knee extension angle was approximately 70 degrees. For both the 70 and 75 degree ladder slants the hip abduction angle was approximately plus or minus 5 degrees. He also found that for shorter subjects both the hip and the knee had to flex more to lift the foot onto the rung. This effect was approximately the same for both ladder slants in the case of the knee but was less for the hip in the case of the 70 degree ladder slant.

Forces and joint moments/muscle activity

Hand/foot force

Lee *et al.* (1994) found that for a 70–75 degree ladder slant the legs served to move the body upward and the hand served primarily to balance the body, particularly when moving from the double to the single foot stance phase. They found that for males the total (two-hand) peak hand force was approximately 25 per cent of body weight and that the peak hand force was somewhat less at the 70 degree angle than at the 75 ladder slant. McIntyre *et al.* (1983) also found that the hands serve primarily to maintain dynamic stability for a 75 degree ladder slant but that as the space between the rungs increases, the hands are used more for propulsive forces to assist the legs. He notes that the one-hand forces range from 4.2 to 9.6 per cent of body weight, the hand forces exerted by the short subjects were higher than those of the tall subjects, and the hand forces of short subjects increased more rapidly as rung separation increased. Ayoub and Bakken (1978) found that the pull force on one hand ranged between 20 and 36 per cent of body weight during vertical ladder ascent.

Bloswick and Chaffin (1990) found that for male subjects the average total force on one hand as a percentage of body weight was 9.3 per cent for 70 degree ladder slant, 11.5 per cent for 75 degree ladder slant, 15.6 per cent for 80 degree ladder slant, and 24.5 per cent for the vertical ladder. They also found that the peak hand force was approximately 30 per cent of body weight during the one-foot stance when using a vertical ladder. This approaches the estimate of 35 per cent of body weight, which was found to be the mean grip strength on a slippery hand rail of 2.2 cm (0.875 in) diameter (Jack *et al.*, 1978). Bloswick and Chaffin (1990) also found that most subjects demonstrated an average preferred hand separation of 32.3 cm (12.7 in) but that short, heavy subjects preferred a significantly wider hand separation of 39.9 cm (15.7 in). This suggests that the generally accepted ladder width standard of 38.1 cm (15 in) is adequate for all but short, heavy climbers. This agrees with Chaffin *et al.* (1978) who found that a ladder width of 40.6 cm (16 in) would provide adequate lateral stability for arm strength to resist the force of the wind.

McIntyre (1979) found that average foot forces for one foot range from 48 to 60 per cent of body weight. Chaffin and Stobbe (1979) found that peak foot forces ranged from a high of 40 per cent in the horizontal direction to 170 per cent of body weight in the vertical direction for vertical ladder climbing. Bloswick and Chaffin (1990) found that for male subjects the total one-foot forces, as a percentage of body weight, were 63.7 per cent for a ladder slanted at 70 degrees, 62 per cent for a ladder slanted at 75 degrees, 59.3 per cent for 80 degrees, and 54.7 per cent for a vertical ladder. They also note that while the peak foot force is highest (approximately 85 per cent of body weight) during the one-foot stance for a ladder slanted at 70 degrees the foot slip potential is highest during the use of vertical ladders where a coefficient of friction in excess of 0.4 may be required to resist a forward slip.

Upper extremity moments

Bloswick and Chaffin (1990) found that the average elbow and shoulder moments varied as a function of ladder slant (as shown in Figure 18.1). In addition they note that during vertical ladder use the peak elbow flexion moment and shoulder extension moments were 45 per cent and 15 per cent of the maximum static moment. Lee *et al.* (1994) note that there may be a potential for localised fatigue at the elbow during long climbs since the peak hand force reached nearly 25 per cent of body weight.

Lower extremity moments

Bloswick and Chaffin (1990) also found that for male subjects the average hip, knee, and ankle moment as a percentage of static maximum varied by ladder slant (as shown in Figure 18.2). They found that the peak hip extensor, knee extensor, and ankle plantar flexion moments were 30 per cent, 15 per cent, and 10 per cent of maximum static moment, respectively, when climbing a ladder slanted at 70 degrees. Ayoub and Bakken (1978) contend that the knee is a limiting articulation, as opposed to the hip. They base this on the fact that hip moment capability is greater than that of the knee and that the knee must assume significant flexion and consequent reduction in moment generation capability. Chaffin *et al.* (1978) note that based on ankle torque (plantar flexion strength) capability the minimum foot clearance behind the ladder rung should be 16.5 cm (6.5 in). Based on ankle plantar flexion strength capability Bloswick and Chaffin (1990) note that this distance should be a minimum of 15.5 cm (6.1 in).

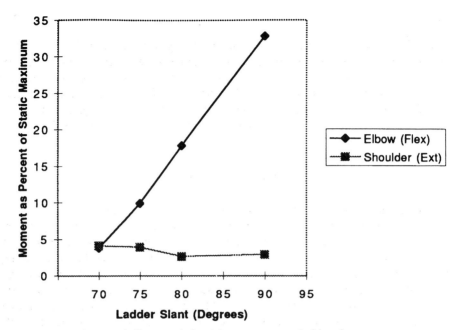

Figure 18.1 Relation of elbow and shoulder moments to ladder slant.

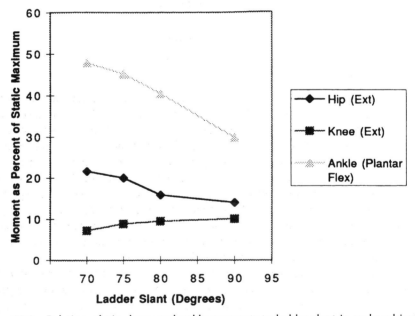

Figure 18.2 Relation of trip, knee and ankle moments to ladder slant in male subjects.

Back

Bloswick and Chaffin (1990) used integrated electromyographic (IEMG) activity of the erector spinae as a measure of low back stress during ladder climbing activities. They found that for males the erector spinae activity was approximately 65 per cent of static maximum and increased slightly as the ladder slant went from 70 degrees to 90 degrees (vertical). They also found that peak erector spinae IEMG activity approached 100 per cent of static maximum as climbing speed increased when using vertical ladders.

Energy consumption/fatigue

Brahler and Blank (1994) note that the whole body ladder climbing exercise on a simulated climbing machine elicited significantly greater maximum oxygen consumption values for collegiate oarswomen than did either treadmill running or rowing ergometry. Lehmann (1962) found that a ladder slanted at 70 degrees required the lowest energy demand per unit of height. Hammer and Schmalz (1992) also found that the time required per unit of height climbed was lowest with a ladder inclination of 70 degrees and consider this angle as 'optimal'. Chaffin *et al.* (1978) propose that rung separations of greater than 35.6 cm (14 in) require a 'fatiguing' exertion. Kamon (1970) found that metabolic efficiency in climbing a 60 degree ladder was higher when using a foot-over-foot pattern than when moving both feet to the same step.

STAIR BIOMECHANICS

Body movement

General description

Templer (1994) provides what may be the most comprehensive discussion of stairways. He notes that the gait on stairs must be defined differently than the gait in level walking where a gait cycle occurs between the heel strike of one foot and the subsequent heel strike of that same foot. On stairs the ball of the foot, as opposed to the heel, tends to be the first point of contact. On stairs the gait cycle must be considered as the cycle between foot contact (toe, foot, or heel) and the subsequent foot contact of the same side of the body. This includes one stance phase and one swing phase. The stance phase begins when the leading foot contacts the step. At midstance the body centre of mass is directly over this foot and starts to become elevated or lowered by concentric or eccentric contractions of the muscles in that leg. The stance phase continues until the weight transfer to the contra-lateral leg allows the foot to be lifted from the step.

The stance phase during stair ascent, as a percentage of gait cycle, has been determined to be 65 per cent (Zachazewski *et al.*, 1993), 64 per cent (males) (McFadyen and Winter, 1988), and 50–60 per cent (females) (Livingston *et al.*, 1991). The stance phase during descent, as a percentage of gait cycle, was 60 per cent (Joseph and Watson, 1967), and 55 per cent of the cycle for stairs slanted at 16.8 degrees, 40 per cent for stairs at 33.7 degrees, and 25 per cent for stairs steeply slanted at 45 degrees (Livingston *et al.*, 1991). McFadyen and Winter (1988) note that it is conceivable that one would change climbing strategies between and within the same stair climbing activity.

Other points of interest relating to stair movement include that by Zachazewski *et al.* (1993) who note that stair descent is a more dynamic process with greater inherent instability than ascent. Livingston *et al.* (1991) note that shorter women climbed with a more rapid cadence than did taller women and that stepping rate increased as stair slant increased. Shiomi (1994) notes that a step pattern where both feet move to the same step before proceeding to the next is more stable than the 'normal' foot-over-foot step pattern.

Body centre of mass/trunk

Krebs *et al.* (1992) note that the deviation of the centre of mass from the centre of pressure is greater during stair descent than ascent and that stair descent requires more balance than does ascent. McFadyen and Winter (1988) note, however, that the body is in a more 'optimal' position (centre of mass closer to the point of support) while walking down stairs.

Krebs *et al.* (1992) note that trunk abduction/adduction range of motion (ROM) and peak trunk flexion substantially exceeded those values during gait and that peak torso flexion during stair climbing was roughly parallel to the 33 degree stair slope. They also note that the trunk frontal plane ROM during stair climbing was greater than that of gait and suggest that it was to clear the swing foot over the step and minimise lower limb flexion requirements. They observed that subjects descended stairs with considerably less maximum trunk flexion than during ascent in order to maintain stability. In an observation of subjects on a stair ergometer, Asplund and Hall (1995) note that during stair climbing ergometry the average trunk flexion was approximately 18 degrees forward from vertical. Cooper *et al.* (1989) found that subjects flexed the trunk approximately 12 degrees with approximately 13 degrees of anterior pelvic inclination during stair climbing. Trunk flexion and pelvic inclination were approximately 0–3 degrees and 0–5 degrees respectively during stair descent.

Extremities

Asplund and Hall (1995) note that during stair climbing ergometry the hip range of motion was 15.2–51.4 degrees flexion, knee 12.7–72.8 degrees flexion, and the total ankle range of motion was 32.4 degrees. In a review of the literature, Livingston *et al.* (1991) note that hip flexion is approximately 42 degrees, knee flexion 83–90 degrees, and ankle plantar flexion 30–40 degrees during stair climbing tasks. In their research, Livingston *et al.* (1991) found that for female subjects the maximum hip flexion angle decreased as the slope of the stair decreased from 38–45 degrees on a 45 degree slanted stair down to 27–35 degrees on a 16.8 degree slanted stair. They also found that during stair climbing hip flexion ranged from 47 to 56 degrees. They also found that subject height was an important factor in determining knee motion during stair climbing. Short subjects had knee flexion angles ranging from 92 to 105 degrees while taller subjects had knee flexion angles ranging from 83 to 96 degrees. They found that subjects used 14–27 degrees of dorsiflexion and 23–30 degrees of plantar flexion at the ankle during stair ascent. They observed that the subjects in their study used approximately 20–35 degrees of dorsiflexion and 20–30 degrees of plantar flexion to perform stair descent as opposed to Andriacchi *et al.* (1980) who observed that males used 40 degrees of dorsiflexion and 40 degrees of plantar flexion during stair descent. Livingston *et al.* (1991) note that subjects appear to adjust to different stair dimensions by varying the flexion extension at the knee rather than that at the ankle or hip.

Foot forces and joint moments/muscle activity

During normal stair ascent and descent the forces on the hands and moments in the upper extremities are minimum. When these forces or moments do exist they tend to result from recovery from slips and falls and are resisted by the grab rails discussed earlier.

Lower extremity moments/foot force

Shiomi (1994) notes that walking up stairs involves a shortening of the muscles during contraction in performing positive work against gravity and that walking down stairs results in negative, or eccentric, work in which the leg extensors (quadriceps femoris) are stretched while resisting gravity. Asplund and Hall (1995) note that stair climbing ergometry also produces concentric muscle contractions throughout the lower extremity. McFadyen and Winter (1988) found that, with the exception of the rectus femoris and gluteus medius muscles, all muscles had greater mean activity for stair ascent compared to descent. Andriacchi *et al.* (1980) found that for male subjects the maximum moments for stair ascent for the ankle, knee, and hip were 137.2 (101.2), 57.1 (42.1), and 123.9 (91.4) Kn (ft lb) and during stair descent 107.5 (79.3), 146.6 (108.1), and 112.5 (83.0) Kn (ft lb), respectively.

Lyons *et al.* (1983) found that climbing stairs produced higher EMG activity in the upper and lower portions of the gluteus maximus, gluteus medius, and extensor fasciae latae muscles than did level walking. Descending stairs required lower muscle activity in these muscles as well as in the semimembranosus long head of the biceps femoris and adductor magnus muscles. They also found that the lower portion of the gluteus maximus is the primary hip extensor for ascending stairs. Shinno (1971) notes the importance of the quadriceps, particularly the vastus lateralis during stair ascent. He also notes that the quadriceps is more active during stair ascent than descent. McFadyen and Winter (1988) indicate that the quadriceps are dominant and the vastus lateralis is most active during propulsion up the stairs; they conclude that the knee extensors play a dominant role in stair climbing assisted by ankle plantar flexion moment. They note that walking up stairs primarily involves concentric contractions of the rectus femoris, vastus lateralis, soleus, and medial gastrocnemius and that walking down the stairs is achieved primarily through eccentric contractions of these same muscles to control the force due to gravity. Shinno (1971) also indicates the importance of the quadriceps muscle in supporting the body weight during the single stance phase of the stair use. He notes that the activity of the extensors is smaller in stair descending than ascending but that the biceps femoris activity is greater during stair descending than ascending. He found that the overall action of the quadriceps muscle is higher going up than while going down stairs and that the knee flexor activity is relatively small in both directions. He also points out that the knee joint is more unstable when going down stairs because the 'screwing home' at the knee joint becomes loose, the quadriceps muscle is passively stretched, and movement speed may be increased by gravity. McFadyen and Winter (1988) note that the soleus is the primary contributor to body elevation after foot contact, although some gastrocnemius activity was observed.

Kowalk *et al.* (1996) found that knee abduction moments ranged from 25 to 45 Km and were statistically smaller than the knee extension moments of 60–85 Km both for stair ascent and descent. They also found that the knee extension moments were greater during stair descent than ascent and that knee adduction moments did not exist. Costigan *et al.* (1993) found that abduction moments were approximately 50 per cent of the maximum found in the study by Kowalk *et al.* (1996). Lyons *et al.* (1983) indicate that limb support in descending stairs depends on hip adduction but not hip extensor activity.

McFadyen and Winter (1988) note that during stair descent energy is absorbed at both the ankle and the knee during foot contact, primarily by the plantar flexors. Loy and Voloshin (1991) found that males walking up and down stairs experienced induced impulsive loading or 'shock waves' in the tibia with an amplitude of 180 per cent and 250 per cent of level walking values, respectively. Zachazewski *et al.* (1993) also note a rapid increase in the vertical ground reaction force at foot contact.

Back

Cooper *et al.* (1989) note that erector spinae muscle activity in males was approximately 25 per cent of MVC during stair climbing and 10 per cent MVC during stair descent. This is compared to approximately 13 per cent MVC during level walking. Asplund and Hall (1995) note electric activity of the lumbar paraspinal muscles did not change significantly during 22 minutes of activity on a stair climbing ergometer.

Energy consumption/fatigue

Templer (1994) notes that the energy expended during stair climbing exceeds that of any other routine daily physical activity and is comparable to heavy physical labour. He notes that for a 70 kg person, the total energy cost of using stairs, while dependent on stair geometry, ranges from 0.548 to 1.12 kcal/metre (vertical) for stair ascent and 0.098 to 0.280 kcal/metre (vertical) for stair descent. He also notes that the total energy cost of vertical ascent decreases as stair slant increases up to about 45 degrees. Steep stairs, however, are often perceived as being more fatiguing because the rate of energy expenditure is higher even though the total energy expended for a given amount of vertical ascent may not be. Ward and Beadling (1970) note that the rate of energy expenditure affects people's judgement more than the total energy expended. Bruce *et al.* (1967), however, note that when normalised for total vertical travel, shallow slanted stairs require less energy than steep stairs. It is also not surprising that they found that the addition of a load to the climber increased the energy consumption for both shallow and steep stairs. Karpovich and Shinning (1971) note that the energy expenditure during stair descent was one-third of that during stair ascent. Using a climbing treadmill (Richardson, 1966) found that energy during stair descent was 59 per cent of stair ascent.

Shiomi (1994) proposes that, when normalised for total vertical movement per unit time, the optimum stepping rate for males is 50–62 steps per minute. He also notes that oxygen consumption increased as movement velocity increased during stair ascent and that oxygen consumption increased with an increase in stepping rate during both stair ascent and stair descent. Shinno (1971) notes that stairs with a 30–35 degree slope are most convenient and that optimal stair height, determined by oxygen consumption is defined as the square root of $R^2 + T^2 = 33$ cm, where R = step height and T = step depth. He determined that the optimum stair has a height of 16.6 cm (6.54 in) and a depth of 28.6 cm (11.26 in) with a slope of approximately 30 degrees. Seidl *et al.* (1989) found that for female subjects the efficiency in stair use, as determined by oxygen uptake, increased approximately 5 per cent over a four-day training period.

In studies of special populations Benn *et al.* (1996) found that for older men (age 64 ± 0.6 years) stair climbing produced greater systolic blood pressure, heart rate, and rate pressure product than did treadmill walking or dynamic weight lifting and that the increases in heart rate, mean arterial pressure, and mean pressure product were extremely rapid and reached very high levels. The rate pressure product was more than twice that recorded in normal walking and 50 per cent greater than during four minutes of uphill walking or weight lifting. In a study of simulated fire-fighting tasks O'Connell et al. (1986) found that stair ascent with a 20.3 cm (8 in) stair elevation at 60 steps per minute for five minutes resulted in 45 per cent of maximum oxygen consumption and 71 per cent of maximum heart rate. When carrying an 86.5 lb pack for five minutes subjects averaged 80 per cent maximum oxygen consumption and 95 per cent maximum heart rate.

CONCLUSIONS/RECOMMENDATIONS

Ladders

When climbing a ladder the whole body centre of mass moves further back (away from the ladder) as the ladder steepness increases. In general, the legs provide power and the hands provide support; however as the ladder steepness increases hand force increases as the hands provide more of the propulsive force and stability. Hand force also increases as the distance between the rungs (rung separation) increases. The force on one hand is a maximum (25–30 per cent of body weight) during the use of vertical ladders and this approaches the 35 per cent maximum grip strength on a slippery hand rail which indicates that there may be some potential for hand slip in this situation. A ladder width of 38.1 cm (15 in) appears to be adequate to accommodate preferred hand separation for most personnel and allow adequate lateral stability to resist wind force.

Foot force approaches a maximum of 85 per cent of body weight when climbing a ladder slanted at 70 degrees; however, foot slip potential is highest during the use of vertical ladders where a coefficient of friction in an excess of 0.4 may be required to resist a forward slip. Average shoulder moment is relatively low (approximately 5 per cent of static maximum) during the use of ladders slanted at 70 to 90 degrees (vertical). Average elbow flexion moment increases from approximately 5 per cent of maximum for 70 degree ladders up to 35 per cent for vertical ladders. When climbing vertical ladders peak shoulder extension and elbow flexion moments were 15 per cent and 45 per cent of static maximum. Peak hip extensor, knee extensor, and ankle plantar flexion moments reached 30 per cent, 15 per cent, and 60 per cent of static maximum, respectively, when climbing a ladder slanted at 70 degrees. Toe clearance behind the ladder must be approximately 16.5 cm (6.5 in) to allow adequate plantar flexion capability during vertical ladder use.

It should be noted that the joint moments, and particularly the maximum joint moments, were cyclic and of less than one second duration. This reduces the potential for localised fatigue except in long periods of climbing.

Average erector spinae activity is approximately 65 per cent of static maximum and increases slightly as the ladder slant goes from 70 to 90 degrees (vertical). Peak erector spinae activity approaches 100 per cent of static maximum during fast climbing of a vertical ladder. This suggests that there may be some potential for low back stress during some ladder climbing activities.

Ladder climbing is a fatiguing physical activity and has been found to be more stressful than either treadmill running or rowing ergometry. Rung separations of 35.6 cm (14 in) are more fatiguing than rung separations of 30.5 cm (12 in). Ladders slanted at 70 degrees require the lowest energy demand per unit of height and lowest climbing time per unit of height. The foot-over-foot climbing pattern is more energy efficient than when both feet are moved to the same step during the climbing activity.

Stairs

There is no clear agreement as to whether the whole body centre of mass deviates more from the foot centre of pressure during stair ascent or descent. Foot forces are higher during stair descent, however, and the impulsive loading may be 250 per cent of level walking during stair descent and 180 per cent during stair ascent. This force is absorbed primarily by the plantar flexors. Trunk abduction/adduction range of motion exceed those experienced during gait. Trunk flexion can approach 30 degrees (stair slant during climbing) but is considerably less during stair descent. Hip flexion ranges from 40 to 55 degrees during stair climbing and decreases as the stair slope decreases. Knee flexion ranges from 83 to 105 degrees with shorter subjects demonstrating the greatest degree of flexion. Ankle dorsiflexion and plantar flexion range of motion appear to range from 15 to 30 degrees in each direction during both stair ascent and descent. People appear to adjust to different stair dimensions by varying the flexion or extension at the knee rather than that at the ankle or hip.

Hand forces in normal use are minimum during both stair ascent and descent. Lower extremity moments and muscle forces are quite complex during stair use. With the exception of the rectus femoris and gluteus medius muscles, all muscles have greater mean activity for ascent as compared to descent and stair climbing produces higher EMG activity in the gluteus maximus, gluteus medius, and extensor fasciae latae than does level walking. Stair ascent primarily involves concentric contractions of the rectus femoris, vastus lateralis, soleus, and medial gastrocnemius with the vastus lateralis playing the most important role. Stair descent is achieved primarily through eccentric contractions of these same muscles to control the force due to gravity. Knee extension moments are higher during stair descent than ascent. Knee abduction moments are somewhat smaller than knee extension moments and knee adduction moments are minimal for stair ascent and descent.

Erector spinae muscle activity is in the same general range as that incurred during level walking and it does not seem to be indicative of a high potential for back stresses during normal stair use.

The energy expended during stair climbing, while not equivalent to ladder climbing, exceeds that of any other routine daily physical activity. While steeper stairs tend to be more energy efficient per vertical distance travelled, they are perceived as being more fatiguing because the rate of energy expenditure is higher. The energy expended during stair descent appears to be one-third to one-half of that expended during that of stair ascent. One study found that the 'optimum' stair from an energy standpoint has a height of 16.6 cm (6.54 in), a depth of 28.6 cm (11.26 in), and a slope of approximately 30 degrees.

ERGONOMIC SIGNIFICANCE

Stair and ladder use generate considerable biomechanical and metabolic stresses on the body. An understanding of design guidelines, user preferences, and the biomechanical and physiological stresses during ladder and stair use will assist in the minimisation of stress and a reduction of injury potential.

References

ANSI (AMERICAN NATIONAL STANDARDS INSTITUTE), 1983, *Rationales for ANSI A14.1-1981 (Wood Ladders), A14.2-1981 (Metal Ladders), and A14.5-1981 (Reinforced Plastic Ladders)*, Des Plaines, IL: American Society of Safety Engineers.

ANSI (AMERICAN NATIONAL STANDARDS INSTITUTE), 1990, *American National Standard for Ladders – Portable Metal – Safety Requirements*, ANSI A14.2-1990, Des Plaines, IL: American Society of Safety Engineers.

ANSI (AMERICAN NATIONAL STANDARDS INSTITUTE), 1992, *American National Standard for Ladders – Fixed – Safety Requirements*, ANSI A14.3-1992, Des Plaines, IL: American Society of Safety Engineers.

ANSI (AMERICAN NATIONAL STANDARDS INSTITUTE), 1994, *American National Standard for Ladders – Portable Wood – Safety Requirements*, ANSI A14.1-1994, Des Plaines, IL: American Society of Safety Engineers.

ANDRIACCHI, T.P., ANDERSSON, G.B.J., FERMIER, R.W., STERN, D. and GALANTE, J.O., 1980, A study of lower-limb mechanics during stair-climbing, *Journal of Bone Joint Surgery*, **62**, 749–757.

ARCHEA, J., COLLINS, B.L. and STAHL, F.I., 1979, *Guidelines for Stair Safety*, NBS Building Science Series 120, Washington, DC: US Department of Commerce.

ASPLUND, D.J. and HALL, S.J., 1995, Kinematics and myoelectric activity during stair-climbing ergometry, *JOSPT*, **22**(6), 247–253.

AXELSSON, P.-O. and CARTER, N., 1995, Measures to prevent portable ladder accidents in the construction industry, *Ergonomics*, **38**(2), 250–259.

AYOUB, M.M. and BAKKEN, G.M., 1978, *An Ergonomic Analysis of Selected Sections in Subpart D, Walking and Working Surfaces*, Service Contract No. B-9-F-8-1320, Institute for Biotechnology, Texas Tech University TX.

BENN, S.J., MCCARTNEY, N. and MCKELVIE, R.S., 1996, Circulatory responses to weight lifting, walking, and stair climbing in older males, *Journal of the American Geriatric Society*, **44**(2), 121–125.

BJÖRNSTIG, U. and JOHNSSON, J., 1992, Ladder injuries: mechanisms, injuries, and consequences, *Journal of Safety Research*, **23**, 9–18.

BLOSWICK, D.S. and CHAFFIN, D.B., 1990, An ergonomic analysis of the ladder climbing activity, *International Journal of Industrial Ergonomics*, **6**, 17–27.

BLOSWICK, D.S. and CROOKSTON, G., 1992, The effect of personal, environmental, and equipment variables on preferred ladder slant, in Kumar, S. (Ed.), *Advances in Industrial Ergonomics and Safety IV*, London: Taylor and Francis, 1015–1020.

BRAHLER, C.J. and BLANK, S.E., 1994, VersaClimbing elicits higher VO_{2MAX} than does treadmill running or rowing ergometry, *Medicine and Science in Sports and Exercise*, July.

BRUCE, F.M., FLOYD, W.F. and WARD, J.S., 1967, Oxygen consumption and heart rate during stair climbing, *Proceedings of the Physiological Society*, 14–15 April, 90–92.

CHAFFIN, D.B. and STOBBE, T.J., 1979, *Ergonomic Considerations Related to Selected Fall Prevention Aspects of Scaffolds and Ladders as Presented in OSHA Standard 29 CFR 1910 Subpart D*, Technical Report, University of Michigan Department of Industrial and Operations Engineering.

CHAFFIN, D.B., MIODONSKI, R., STOBBE, T., BOYDSTUN, L. and ARMSTRONG, T., 1978, *An Ergonomic Basis for Recommendations Pertaining to Specific Sections of OSHA Standard, 29CFT Part 1910, Subpart D – Walking, and Working Surfaces*, Technical Report, University of Michigan Department of Industrial and Operations Engineering.

COOPER, J., QUANBURY, A., GRAHAME, R. and DUBO, H., 1989, Trunk kinematics and trunk muscle EMG activity during five functional locomotor types, *CJOT*, **56**(3), 120–127.

COSTIGAN, P.A., WYSS, U.P., LI, J., COOKE, T.V.D. and OLNEY, S.J., 1993, Forces and moments at the knee during stairclimbing, *Proceedings of the XIVth Congress International Society of Biomechanics*, Paris, France, pp. 288–289.

DANIELSSON, K., 1987, *Improve Safety*, Stockholm, Sweden: Swedish Consumer Institute (in Swedish).

DEWAR, M.E., 1977, Body movements in climbing a ladder, *Ergonomics*, **20**(1), 67–86.

DIFFRIENT, N., TILLEY, A.R. and HARMAN, D., 1991, *Humanscale 7/8/9*, Cambridge, MA: MIT Press.

HÄKKINEN, K.K., PESONEN, J. and RAJAMÄKI, E., 1988, Experiments on safety in the use of portable ladders, *Journal of Occupational Accidents*, **10**, 1–19.

HAMMER, W. and SCHMALZ, U., 1992, Human behaviour when climbing ladders with varying inclinations, *Safety Science*, **15**, 21–38.

IRVINE, C.H. and VEJVODA, M., 1977, An investigation of the angle of inclination for setting non-self-supporting ladders, *Professional Safety*, July, 34–39.

JACK, E., ESTES, H. and GRACE, P., 1978, *Operator Strength*, Ford Operator Safety Office.

JOSEPH, J. and WATSON, R., 1967, Telemetering electromyography of muscles used in walking up and down stairs, *Journal of Bone and Joint Surgery*, **49B**(4).

KAMON, E., 1970, Negative and positive work in climbing a laddermill, *Journal of Applied Physiology*, **29**, 1–5.

KARI, H.K., JUSSI, P. and ERKKI, R., 1988, Experiments on safety in the use of portable ladders, *Journal of Occupational Accidents*, **10**(1), 1–19.

KARPOVICH, P. and SHINNING, W., (1971), *Physiology of muscular activity*, 7th edn, Philadelphia: Saunders, pp. 294–295.

KINOSHITA, K., KAWAJIRI, Y. and NAGATA, H., 1984, *Experimental Study on Optimum Dimensions of Vertical Fixed Ladders*.

KOWALK, D.L., DUNCAN, J.A. and VAUGHAN, C.L., 1996, Abduction–adduction moments at the knee during stair ascent and descent, *Journal of Biomechanics*, **29**(3), 383–388.

KREBS, D.E., WONG, D., JEVSEVAR, D., RILEY, P.O. and HODGE, W.A., 1992, Trunk kinematics during locomotor activities, *Physical Therapy*, **72**(7), 505–514.

LEE, Y.-H., CHENG, C.-K. and TSUANG, Y.-H., 1994, Biomechanical analysis in ladder climbing: the effect of slant angle and climbing speed, *Proceedings of the National Science Council, ROC Part B: Life Sciences*, **18**(4), 170–178.

LEHMANN, G., 1962, Praktische Arbeitsphysiologie. Neuauflage: Rohmert, W., Rutenfranz, J. (Hrsg.), 1983. Praktische Arbeitsphysiologie, G. Thieme Verlag, Stuttgart.

LIVINGSTON, L.A., STEVENSON, J.M. and OLNEY, S.J., 1991, Stairclimbing kinematics on stairs of differing dimensions, *Arch Phys Med Rehabil*, **72**, 398–402.

LOY, D.J. and VOLOSHIN, A.S., 1991, Biomechanics of stair walking and jumping, *Journal of Sports Sciences*, **9**, 137–149.

LYONS, K., PERRY, J., GRONLEY, J.K., BARNES, L. and ANTONELLI, D., 1983, Timing and relative intensity of hip extensor and abductor muscle action during level and stair ambulation, *Physical Therapy*, **63**(10), 1597–1605.

MALMROS, E., 1986, *Ladder Accidents 1984*, Stockholm, Sweden: National Board of Occupational Safety and Health.

MCFADYEN, B.J. and WINTER, D.A., 1988, An integrated biomechanical analysis of normal stair ascent and descent, *Journal of Biomechanics*, **21**(9), 733–744.

MCINTYRE, D.R., 1979, The Effects of Rung Spacing on the Mechanics of Ladder Ascent, dissertation, University of Oregon.

MCINTYRE, D.R., 1983, Gait patterns during free choice ladder ascents, *Human Movement Science*, **2**, 187–195.

MCINTYRE, D.R., SMITH, M.A. and JACKSON, A.W., 1983, The effects of shoe type on the stability and propulsive efforts of the lower limbs during ladder ascents, *Human Movement Science*, **2**, 57–65.

NATIONAL SAFETY COUNCIL, 1994, *Accident Facts*, 1994 Edition, Itasca, IL: NSC.

O'CONNELL, E.R., THOMAS, P.C., CADY, L.D. and KARWASKY, R.J., 1986, Energy costs of simulated stair climbing as a job-related task in fire fighting, *Journal of Occupational Medicine*, **28**(4), 282–284.

OREGON DEPARTMENT OF CONSUMER AND BUSINESS SERVICES, 1997, *Oregon Workers' Compensation Claims Characteristics – Calendar Year 1995*, Salem, OR: ODCBS.

PAULS, J.L., 1985, Review of stair-safety research with an emphasis on Canadian studies, *Ergonomics*, **28**(7), 999–1010.

RICHARDSON, M., 1966, Physiological responses and energy expenditures of women using stairs of three designs, *Journal of Applied Physiology*, **21**, 1078–1082.

SAFETY SCIENCES, 1978, *Occupational Fall Accident Patterns Supplementary Data*, contract no. 210-75-0017, prepared for National Institute for Occupational Safety and Health.

SEIDL, C., MONTGOMERY, D. and REID, G., 1989, Stair stepping efficiency of mentally handicapped and nonhandicapped adult females, *Ergonomics*, **32**(5), 519–526.

SHINNO, N., 1971, Analysis of knee function in ascending and descending stairs, *Medicine and Sport*, **6**, 202–207.

SHIOMI, T., 1994, Effects of different patterns of stairclimbing on physiological cost and motor efficiency, *Journal of Human Ergology*, **23**, 111–120.

SNYDER, R.G., 1977, *Occupational Falls*, report no. UM-HSRI-77-51, National Institute for Occupational Safety and Health.

TEMPLER, J.A., 1994, *The Staircase: Studies of Hazards, Falls, and Safe Design*, Cambridge, MA: MIT Press.

UNFALLSTATISTIK DET GESETZLICHEN UNFALLVERSICHERUNG IN DER BUNDESREPUBLIK DEUTSCHLAND, 1984, (Annual Report on Occupational Injuries), Hauptergebnisse fur Arbeit und Sozialordnung, Bonn, Germany.

WARD, J.S. and BEADLING, B., 1970, Optimum dimensions for domestic stairways: a preliminary study, *Architects Journal*, 5 July.

ZACHAZEWSKI, J.E., RILEY, P.O. and KREBS, D.E., 1993, Biomechanical analysis of body mass transfer during stair ascent and descent of healthy subjects, *Journal of Rehabilitation Research and Development*, **30**(4), 412–422.

CHAPTER NINETEEN

Slips and falls

RAOUL GRÖNQVIST

INTRODUCTION

The causality of slips, trips and falls is not yet fully understood. Before effective prevention strategies can be put into practice one must clarify the accident and injury mechanisms involved. The chain or network of events – constituting exposure to hazards, initiation of hazardous incidents, and final injury – should and can be identified using epidemiological principles and methodologies (Hernberg, 1992).

Risk-assessment models have been developed to predict the risk of slipping and to scrutinise the causes of slips and falls. A model based on artifical neural networks for predicting the dynamic coefficient of friction as a function of six independent measurement variables (Twomey et al., 1995), and the elaborated friction model for slipping (Grönqvist, 1995) are examples of models which are focused on certain limited elements. Lehto and Miller (1987), on the contrary, described an expert system for performing generic safety analysis and extended it with empirical data on the prediction of slipping safety. Fendley et al. (1995) recently developed a comprehensive slip-prediction model based on ratiometric analysis and thresholded dimensionless numbers.

Injuries are predictable entities with known extrinsic and intrinsic risk factors (Smith, 1987). The primary extrinsic risk factor for falls initiated by slipping is by definition poor grip or low friction between the foot (footwear) and substrate (floor, pavement, etc.). The question whether the risk of falling and injury initiated by a slip or trip is more related to a constantly low (slip) or high (trip) friction or an unexpected, sudden change in friction still remains to be solved. A fact is that an unexpected fall is a very hasty event, which lasts only 0.6 to 0.7 seconds until an outstretched hand, or the pelvis or trunk will be impacting the ground (Robinovitch et al., 1996). Other risk factors for slips, trips and falls are related to, for example, insufficient lighting, uneven surfaces, incomplete design of stairs and floors, poor housekeeping, load carrying, inadequate control of posture, ageing, dizziness, vestibular disease, peripheral neuromuscular dysfunction, diabetes, osteoporosis, alcohol intake, and use of antianxiety drugs (Alexander et al., 1992; Davis, 1983; Era et al., 1997; Fothergill et al., 1995; Honkanen, 1983; Jackson and Cohen, 1995; Malmivaara et al., 1993; Nagata, 1993; Pyykkö et al., 1988; Saarela, 1991; Sorock, 1988; Sorock and Labiner, 1992; Templer et al., 1985; Tideiksaar, 1990; Waller, 1978). Many of the risk factors for falls are interrelated and can have cumulative effects.

The main consequences of slipping and tripping accidents are either falls on the same level, falls from a higher to a lower level, or staggerings with recovery of balance but causing, for instance back overexertion or body contact with moving or stationary objects (Strandberg and Lanshammar, 1981). Manning *et al.* (1988) differentiated between various initiating events for falls and used the term 'underfoot accident' for fall injuries and some special types of injuries (e.g. to the lumbar spine) initiated by slipping (62 per cent), tripping (17 per cent), twisting of foot or ankle (12 per cent), treading on air (2 per cent), etc., where the first unforeseen event was an interaction between the victim's foot and the substrate. Sacher (1996) made an attempt to define some common misstep mechanisms during human walking from the viewpoint of forensic biomechanics. He distinguished these by the mode of initiation (slip, trip or stumble) and termination (e.g. direction of fall and nature of injury).

The focus of this chapter is on the biomechanics and prevention of accidents and injuries initiated by foot slip-ups. Other likely causes of falls like trips and stumbles, and missteps on stairs are mostly not dealt with but their biomechanics have been discussed elsewhere, for example by Grabnier *et al.* (1993), Eng *et al.* (1994), and Simoneau *et al.* (1991). The following areas and topics are covered here: mechanics and dynamics of slipping, basic features of the tribosystem of the interacting surfaces (feet, shoes, floors, etc.) and contaminants (water, oil, dirt, snow, etc.), risk-assessment of slips and falls, criteria for safe friction and locomotion, measurement principles and techniques for the assessment of slip resistance, and validity of test instruments. The ergonomic significance of the material presented is also discussed.

THE CONCEPT OF SLIP RESISTANCE

The following definitions for the terms 'slipping' and 'slip resistance' apply here:

> *Slipping* is a sudden loss of grip, resulting in sliding of the foot on a surface due to a lower coefficient of friction than that required for the momentary activity, often in the presence of liquid or solid contaminants (Grönqvist, 1995).

> *Slip resistance* refers to static, transitional and kinetic frictional properties of underfoot surfaces and foot/footwear during relative motion in actual conditions of wear; friction due to adhesion tends to dominate during static posture, standing, pushing and pulling, and at the moment of a slip start, whilst both adhesional and hysteretic friction play a role during dynamic locomotion without and with carrying loads, and at continuation of a slip after initiation (Grönqvist, 1997).

Three complementary models for assessing the risk of foot slippage and for determining the slip resistance of shoes and floors will be presented: a general concept model (Figure 19.1), a flowchart friction model (Figure 19.2), and a biomechanical parameter model (Figure 19.6). These models can be applied independently or successively.

MECHANICS AND DYNAMICS OF SLIPPING

Walking

During walking one is often totally unaware of the fact that slight sliding between the footwear and the substrate occurs even in dry non-slippery conditions in the very

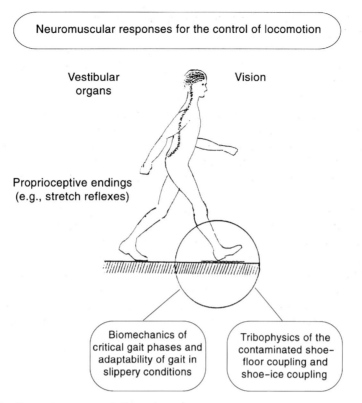

Figure 19.1 General concept of slip resistance.

beginning of the heel contact at landing (Perkins and Wilson, 1983; Strandberg and Lanshammar, 1981). Leamon and Son (1989) used the term microslip, also used by Perkins (1978), for slip incidents at heel contact on dry non-slippery surfaces. The lengths of such microslips were less than 1 cm. Leamon and Li (1990) determined the tendency of human subjects to such microslips on a slippery surface. They then redefined the term microslip to cover a range of slip distances from zero to 3 cm. Their data indicated that any distance less than 3 cm would only be detected on 50 per cent of occasions, and that a slip distance in excess of 3 cm would be perceived as a slippery condition.

Strandberg and Lanshammar (1981) studied the dynamics of human slipping in order to achieve biomechanical data for the prevention of slipping accidents. They simulated unexpected heel slip-ups when approaching a force plate which was lubricated with water and detergent in 76 trials (61 per cent) out of 124. The trials were categorised into two main groups, grips (85 trials) and skids (39 trials). The skids were then split into two categories, slip-sticks (16 trials) and falls (23 trials), while the slip-sticks were finally differentiated into mini-, midi- and maxi-slips. In the mini-slips the subjects were unaware of the sliding motion, in the midi-slips no apparent gait disturbances were observed, but in the maxi-slips compensatory swing-leg and arm motions occurred. The peak sliding velocity was above walking speed (1 to 2 m s^{-1}) in the skids that resulted in a fall, but did not normally exceed 0.5 m s^{-1} in the remaining skids called slip-sticks, where the subjects were able to regain balance. Strandberg and Lanshammar concluded that a slip was likely to result in a fall if the sliding exceeded 0.1 m in distance or 0.5 m s^{-1} in velocity. The average critical slip motion started 50 ms after heel contact, when the vertical load was about 60 per cent of body weight, acting typically at the heel rear edge.

Morach (1993) found in human slipping experiments on contaminated (oil, glycerine, and water) floors that the horizontal foot velocity in forward direction prior to heel contact varied between 0.3 m s^{-1} and 2.75 m s^{-1} depending on the type of slip, i.e., slip start after a short (more than 26 ms) static position (106 trials), immediate (during less than 6 ms) slip start (300 trials), and unclear (6 to 26 ms) slip start (112 trials). The highest velocities at slip start and during slipping were 2.5 m s^{-1} and occurred on a steel floor with oil as lubricant, when there was an immediate slip start after heel touch-down. The average walking speed was approximately 1.5 m s^{-1} in all the above experiments. Morach's findings suggest that a higher minimum sliding velocity (1.0 m s^{-1}) than that proposed by Strandberg and Lanshammar should be used when assessing the slip resistance properties of shoes and floors, particularly in the presence of oil. His findings also suggest a higher heel pitch angle of 15 to 20 degrees for simulation of slipping at heel landing and a shorter contact time of 30 to 60 ms.

Hirvonen et al. (1994) studied unexpected trunk movements during foot slip-ups of 20 male volunteers, who walked at two speeds (normal and race walking) along a horizontal track. They reported that the peak acceleration levels of the trunk increased significantly in the slipping incidents compared to normal or race walking without slipping, both in antero-posterior and medio-lateral directions. The peak accelerations varied from 0.5 to 4.5 g (1g = 9.81 m s^{-2}) during slipping, whilst the accelerations were typically less than 0.5 g during walking without slipping. The mean peak accelerations of the trunk during the sudden and unexpected slipping incidents that occurred at normal and race walking speeds were 1.3 g for the antero-posterior and 1.0 g for the medio-lateral direction.

Biomechanical slipping experiments were carried out and heel dynamics was studied at the Finnish Institute of Occupational Health during a collaborative European research project (M&T Slip Resistance Shoes, 1996). Volunteers walked over a horizontal slipping track at a cadence of 100 steps per minute, corresponding to a walking velocity of 1.2–1.4 m s^{-1}. The track was covered with a slip-resistant rubber carpet in order to facilitate normal walking. The downward vision of the subjects was restricted using special spectacles, since the objective was to study unexpected heel slip-ups when approaching a force platform on the track. The force plate was covered with a stainless steel floor, which was either dry or lubricated (glycerol, diluted glycerol, or wiped glycerol) in order to create unexpectedness and different slip or non-slip conditions. Of the 129 trials with five male subjects wearing six types of safety shoes, 12 trials for two subjects were randomly selected for further analysis and compilation of Table 19.1. These 12 trials were judged to be representative for the test condition with glycerol (85.0–91.5 per cent wt) as lubricant.

Two reference walking trials, where the same two subjects as above stepped unexpectedly onto a non-slippery, dry surface of stainless steel, were also analysed. In these dry trials only two of the variables in the column 'potential slip start' changed significantly compared to Table 19.1 whereas no changes were observed for the column 'approaching heel contact'; the vertical upward heel velocity during 60 ms after heel landing increased to 0.15 ± 0.04 m s^{-1} and the heel pitch angle increased to 14 ± 2 degrees. These changes indicated that immediate sensory feedback affected gait at heel contact (i.e. a protective gait strategy), when the floor surface was lubricated and slippery. The heel impact velocity and the foot inclination angle were reduced in comparison to the dry condition, but the vertical force and the horizontal heel velocity remained unaffected.

Table 19.1 Dynamics of the approaching heel contact, the potential slip start, and the slip continuation after initiation during normal walking when subjects stepped unexpectedly onto a slippery surface of stainless steel contaminated with glycerol 85.0–91.5% wt.

Variable	Approaching heel contact (during 60 ms before landing)	Potential slip start (during 60 ms after landing)	Slip continuation after initiation (from 60 to 200 ms after landing)
Vertical force (N)	Approx. 0[a]	Approx. 250[b]	Approx. 550
Vertical heel velocity (ms^{-1})	-0.17 ± 0.05[c]	0.08 ± 0.02	Approx. 0
Horizontal heel velocity (ms^{-1})	1.03 ± 0.16	0.18 ± 0.19	0.27 ± 0.32
Range of horizontal velocities (ms^{-1})	0.74–1.32	-0.26–0.37[d]	-0.03–1.20[d]
Peak horizontal velocity (ms^{-1})	Not calculated	Not calculated	0.48 ± 0.53
Range of peak horizontal velocity (ms^{-1})	Not calculated	Not calculated	-0.04–2.07[d]
Heel pitch angle (degrees)	32 ± 4	7 ± 3	6 ± 5[e]
Range of heel pitch angles (degrees)	22–37	3–13	0–18[e]
Slip length (mm)	Not relevant	16 ± 4	27 ± 47
Range of slip lengths (mm)	Not relevant	9–22	4–168

Average value, range and one standard deviation of each variable are given for 12 walking experiments with two young and healthy male subjects wearing six different types of safety footwear (from M&T Slip Resistance Shoes, 1996).
[a] End of swing phase.
[b] Beginning of stance phase.
[c] Negative value means movement downwards (heel descent).
[d] Negative value means movement backwards (heel rotation).
[e] Heel pitch angle at peak horizontal velocity.

Load carrying

Redfern and Rhoades (1996) reported experimental results concerning heel dynamics of individuals during load carrying (boxes of varying weights up to 13.5 kg) at three different walking cadences (70, 90, and 100 steps per minute). The surface condition studied was probably dry, but some microslips occurred during the experiments after heel contact. The horizontal (forward) heel velocity decreased from a pre-heel contact maximum of 4.5 m s^{-1} at the end of swing phase to between 0.14 and 0.24 m s^{-1} at heel contact in the beginning of stance phase. The heel pitch angle at heel touch-down was between 20 and 25 degrees and then decreased to foot flat within about 100 ms after contact. The heel came to a complete stop during microslip conditions about 100 ms after the impact.

Carrying loads showed, according to Redfern and Rhoades (1996), the same dynamic qualities as normal walking, and they concluded that load carrying had only minor effects on the heel movement parameters. Recently, Myung and Smith (1997) argued that this was true only for dry conditions while oily floors significantly affected those parameters. They recorded for oily vinyl and plywood floors horizontal heel landing velocities of at least 0.6 to 1.4 m s^{-1} during load carrying experiments with ten young male subjects. They also found that stride length was in general slightly reduced as floor slipperiness and load carrying levels increased.

TRIBOPHYSICS OF SLIPS AND FALLS

Footwear–contaminant–floor tribosystem

For elastomeric friction of rubberlike polymers (shoe solings) on dry surfaces, the total frictional coefficent (μ) due to adhesion and hysteresis depends on contact pressure according to the equation (Moore, 1972):

$$\mu = K_1 \ (E'/p^r + K_2 \ (p/E')^n) \tan \delta \qquad (19.1)$$
 adhesion $\quad$ hysteresis

In this equation tan δ is the tangent modulus of the elastomer, defined as the ratio of energy dissipated (E'') to energy stored (E') per cycle. The normal pressure is p, K_1 and K_2 are constants, r is an exponent less than 1 and n an exponent equal to or greater than 1. Moore (1975) later added the term s, i.e., the effective shear strength of the sliding interface, into the adhesion component (the term shear stress, τ, was used by Oksanen (1983), see Equation 19.5). Equation 19.1 is thus modified as follows:

$$\mu = K_1 \ (s \ (E'/p^r) + K_2 \ (p/E')^n) \tan \delta \qquad (19.2)$$
 adhesion $\qquad$ hysteresis

Kummer (1966) showed that both these components of rubber and elastomer friction are manifestations of the same basic viscoelastic energy dissipation mechanism. Adhesion is caused by a dissipative stick–slip process on a molecular level, whilst hysteresis is the ability of elastomers to store elastic energy. When the stress is removed during travel across a rigid surface, elastomers do not return completely from their deformed to their original shape. The deformation frequency is defined as the sliding velocity divided by distance between surface asperities of the rigid surface (Moore, 1972). Thus, the hysteresis component of friction increases on finer surfaces; however, under lubricated conditions the requirements of drainage put a lower limit on the size of surface asperities.

Strandberg (1985) pointed out that under lubricated conditions similar mechanisms to the ones that are valid for a rolling pneumatic tyre on a wet roadway (Moore, 1975) determine walking friction too: the squeeze-film process and drainage capability of the shoe–floor contact surface; the draping of the shoe heel and sole about the asperities of the underfoot surface (deformation, hysteresis); and the true contact between the surfaces (traction, adhesion). Since draping is time-dependent, slower sliding velocities permit a greater draping effect than higher velocities. Hence, a distinctly higher coefficient of adhesional friction is ensured at slow velocities. Hysteretic friction, on the contrary, is small in the low-speed range, but increases as sliding velocity and deformation frequency increase (Moore, 1972).

The tribophysics of human slipping have been discussed by Tisserand (1985), Proctor and Coleman (1988), and Leclercq et al. (1995). The classical squeeze-film theory of Reynolds states that the generation of hydrodynamic pressure and load support in the lubricant film is a function of wedge, stretch and squeeze terms (Moore, 1972). Hence, Reynolds' theory takes into account the vertical squeezing motion, as well as the tangential sliding motion and its gradient. The effect of the squeeze term has been scrutinised by Strandberg (1985) and the effect of the wedge term by Proctor and Coleman (1988). The stretch contribution has not yet been discussed in the context of human slipping, though it is considered important for rubbers and elastomeric materials.

The equation for the squeeze term, according to Strandberg (1985) is:

$$h^2 = (K \ u \ A^2)/(F_N \ t) \qquad\qquad (19.3)$$

where,

h is height of the wear surface element above flooring (film thickness)
u is viscosity of the fluid
A is contact area between the surfaces
F_N is normal force
t is descending time.

According to this model by Strandberg, the height of the wear surface element above the floor surface when a shoe vertically descends in a fluid film depends on the viscosity of the fluid, the contact area between the surfaces, the vertical load, and the descending time. The lubricant drainage time for a specified fluid viscosity, normal load and fluid film thickness becomes four times longer when the contact area is doubled. A long drainage time, on the contrary, increases the actual risk of slipping, because the time available to prevent a forward slip after heel contact is very short, only a few tenths of a second (Strandberg and Lanshammar, 1981). Hence, adequate frictional forces may not be produced between the shoe heel and a smooth lubricated walking surface quickly enough to prevent slipping and falling.

Leclercq et al. (1993) confirmed the above observation concerning the descending time (t) in Equation 19.3 by adjusting the rolling speed of the test wheel of the PFT (portable friction tester) device. When the rolling speed was decreased, t increased and h decreased so that adhesional friction became possible. Greater adhesion then contributed to a higher kinetic coefficient of friction between the test wheel and the substrate.

The equation for the wedge term, according to Proctor and Coleman (1988) is:

$$h^2 = (0.066 \ u \ l^3)/F_N \ v \qquad\qquad (19.4)$$

where,

h is film thickness of the fluid
u is viscosity of the fluid
l is length of slider (a square slider is assumed)
v is velocity of sliding
F_N is normal force.

Proctor and Coleman called this the hydrodynamic squeeze-film model. Its principle of operation is the tapered wedge, and it shows that for a specific viscosity, vertical load and slider dimensions, the film thickness varies as the square root of the sliding velocity. The model especially emphasises the importance of reducing the sliding velocity during a slip in order to minimise the lubricant film thickness, and then to obtain good contact and grip between the shoe sole and floor.

Footwear–ice tribosystem

Bowden and Hughes (1939) have shown that the very low friction between ice and other materials is due to a water layer formed by frictional heating. However, ice is not always slippery (Petrenko, 1994); the ice friction coefficient can assume both very small values ($\mu < 0.01$), at high temperatures ($-1°C$) and high velocities ($3 \ m \ s^{-1}$), or very large values ($\mu = 0.67$), at low temperatures ($-40°C$) and low velocities ($0.01 \ cm \ s^{-1}$). The viscoelastic nature of ice friction has been discussed by Moore (1975). The frictional mechanisms in the footwear–ice interface are mostly adhesional, but the properties of the interface layer in ice and snow friction are still poorly known (Makkonen, 1994).

In general, the properties of ice, e.g., temperature, structure and hardness, as well as the thickness of the water layer, seem to determine the friction during a slip to a greater extent than the viscoelastic properties of rubber or polymers (Gnörich and Grosch, 1975; Roberts, 1981). Low hysteresis and low hardness, which are in many cases interrelated, seem to be necessary properties of a rubber to improve friction on ice (Ahagon et al., 1988).

Assuming that the frictional force, F_μ, in the footwear–ice interface is caused only by viscous shear in a water layer (other phenomena such as scratch formation are omitted) the following equation (Oksanen, 1983) is obtained:

$$F_\mu = \tau \, A = u_o \, v/d \, A \tag{19.5}$$

where,

τ is shear stress
A is contact area
u_o is viscosity of water
v is velocity of sliding
d is thickness of the water layer.

The coefficient of friction, μ, is then:

$$\mu = F_\mu/F_N = (u_o \, v/d \, A)/F_N \tag{19.6}$$

where F_N is normal force.

Near the melting point of ice the friction seems to be governed particularly by ice flow and melting (Roberts and Richardson, 1981). Ionic impurities in ice lower its melting point, thereby forming liquid brine at the surface which has an essential lowering effect on adhesional friction. Warm ice is also sensitive to high pressure effects at heel strike in gait. At high pressure points ice will either flow to relieve the pressure or melt. Both phenomena tend to lower the coefficient of friction when the temperature of ice is warmer than $-10°C$.

Friction model for slipping

A flowchart friction model for slipping is presented in Figure 19.2 (Grönqvist, 1995). This model complements the previously presented general concept of slip resistance and it takes into account the drainage capability of the shoe–floor contact surface (squeeze-film processes), the draping of the shoe bottom about the asperities of the floor surface (deformation and damping), and finally the true contact between the interacting surfaces (traction). The squeeze-film processes, occurring between the shoe and the walking surface immediately after first contact at heel touch-down, can be considered as the most important single phenomenon affecting pedestrian safety in slippery, contaminated conditions. The key point in injury prevention is therefore the drainage capability of walkways, floorings and footwear solings. If the drainage after heel landing fails or is too slow due to hydrodynamic load support and elastohydrodynamic effects, then the development of any frictional forces will be incomplete. Its immediate consequence will be an unstable

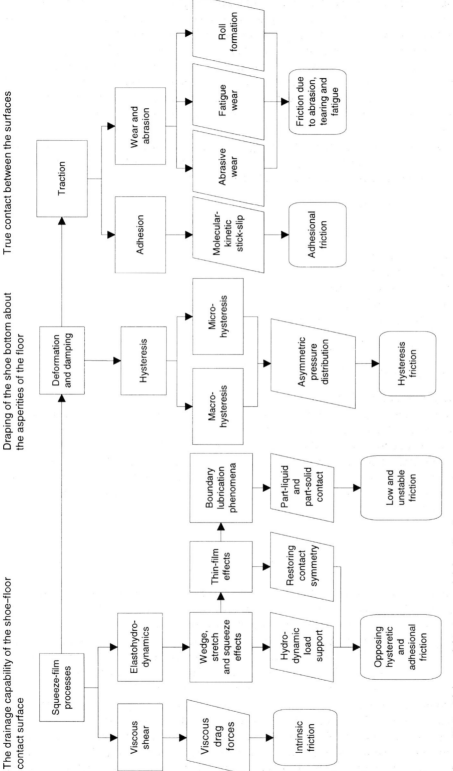

The drainage capability of the shoe–floor contact surface

Draping of the shoe bottom about the asperities of the floor

True contact between the surfaces

Figure 19.2 Elaborated friction model for slipping.

situation with increased risk of slipping and falling. However, if draping occurs then adequate frictional forces may develop due to deformation (macro- and microhysteresis) and may even result in true molecular contact (adhesion and wear) between the interacting surfaces.

RISK ASSESSMENT OF SLIPS AND FALLS

Control and adaptability of gait

Humans rely on numerous sensomotoric systems to maintain upright static posture and dynamic balance during locomotion. The sensory input from vestibular organs, vision, proprioceptive receptors (muscle spindles, stretch reflexes), and exteroceptive tactile cues (pressure) are rapidly and accurately processed by the central nervous system (Claussen, 1986; Nienstedt et al., 1986). When posture and balance are challenged, for instance during a sudden slip or trip, then a coordinated neuromuscular motor response is needed to re-establish the balance and to avoid a fall and subsequent injury. This motor control aims at regulating more than 700 muscles in a multi-link system including more than 200 degrees of freedom (Era et al., 1997).

Oscillations in posture during normal quiet standing and sudden perturbation are generally assumed to reflect the balancing abilities. Vestibular influx governs normally 65 per cent of the body sway during sudden perturbation, whilst 35 per cent is accounted for by visual and proprioceptive influx (Pyykkö et al., 1990). Stretch reflexes in joints and muscles and tactile cues from pressoreceptors seem to operate in the early prevention of falls. Any protective responses to sudden perturbations will be incomplete if these do not function properly. Since ageing is one of the main reasons for defective coactivation of functional stretch reflexes, the very elderly rely mostly on slower (latency 120–200 ms) visual control of balance, which thus contribute to an increased risk of slipping, tripping and falling (Pyykkö et al., 1990). Latencies for corrective reflex responses for healthy young men in the recovery from tripping have been reported to be 60–140 ms, indicating that quick polysynaptic pathways were involved (Eng et al., 1994). This study suggested that balance control during locomotion involves specific movement patterns in response to a tripping perturbation.

Protective gait adaptations are aimed at regulating gait in hazardous, for example slippery, conditions. Experimental walking trials reviewed by Andres et al. (1992) have shown that subjects can adapt to walking continuously over very slippery surfaces. This adaptation takes place in essentially a one step cycle after becoming aware of the slipperiness of the surface being approached. Llewellyn and Nevola (1992) reported the results of trials where subjects adapted their gait under low-friction conditions by adopting a protective strategy, which involved the combined effect of force and postural changes of the early stance. The subjects took shorter steps and increased their knee flexion, which in combination reduced the vertical acceleration and the forward velocity of the body.

Perception of slipperiness

The risk of slipping and falling seems to depend to a great extent on a person's subjective awareness of the potential slipperiness of the actual conditions. Probably it is easier to adapt one's gait when a slippery condition is steady than when rapid, unexpected changes in slipperiness occur. However, no accident or injury statistics are available to confirm this hypothesis. On the contrary, it has been shown by Merrild and Bak (1983) that certain high-risk winter days can cause an enormous increase of pedestrian injuries due to falls initiated by slipping.

Vision may be the only sensory mode allowing a person to predict the potential slipperiness of a surface before stepping onto it. Proprioceptive (e.g. stretch reflexes) and other control systems (e.g. pressoreceptors) seem to require that one already has walked on a slippery surface and felt it, in order to acquire the feedback to properly adapt one's gait. Visual control may lead to several avoidance and accommodation strategies of gait when challenging conditions are encountered. Vision regulates step length and width, direction of gait, walking velocity, and orientation of limbs, etc. (Patla, 1991), but since visual control is slower than proprioceptive control, it cannot be solely relied upon in sudden perturbations like slips and trips.

Critical gait phases

Winter (1991) mentions five major motor functions during the gait cycle in order to achieve safe and efficient propulsion of the body. These functions, which are independent of whether one walks or runs, are the maintenance of support of the upper body during stance, the maintenance of upright posture and balance of the total body, the control of foot trajectory to achieve safe ground clearance and gentle heel or toe landing, the generation of mechanical energy to maintain the present forward velocity or to increase the forward velocity, and finally the absorption of mechanical energy for shock absorption and stability or to decrease the forward velocity of the body.

From the slipping point of view there are two critical gait phases in walking; heel contact and toe-off (Perkins, 1978; Skiba *et al.*, 1983; Strandberg and Lanshammar 1981). The heel contact causes a forward slip on the leading foot, whereas the toe-off causes a backward slip on the sole forepart, which can be more easily counteracted by stepping forwards with the leading foot (Figure 19.3). It is therefore considered less dangerous than the heel slip. The forward slip starting at heel contact, on the contrary, would very likely result in a dangerous fall backwards due to the fact that the forward momentum maintains the body weight on the slipping foot and permits the sliding movement to continue until a fall.

CRITERIA FOR SAFE FRICTION

Minimum friction requirement

Walking is regarded as safe when the coefficient of friction (μ) is greater than the ratio of the horizontal (F_H) and vertical (F_V) force components applied to the ground (Carlsöö, 1962):

$$\mu > F_H/F_V \tag{19.7}$$

The frictional force (F_μ), on the other hand, is directly proportional to the normal force (F_N) according to the classic laws of friction:

$$F_\mu = \mu \, F_N \tag{19.8}$$

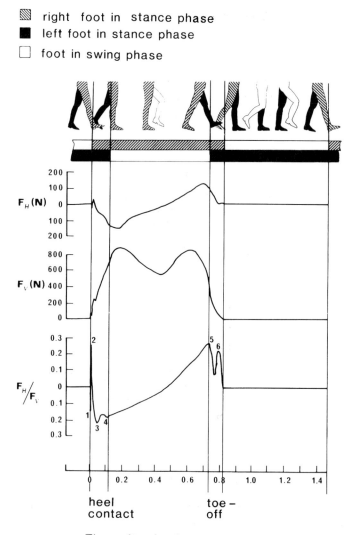

Figure 19.3 Gait phases in normal level walking with typical horizontal (F_H) and vertical force (F_V) components and their ratio, F_H/F_V, for one step (right foot). Critical from the viewpoint of slipping are the heel contact (peaks 3 and 4) and the toe-off (peaks 5 and 6) phases.

These two equations can be combined to give:

$$F_\mu/F_N > F_H/F_V \qquad (19.9)$$

Consequently, if the sizes of the horizontal and vertical force components applied to the ground during walking and the coefficient of friction for the actual tribosystem are known, then it is possible to evaluate whether this system is potentially slippery and hazardous (Figure 19.4). A transverse force component has been ignored here (level walking assumed), but should be added to these equations in slip situations where the transverse component plays a role.

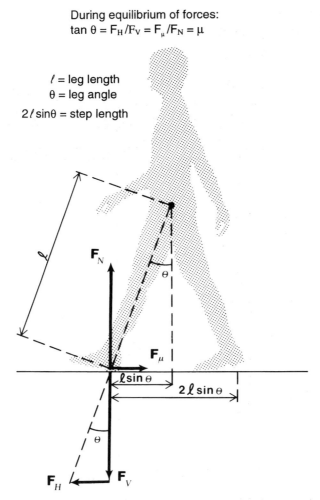

During equilibrium of forces:
$$\tan \theta = F_H/F_V = F_\mu/F_N = \mu$$

l = leg length
θ = leg angle
$2l\sin\theta$ = step length

Figure 19.4 Frictional (F_μ) and normal force (F_N) vectors versus horizontal (F_H) and vertical force (F_V) vectors during heel contact phase.

Friction demands in various activities

The friction demand, based on human experiments during normal level walking has been found to be between 0.15 and 0.30 (Bring 1982; Perkins, 1978; Strandberg and Lanshammar 1981). Strandberg and Lanshammar (1981) measured the friction use peak, F_H/F_V, approximately 0.1 s after heel contact. The peak F_H/F_V was on the average 0.17 when there was no skidding between the shoe and the floor (grip), 0.13 when the subject was unaware of the sliding motion or regained balance (slip-stick), and 0.07 when the skid resulted in a fall. Kinetic friction properties seemed to be more important than the static ones, because in most of their experiments the heel slid upon heel contact even without any lubricant.

Strandberg (1983a) favoured 0.20 as a safe limit value for the kinetic coefficient of friction in level walking. He nevertheless pointed out that the adequate value depends on gait characteristics and the way of measurement. He found that friction properties were most important for preventing falls at sliding velocities below 0.5 m s^{-1}. Static friction values for safe walking that were proposed in the United States in the mid-1970s range from 0.40 to 0.50 (Brungraber, 1976). These values are contradictory to the actual friction demand based on human walking experiments on a level surface, and thus may be more an indication of practical eligibility.

Coefficient of friction limit values should be correlated to the normal variability of human gait characteristics. Walking speed, stride length, and anthropometric parameters, etc., may greatly affect the friction demand during locomotion (Andres et al., 1992; Carlsöö, 1962; James, 1983; Myung et al., 1992). Depending on the type of movement (level walking, and walking on stairs or ramp) James (1980) referred to limit values between 0.15 and 0.40. Harper et al. (1967) and Skiba et al (1983) referred to limit values between 0.30 and 0.60 during stopping of motion, curving and walking on a slope. Later Skiba (1988) defined that the safety limit for the kinetic coefficient of friction, based on the forces measured during human walking and the social acceptance of the risk of slipping, would be 0.43 at sliding speeds of at least 0.25 m s^{-1}. At heel contact in running gait the peak F_H/F_V is typically slightly greater (about 0.30) compared to walking, and the difference between running and walking is even greater at toe-off, when the force ratio peak is about 0.45 (Vaughan, 1984).

Buzcek et al. (1990) emphasised that the slip resistance needs for the mobility disabled are greater than for able-bodied persons. Their study indicated that the required coefficient of friction near touch-down for the unaffected side of the mobility disabled was significantly higher (average 0.64) than for the able-bodied (average 0.31) regardless of the speed (slow or fast) of walking, whereas no difference was observed for the push-off phase.

Grieve (1983) studied static friction demands for avoiding slipping during manual exertion (lifting, pushing, and pulling) and found that static manual exertion can create unavoidable slip-ups due to high frictional requirements (even > 1) in some conditions. He concluded that more efforts should be concentrated to the events which follow the foot slip-up.

An important point of interest which has not received enough attention when trying to set limit values for safe friction is that the suggested friction demands ('friction use' or 'required' friction) have not been related to the duration of the friction value. Just the magnitude of peak values have been mostly referred to, which is a significant drawback, and could lead to an overestimation regarding the friction demand during various types of movement (walking, running, stopping, etc.) and various activities (pushing and pulling, load carrying, etc.). When comparing subjective friction utilisation ratios and objective apparatus-based coefficient of friction values, Grönqvist (1995) defined the exact time-interval (100–150 ms after heel contact) for calculating friction values (Figure 19.5).

MEASUREMENT OF SLIP RESISTANCE

Main test principles

Slip resistance can be determined quantitatively by the coefficient of friction between the interacting surfaces, but there has been much debate on how to measure it correctly (Grönqvist, 1995; James, 1983; Strandberg, 1985). Traditionally, either static or kinetic (dynamic) coefficient of friction measurements have been used to predict pedestrian slip resistance. Static friction has been regarded important for causing a slip to start and kinetic friction for the continuation of a slip after initiation. Nevertheless, criticism against

Friction utilisation ratio, F_H/F_V

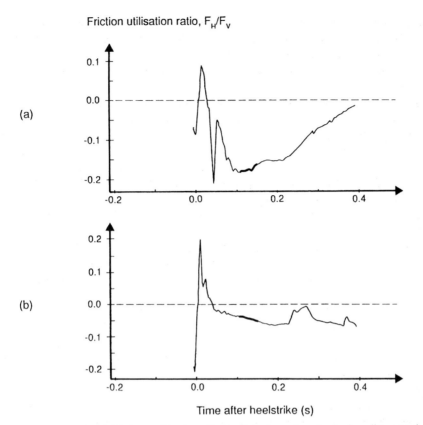

(a)

(b)

Time after heelstrike (s)

Figure 19.5 Example of friction utilisation, F_H/F_V, data from two typical walking trials; **(a)** good grip (0.18) and **(b)** poor grip (0.04). The time-interval for computing the force data, 0.10–0.15 s from heel contact, is marked bold. Force ratios forward in the walking direction are represented by negative values.

static friction measurements of rubberlike viscoelastic materials may be raised because any frictional force applied to them will produce some creep, i.e., motion (Rabinowicz, 1956). Support for both the static and the kinetic coefficient of friction as a predictor of slipperiness of floors and footwear has been reported (Grönqvist, 1995). Besides translational friction, rotational friction properties have also been found to be useful for slip prediction in the context of various sports and sport surfaces (Nigg and Yeadon, 1987).

A fully developed slip condition may require the determination of steady-state kinetic friction, which is produced only after some time-delay from the slip start, whilst the static friction is limited to the slip start before any detectable motion. The transitional behaviour of the coefficient of friction between those two extremes has evoked little interest, though some of the current test instruments may measure that property (Grönqvist, 1997). The transitional period after the slip initiation is typically very short (less than 250 ms) when slipping at heel touch-down, and it seems to reflect well the squeeze-film phenomena during early stance foot slip-ups on contaminated surfaces.

For distinguishing between various principles of measurement one must consider direct and indirect friction measurements, lubricated and non-lubricated friction tests, laboratory and portable on-site measurement methods, apparatus-based and subjective evaluation methods, and floor and footwear test methods. The following principles of operation are often referred to in the context of slip resistance measurement (Grönqvist,

Table 19.2   Examples of portable test devices for assessing floor slipperiness.

Operating principle (output quantity)	Name of device	Criterion for slip resistance	Special remarks
Drag/towed-sled (force)	1. Bigfoot 2. Drag sled tester, PTI-DST 3. Schuster 4. Model 80 5. Horizontal pull slipmeter, HPS 6. Tortus 7. Floor slide control 2000	Static COF[1,2,3,4,5] Steady-state kinetic COF[3,4,5,6,7]	Manually pulled[1,2,3,4] Electrically driven[5,6,7] Uncontrolled normal force application time[1,2,3,4,5,6,7] Low normal pressure[1,2,3,4,5,6,7] Uncontrolled velocity[3,4] Low controlled velocity[5,6,7] Long test distance[3,4,5,7] Short test distance[6] Sensitive to surface nonuniformities[5,6] Operator-dependent[1,2,3,4]
Pendulum striker (loss of energy)	8. British portable skid tester, BPST 9. RRL skid tester 10. Sigler	Transitional kinetic COF[8,9,10]	Uncontrolled normal force application time[8,9,10] High uncontrolled velocity[8,9,10] Short test distance[8,9,10] Incapable of testing raised profiled floors[8,9,10]
Articulated-strut/ inclined leg (angle of inclination)	11. Carlsöö-Mayr 12. Pangels 13. Brungraber M1 14. Brungraber M2 15. Ergodyne	Static COF[11,12,13,14,15] Transitional kinetic COF[14]	Manually pushed[11] Mechanically loaded[12,13,14] Instantaneous actuation[15] Long uncontrolled normal force application time[11,12,13] Short uncontrolled normal force application time[14,15] Low normal pressure[11,12,13,14,15] Short test distance[14] Operator-dependent[11,13]
Braked-wheel/ skiddometer (axle torque using various slip ratios)	16. Portable friction tester, PFT 17. FIDO (pre-proto-type of PFT)	Steady-state kinetic COF[16,17]	Manually pushed[16,17] Long uncontrolled normal force application time[16,17] Controlled velocity[16,17] Long test distance[16,17] Operator-dependent[16,17]

The index numbers in the table refer to appropriate test devices.
(From Andres and Chaffin, 1985; English, 1992; Harris and Shaw, 1988; Jung and von Diecken, 1992; Kulakowski *et al.*, 1989; Proctor, 1993; Proctor and Coleman, 1988; Skiba, 1984; Skiba *et al.*, 1994; Strandberg, 1983b).

1995; James, 1980; Proctor, 1993; Skiba, 1984): drag type or towed-sled devices, pendulum strikers, articulated-strut devices, braked-wheels or skiddometers, turntables or rotating discs, and gait simulators. The output quantity according to these different principles is typically force, torque, loss of energy, inclination angle, or rolling resistance. Examples of portable test instruments for assessing on-site floor slipperiness are given in Table 19.2.

A number of purely subjective methods (e.g. paired comparison tests) or partly subjective and partly objective methods (e.g. ramp tests) have also been used to assess slip resistance. Human subjects are capable of differentiating the slipperiness of floors (Chiou et al., 1996; Myung et al., 1993; Swensen et al., 1992) and footwear (Nagata, 1989; Strandberg et al., 1985; Tisserand, 1985) in various dry, wet and contaminated conditions. Cohen and Cohen (1994a, 1994b) pointed out that tactile sliding resistance cues are the most sensitive predictors of the coefficient of friction under various experimental conditions, but particularly on wet surfaces. Leamon and Son (1989) and Myung et al. (1992) have suggested that measuring microslip length or slip distance during slipping incidents might be a better means to predict slip resistance than the traditional friction measurement techniques.

Measurement techniques

A variety of techniques are currently available for measuring slip resistance of shoes and floors (Bring, 1964; Brungraber, 1976; James, 1980; Strandberg, 1983b). About 70 types of slip resistance measurement devices were found in the literature by Strandberg (1983b), but Strandberg and Lanshammar (1981) found surprisingly little support in their biomechanical skidding data for the most common measurement principles. Since some of the techniques represent several operational modes of testing slip resistance, the number of different test methods is in fact considerably greater. Strandberg (1983b) pointed out that neither the measurement methods themselves nor their outputs should be accepted without examination of their inherent slip resistance definition based on tribology and biomechanics. After his review a number of new test devices have been presented in the literature (Grönqvist, 1995), but few devices seem to meet even the minimum criteria for validity, consistency, repeatability and precision.

Biomechanical measurement parameters

For assessing slip resistance, any test instrument based on friction measurement should meet the criteria in Figure 19.6. The first is the capability to measure static, transitional kinetic, and steady-state kinetic friction properties of the interacting surfaces and the contaminants. The second is the possibility for two optional modes of operation, i.e., impact (dynamic loading) and non-impact (static loading) testing. The third is the flexibility for selecting relevant measurement parameters, such as the normal force build-up time and rate, normal force and pressure, sliding velocity, and contact time prior to and during friction measurement.

A dynamic loading test condition, typical for heel contact in normal walking, has received too little attention in many current slip testing devices. Only the pendulum strikers, some gait simulators, and some articulated-strut devices produce an impact at the moment when the coefficient of friction is measured. However, the impact forces produced are mostly poorly defined and do not correspond to normal gait, where the heel touch-down is characterised by collision-type contact forces (Cappozzo, 1991).

Test methods applying static loading, i.e., static or kinetic coefficient of friction testing without impact, tend to lead to a poorer separation of the interacting surfaces due to lower hydrodynamic pressure generation in the contaminant-film (Moore, 1972). Therefore, they will produce higher coefficient of friction values than the methods applying impact

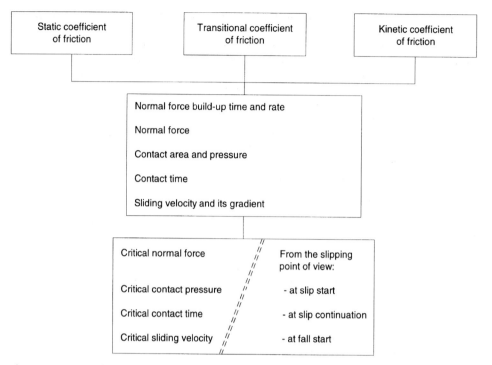

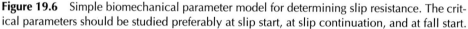

Figure 19.6   Simple biomechanical parameter model for determining slip resistance. The critical parameters should be studied preferably at slip start, at slip continuation, and at fall start.

loading when test conditions are the same. Non-impact measurement techniques underestimate the real risk of slipping, particularly when wet, oily or greasy conditions are encountered.

The measurement parameters and their ranges should reflect the biomechanics and tribophysics of actual slipping incidents. The normal force build-up rate must be at least 10 kN s^{-1}, the normal pressure between the interacting surfaces from 0.1 to 0.6 MPa, the sliding velocity between zero and 1.0 m s^{-1}, and the time of contact prior to and during the coefficient of friction computation between 50 and 800 ms (Table 19.3).

ERGONOMIC SIGNIFICANCE

Injuries and fatalities due to falls

The human and economic dimensions of slip, trip and fall injuries at work, in the home and during leisure-time activities are overwhelming. Falls account for 17 per cent of all work-related injuries and 12 per cent of worker fatalities in the United States (Leamon and Murphy, 1995). The incidence rates for falls and workers' compensation claims were found to be highest for young (less than 25 years) and old (over 65 years) workers. According to the same source, falls represented about 9 per cent of all fatal injuries and 33 per cent of all hospitalised injuries in the USA in 1985, whilst the total lifetime cost of these injuries was estimated at $37.3 billion. Englander *et al.* (1996) reported that the direct costs of fall injuries in the USA increased dramatically with advancing age of the

Table 19.3 Relevant biomechanical measurement parameters and their ranges during slipperiness evaluations.

Measurement parameter	Relevant range	Remarks
Normal force build-up time (rate)	50–150 ms (10 kN s^{-1})	At heel contact
Normal pressure during coefficient of friction computation	0.1–0.6 MPa	From heel contact to midstance
Horizontal force build-up time (rate)	50–150 ms (1.5 kN s^{-1})	At heel contact
Horizontal velocity during coefficient of friction computation	0–1.4 m s^{-1}	From static to kinetic friction
Contact time prior to coefficient of friction computation	50–150 ms	When normal force is built-up
Contact time during coefficient of friction computation	50–800 ms	Transitional to steady-state kinetic friction properties

(From Bring, 1982; Chaffin *et al.*, 1992; Grönqvist, 1995, 1997; Morach, 1993; M&T Slip Resistance Shoes, 1996; Myung and Smith, 1997; Perkins, 1978; Proctor and Coleman, 1988; Skiba *et al.*, 1983; Strandberg and Lanshammar, 1981; Tisserand, 1985).

Table 19.4 Fatality rates of all accidents and falling accidents for men and women due to slips and trips on the same level and from a higher to a lower level at work, in the home and during leisure-time in Finland.

Type of accident	Fatality rate; number of fatalities per 100 000 people					
	1980		1988		1992	
	Men	Women	Men	Women	Men	Women
All accidents	66.1	24.3	82.4	33.2	74.0	34.5
Falls	11.8	11.2	15.2	15.6	17.6	15.4

(From Heiskanen and Koskela, 1994).

victim, and that the overall total cost of fall injuries in 1995 was estimated at $64.4 billion. This total cost was expected to increase by about one third until the year 2020.

The ageing of the Finnish population has caused the number and severity of slips, trips and falls on the same level and from a higher to a lower level to increase gradually. The current picture of all kinds of unintentional fatal injuries in Finland is dominated by falls, which in 1993 accounted for about 34 per cent (Heiskanen and Koskela, 1994). The fatality rate, i.e. the annual number of fatal injuries per 100 000 people, has been increasing since 1980 for both men and women (Table 19.4). This is worrisome particularly since this trend has been estimated to continue in the future. For men about 24 per cent of all fatalities due to injuries at work, in the home, and during leisure-time and for women about 45 per cent were caused by falls in 1992 in Finland (Heiskanen and Koskela, 1994). The fatality rate due to slips, trips and falls is greatly increasing by age, for men from the age of 25 (fatality rate 4.4) and for women from the age of 45 (2.5), whereas the fatality rates of the elderly (over 75 years) was as high as 211 for men and 159 for women.

Loading on the musculoskeletal system

Slips and trips may, besides causing injuries, also contribute to mechanical loading on the musculoskeletal system. Sudden, unexpected corrective body movements made to restore balance and to prevent a fall can create substantial muscle forces and harmful loading on the spine (Lavender *et al.*, 1988). Manning and Shannon (1981) and Manning *et al.* (1984) reported that slipping was a common cause of low-back pain and disability in a car factory. Slips and trips can lead to quick transitions of shear forces between shoes and floors during manual exertion (lifting, pushing, pulling, and load carrying), which may sometimes create unavoidable mechanical load on the musculoskeletal system. However, the amount of sudden unexpected strain needed to cause irreversible damage in the low back due to a slip or trip has not yet been clarified.

Fatigue of the lower extremities due to too low or too high friction is another common and important ergonomic aspect which is worth more attention in the future. Moderate changes of slip resistance characteristics of adjacent floor areas are probably very important for the prevention of fatigue and disorders of the lower extremities. For controlling that kind of transitions in floorings and in conditions, one needs to measure friction as comprehensively as possible, for example, by regularly checking static, transitional, and kinetic friction properties of floors and shoes *in situ*.

Floorings and footwear

Flooring and footwear manufacturers need more support for designing new and safer products. Specific materials and specific design of products should be favoured for hazardous environments (indoor, outdoor, wet areas, ice, etc.) instead of purely general solutions. Adequate guidelines for the selection of antislip and antitrip materials and proper ergonomic design guidelines for ensuring slip and fall protection should be the ultimate goal in slipping accident and injury prevention. Since contaminant removal is one of the key factors for achieving such a goal, one should not underestimate the vital importance of various housekeeping and maintenance strategies.

Specific product safety standards (e.g. contaminant and task related standards) should be developed for both floorings and footwear in parallel with those standards that already exist. Slip resistance test instruments ought to be validated against biomechanical trials in conditions for which they are intended to be applied. Existing slipping safety guidelines and classification systems for floorings and footwear need to be scrutinised and further elaborated.

References

AHAGON, A., KOBAYASHI, T. and MISAWA, M., 1988, Friction on ice, *Rubber Chemistry and Technology*, **61**, 14–35.

ALEXANDER, N.B., SHEPHARD, N., MIAN JU GU and SCHULTZ, A., 1992, Postural control in young and elderly adults when stance is perturbed: kinematics, *Journal of Gerontology*, **47**, M79–M87.

ANDRES, R.O. and CHAFFIN, D.B., 1985, Ergonomic analysis of slip-resistance measurement devices, *Ergonomics*, **28**, 1065–1079.

ANDRES, R.O., O'CONNOR, D. and ENG, T., 1992, A practical synthesis of biomechanical results to prevent slips and falls in the workplace, in Kumar, S. (Ed.), *Advances in Industrial*

Ergonomics and Safety IV, Proceedings of the Annual International Industrial Ergonomics and Safety Conference, London: Taylor & Francis, pp. 1001–1006.

BOWDEN, F. and HUGHES, T., 1939, The mechanism of sliding friction on ice and snow, *Proc R Soc London A*, **172**, 280–297.

BRING, C., 1964, Friktion och halkning (Friction and slipping), Rapport 112, Statens råd för byggnadsforskning, Stockholm: Bertil Carsslon Skrivbyrå AB (in Swedish with English text).

BRING, C., 1982, *Testing of Slipperiness: Forces Applied to the Floor and Movements of the Foot in Walking and in Slipping on the Heel*, Document D5: 1982, Stockholm: Swedish Council for Building Research.

BRUNGRABER, R.J., 1976, *An Overview of Floor Slip-Resistance Research with Annotated Bibliography*, National Bureau of Standards, NBS Technical Note 895, Washington: US Department of Commerce.

BUZCEK, F.L., CAVANAGH, P.R., KULAKOWSKI, B.T. and PRADHAN, P., 1990, Slip resistance needs of the mobility disabled during level and grade walking, in Gray, B.E. (Ed.), *Slips, Stumbles, and Falls: Pedestrian Footwear and Surfaces*, ASTM STP 1103, Philadelphia: American Society for Testing and Materials, pp. 39–54.

CAPPOZZO, A., 1991, The mechanics of human walking, in Patla, A.E. (Ed.), *Adaptability of Human Gait. Implications for the Control of Locomotion*, Amsterdam: Elsevier Science Publishers BV (North-Holland), pp. 167–186.

CARLSÖÖ, S., 1962, A method for studying walking on different surfaces, *Ergonomics*, **5**, 271–274.

CHAFFIN, D.B., WOLDSTAD, J.C. and TRUJILLO, A., 1992, Floor/shoe slip resistance measurement, *American Industrial Hygiene Association Journal*, **53**, 283–289.

CHIOU, S., BHATTACHARYA, A. and SUCCOP, P.A., 1996, Effect of workers' shoe wear on objective and subjective assessment of slipperiness, *American Industrial Hygiene Association Journal*, **57**, 825–831.

CLAUSSEN, C.-F., 1986, Ein einfacher, objectiver und quantitativer Gleichgewichtstest für die Praxis, *Forschungsbericht Cranio-Corpo-Graphie (CCG)*, Sankt Augustin: Hauptverband der gewerblichen Berufsgenossenschaften e.V. (in German).

COHEN, H.H. and COHEN, M.D., 1994a, Psychophysical assessment of the perceived slipperiness of floor tile surfaces in a laboratory setting, *Journal of Safety Research*, **25**, 19–26.

COHEN, H.H. and COHEN, M.D., 1994b, Perceptions of walking surface slipperiness under realistic conditions, utilizing a slipperiness rating scale, *Journal of Safety Research*, **25**, 27–31.

DAVIS, P.R., 1983, Human factors contributing to slips and falls, *Ergonomics*, **26**, 51–59.

ENG, J.J., WINTER, D.D. and PATLA, A.E., 1994, Strategies for recovery from a trip in early and late swing during human walking, *Experimental Brain Research*, **102**, 339–349.

ENGLANDER, F., HODSON, T.J. and TERREGROSSA, R.A., 1996, Economic dimensions of slip and fall injuries, *Journal of Forensic Science*, **41**, 733–746.

ENGLISH, W., 1992, What effect will new federal regulations have on pedestrian safety? *Professional Safety*, **37**, 16–22.

ERA, P., SCHROLL, M., YTTRING, H., GAUSE-NILSSON, I., HEIKKINEN, E. and STEEN, B., 1997, Postural balance and its sensory-motor correlates in 75 year-old men and women: a cross-national comparative study, *Journal of Gerontology*, **51A**, M53–M63.

FENDLEY, A., MARPET, M.I. and MEDOFF, H., 1995, The friction-related component of a comprehensive slip-prediction model. Part II: Use of ratiometric analysis and thresholded dimensionless numbers, in Mukherjee, D.P. (Ed.), *Proceedings of the 1995 Fourteenth Southern Biomedical Engineering Conference*, Shreveport, LA, pp. 162–165.

FOTHERGILL, J., O'DRISCOLL, D. and HASHEMI, K., 1995, The role of environmental factors in causing injury through falls in public places, *Ergonomics*, **38**, 220–223.

GNÖRICH, W. and GROSCH, K.A., 1975, The friction of polymers on ice, *Rubber Chemistry and Technology*, **48**, 527–537.

GRABNIER, M.D., KOH, T.J., LUNDIN, T.M. and JAHNIGEN, D.W, 1993, Kinematics of recovery from a stumble, *Journal of Gerontology*, **48**, M97–M102.

GRIEVE, D.W., 1983, Slipping due to manual exertion, *Ergonomics*, **26**, 61–72.

GRÖNQVIST, R., 1995, A dynamic method for assessing pedestrian slip resistance, *People and Work*, Research report 2, Helsinki: Finnish Institute of Occupational Health.

GRÖNQVIST, R., 1997, On transitional friction measurement and pedestrian slip resistance, in Seppälä, P., Luopajärvi, T., Nygård C.-H. and Mattila, M. (Eds), *From Experience to Innovation, Vol. 3, Proceedings of the 13th Triennial Congress of the International Ergonomics Association*, Helsinki: Finnish Institute of Occupational Health, pp. 383–385.

HARPER, F.C., WARLOW, W.J. and CLARKE, B.L., 1967, *The Forces Applied to the Floor by the Foot in Walking. Part II. Walking on a Slope. Part III. Walking on Stairs*, National Building Studies, Research Paper 32, London: Ministry of Technology.

HARRIS, G.W. and SHAW, S.R., 1988, Slip resistance of floors: users' opinions, Tortus instrument readings and roughness measurement. *Journal of Occupational Accidents*, **9**, 287–298.

HEISKANEN, M. and KOSKELA, K., 1994, Tapaturmat Suomessa vuosina 1980–1993 (Accidents in Finland during 1980–1993), *Sosiaali-ja terveysministeriön julkaisuja* 1994: 7, Helsinki: Painatuskeskus Oy (in Finnish).

HERNBERG, S., 1992, *Introduction to Occupational Epidemiology*, Chelsea, Michigan: Lewis Publishers.

HIRVONEN, M., LESKINEN, T., GRÖNQVIST, R. and SAARIO, J., 1994, Detection of near accidents by measurement of horizontal acceleration of the trunk, *International Journal of Industrial Ergonomics*, **14**, 307–314.

HONKANEN, R., 1983, The role of alcohol in accidental falls, *Journal of Studies on Alcohol*, **44**, 231–245.

JACKSON, P.L. and COHEN, H.H., 1995, An in-depth investigation of 40 stairway accidents and the stair safety literature, *Journal of Safety Research*, **26**, 151–159.

JAMES, D.I., 1980, A broader look at pedestrian friction, *Rubber Chemistry and Technology*, **53**, 512–541.

JAMES, D.I., 1983, Rubber and plastics in shoes and flooring: the importance of kinetic friction, *Ergonomics*, **26**, 83–99.

JUNG, K. and VON DIECKEN, U., 1992, Rutschhemmung von verlegten Bodenbelägen – eine kritische Betrachtung über ein von Ort einsetzbares Messgerät, *Die Berufsgenossenschaft*, Heft 7, 1–5.

KULAKOWSKI, B.T., BUZEC, F.L., CAVANAGH, P.R. and PRADHAN, P., 1989, Evaluation of performance of three slip resistance testers, *Journal of Testing and Evaluation*, **17**, 234–240.

KUMMER, H.W., 1966, *Unified Theory of Rubber and Tire Friction*, Engineering Research Bulletin B-94, Pennsylvania: The Pennsylvania State University.

LAVENDER, S.A., SOMMERICH, C.M., SUDHAKER, L.R. and MARRAS, W.S., 1988, Trunk muscle loading in non-sagittally symmetric postures as a result of sudden unexpected loading conditions, in *Proceedings of the Human Factors Society 32nd Annual Meeting*, Vol. 1, pp. 665–669, Santa Monica: The Human Factors Society, CA Anaheim, October.

LEAMON, T.B. and LI, K.-W., 1990, Microslip length and the perception of slipping, presentation at the 23rd International Congress on Occupational Health, Montreal, Canada, September.

LEAMON, T.B. and MURPHY, P.L., 1995, Occupational slips and falls: more than a trivial problem, *Ergonomics*, **38**, 487–498.

LEAMON, T.B. and SON, D.H., 1989, The natural history of a microslip, in Mital, A. (Ed.), *Advances in Industrial Ergonomics and Safety I, Proceedings of the Annual International Industrial Ergonomics and Safety Conference*, London: Taylor & Francis, pp. 633–638.

LECLERCQ, S., TISSERAND, M. and SAULNIER, H., 1993, Quantification of the slip resistance of floor surfaces at industrial sites. Part I. Implementation of a portable device, *Safety Science*, **17**, 29–39. Part II. Choice of optimal measurement conditions, *Safety Science*, **17**, 41–55.

LECLERCQ, S., TISSERAND, M. and SAULNIER, H., 1994, Slip-resistant footwear: a means for the prevention of slipping, in Aghazadeh, F. (Ed.), *Advances in Industrial Ergonomics and Safety VI. Proceedings of the Annual International Industrial Ergonomics and Safety Conference*, London: Taylor & Francis, pp. 329–337.

LECLERCQ, S., TISSERAND, M. and SAULNIER, H., 1995, Tribological concepts involved in slipping accident analysis, *Ergonomics*, **38**, 197–208.

LEHTO, M.R. and MILLER, J.M., 1987, Scientific knowledge acquisition during the extension of GSA: an expert system for generic safety analysis, *International Journal of Industrial Ergonomics*, **2**, 61–75.

LLEWELLYN, M.G.A. and NEVOLA, V.R., 1992, Strategies for walking on low-friction surfaces, in Lotens, W.A., Havenith, G. (Eds), *Proceedings of the Fifth International Conference on Environmental Ergonomics*, pp. 156–157, Maastricht.

MAKKONEN, L., 1994, Application of a new friction theory to ice and snow, *Annals of Glaciology*, **19**, 155–157.

MALMIVAARA, A., HELIÖVAARA, M., KNEKT, P., REUNANEN, A. and AROMAA, A., 1993, Risk factors for injurious falls leading to hospitalization or death in a cohort study of 19 500 adults, *American Journal of Epidemiology*, **138**, 384–394.

MANNING, D.P. and SHANNON, H.S., 1981, Slipping accidents causing low-back pain in a gearbox factory, *Spine*, **6**, 70–72.

MANNING, D.P., MITCHELL, R.G. and BLANCHFIELD, L.P., 1984, Body movements and events contributing to accidental and nonaccidental back injuries, *Spine*, **9**, 734–739.

MANNING, D.P., AYERS, I., JONES, C., BRUCE, M. and COHEN, K., 1988, The incidence of underfoot accidents during 1985 in a working population of 10 000 Merseyside people, *Journal of Occupational Accidents*, **10**, 121–130.

MERRILD, U. and BAK, S., 1983, An excess of pedestrian injuries in icy conditions: a high-risk fracture group – elderly women, *Accident Analysis & Prevention*, **15**, 41–48.

MOORE, D.F., 1972, The friction and lubrication of elastomers, in Raynor, G.V. (Ed.), *International Series of Monographs on Material Science and Technology*, Vol. 9, Oxford: Pergamon Press.

MOORE, D.F., 1975, *The Friction of Pneumatic Tyres*, Amsterdam: Elsevier Scientific Publishing Company.

MORACH, B., 1993, Quantifierung des Ausgleitvorganges beim menschlichen Gang unter besonderer Berücksichtigung der Aufsetzphases des Fusses, Fachbereich Sicherheits-technik der Bergischen Universität – Gesamthochschule Wuppertal, Wuppertal (in German).

M&T SLIP RESISTANCE SHOES, 1996, Development of a Test Method for Measuring the Slip Resistance of Protective Footwear, unpublished progress report no. 2 for the Commission of the European Communities, Contract no. MAT1 CT 940 059.

MYUNG, R. and SMITH, J.L., 1997, The effect of load carrying and floor contaminants on slip and fall parameters, *Ergonomics*, **40**, 235–246.

MYUNG, R., SMITH, J.L. and LEAMON, T.B., 1992, Slip distance for slip/fall studies, in Kumar, S. (Ed.), *Advances in Industrial Ergonomics and Safety IV, Proceedings of the Annual International Industrial Ergonomics and Safety Conference*, London: Taylor & Francis, pp. 983–987.

MYUNG, R., SMITH, J.L. and LEAMON, T.B., 1993, Subjective assessment of floor slipperiness, *International Journal of Industrial Ergonomics*, **11**, 313–319.

NAGATA, H., 1989, The methodology of insuring the validity of a slip-resistance meter, in *Proceedings of the International Conference on Safety*, pp. 33–38, Tokyo: Metropolitan Institute of Technology, August.

NAGATA, H., 1993, Fatal and non-fatal falls – a review of earlier articles and their developments, *Safety Science*, **16**, 379–390.

NIENSTEDT, W., HÄNNINEN, O., ARSTILA, A. and NIENSTEDT, I., 1986, Fysiologian ja anatomian perusteet (The basics of physiology and anatomy), Porvoo: WSOY, 3. edition (in Finnish).

NIGG, B.M. and YEADON, M.R., 1987, Biomechanical aspects of playing surfaces, *Journal of Sports Sciences*, **5**, 117–145.

OKSANEN, P., 1983, *Friction and Adhesion of Ice*, Publications 10, Espoo: Technical Research Centre of Finland.

PATLA, A.E., 1991, Visual control of human locomotion, in Patla, A.E. (Ed.), *Adaptability of Human Gait: Implications for the Control of Locomotion*, Amsterdam: Elsevier Science Publishers BV (North-Holland), pp. 55–97.

PERKINS, P.J., 1978, Measurement of slip between the shoe and ground during walking, in Anderson, C., Senne, J. (Eds), *Walkway Surfaces: Measurement of Slip Resistance*, ASTM STP 649, Baltimore: American Society for Testing and Materials, Baltimore, pp. 71–87.

PERKINS, P.J. and WILSON, P., 1983, Slip resistance testing of shoes – new developments, *Ergonomics*, **26**, 73–82.

PETRENKO, V.F., 1994, The effect of static electric fields on ice friction, *Journal of Applied Physics*, **76**, 1216–1219.

PROCTOR, T.D., 1993, Slipping accidents in Great Britain – an update, *Safety Science*, **16**, 367–377.

PROCTOR, T.D. and COLEMAN, V., 1988, Slipping, tripping and falling accidents in Great Britain – present and future, *Journal of Occupational Accidents*, **9**, 269–285.

PYYKKÖ, I., AALTO, H., STARCK, J., MEYER, B. and MAGNUSSON, M., 1988, Postural control in bilateral vestibular disease, in Claussen, C.-F., Kirtane, M.V. and Schlitter, K. (Eds), *Vertigo, Nausea, Tinnitus and Hypoacusia in Metabolic Disorders*, Elsevier Science Publishers BV, Biomedical Division, pp. 473–476.

PYYKKÖ, I., JÄNTTI, P. and AALTO, H., 1990, Postural control in elderly subjects, *Age and Ageing*, **19**, 215–221.

RABINOWICZ, E., 1956, Stick and slip. *Scientific American*, **194**, 109–118.

REDFERN, M.S. and RHOADES, T.P., 1996, Fall prevention in industry using slip resistance testing, in Bhattacharya, A. and McGlothlin, J.D. (Eds), *Occupational Ergonomics, Theory and Applications*, New York–Basel–Hong Kong: Marcel Dekker Inc., pp. 463–476.

ROBERTS, A.D., 1981, Rubber-ice adhesion and friction, *Journal of Adhesion*, **13**, 77–86.

ROBERTS, A.D. and RICHARDSON, J.C., 1981, Interface study of rubber-ice friction, *Wear*, **67**, 55–69.

ROBINOVITCH, S.N., HSIAO, E., KEARNY, M. and FRENK, V., 1996, Analysis of Movement Strategies During Unexpected Falls, presentation at the 20th Annual Meeting of the American Society of Biomechanics, Atlanta, Georgia, October.

SAARELA, K.-L., 1991, *Promoting Safety in Industry: Focus on Informational Campaigns and Participative Programs*, Helsinki: University of Technology.

SACHER, A., 1996, The application of forensic biomechanics to the resolution of unwitnessed falling accidents, *Journal of Forensic Science*, **41**, 776–781.

SIMONEAU, G.G., CAVANAGH, P.R., ULBRECHT, J.S., LEIBOWITZ, H.W. and TYRRELL, R.A., 1991, The influence of visual factors on fall-related kinematic variables during stair descent by older women, *Journal of Gerontology*, **46**, M188–M195.

SKIBA, R., 1984, Geräte zur Bestimmung der Reibung zwischen Schuh und Fussboden unter berücksichtigung des menschlichen Ganges, *Kautschuk+Gummi Kunststoffe*, **37**, 509–514 (in German with English summary).

SKIBA, R., 1988, Sicherheitsgrenzwerte zur Vermeidung des Ausgleitens auf Fussböden, *Zeitschrift für Arbeitswissenschaft*, **14**, 47–51 (in German with English summary).

SKIBA, R., BONEFELD, X. and MELLWIG, D., 1983, Voraussetzung zur Bestimmung der Gleitsicherheit beim menschlichen Gang, *Zeitschrift für Arbeitswissenschaft*, **9**, 227–232 (in German with English summary).

SKIBA, R., SCHEIL, M. and WINDHÖVEL, U., 1994, Vergleichsuntersuchung zur Instationären Reibzahlsmessung auf Fussböden, *Forschung Fb 701*, Dortmund: Bundesanstalt für Arbeitsschutz (in German with English summary).

SMITH, G.S., 1987, Injuries as a preventable disease: the control of occupational injuries from the medical and public health perspective, *Ergonomics*, **30**, 213–220.

SOROCK, G.S., 1988, Falls among the elderly: epidemiology and prevention, *American Journal of Preventive Medicine*, **4**, 282–288.

SOROCK, G.S. and LABINER, D.M., 1992, Peripheral neuromuscular dysfunction and falls in a elderly cohort, *American Journal of Epidemiology*, **136**, 584–591.

STRANDBERG, L., 1983a, On accident analysis and slip-resistance measurement, *Ergonomics*, **26**, 11–32.

STRANDBERG, L., 1983b, Ergonomics applied to slipping accidents, in Kvålseth, T.O. (Ed.), *Ergonomics of Workstation Design*, Butterworth & Co, pp. 201–228.

STRANDBERG, L., 1985, The effect of conditions underfoot on falling and overexertion accidents, *Ergonomics*, **28**, 131–147.

STRANDBERG, L. and LANSHAMMAR, H., 1981, The dynamics of slipping accidents, *Journal of Occupational Accidents*, **3**, 153–162.

STRANDBERG, L., HILDESKOG, L. and OTTOSON, A.-L., 1985, Footwear friction assessed by walking experiments, *VTIrapport 300 A*, Linköping: Väg- och trafikinstitutet.

SWENSEN, E., PURSWELL, J., SCHLEGEL, R. and STANEVICH, R., 1992, Coefficient of friction and subjective assessment of slippery work surfaces, *Human Factors*, **34**, 67–77.

TEMPLER, J., ARCHEA, J. and COHEN, H.H., 1985, Study of factors associated with risk of work-related stairway falls, *Journal of Safety Research*, **16**, 183–196.

TIDEIKSAAR, R., 1990, The biomedical and environmental characteristics of slips, stumbles, and falls in the elderly, in Gray, B.E. (Ed.), *Slips, Stumbles, and Falls: Pedestrian Footwear and Surfaces*, ASTM STP 1103, Philadelphia: American Society for Testing and Materials, pp. 17–27.

TISSERAND, M., 1985, Progress in the prevention of falls caused by slipping, *Ergonomics*, **28**, 1027–1042.

TWOMEY, J.M., SMITH, A.E. and REDFERN, M.S., 1995, A predictive model for slip resistance using artificial neural networks, *IIE Transactions*, **27**, 374–381.

VAUGHAN, C.L., 1984, Biomechanics of running gait, *CRC Critical Reviews in Biomedical Engineering*, **12**(1), 1–48.

WALLER, J.A., 1978, Falls among the elderly – human and environmental factors, *Accident Analysis & Prevention*, **10**, 21–33.

WINTER, D.A., 1991, *The Biomechanics and Motor Control of Human Gait: Normal, Elderly, and Pathological*, second edition, University of Waterloo, Canada.

Index